AF520507

Textbook of

Nutrition

for GNM Nursing Students

(As per the INC Syllabus for GNM)

Textbook of

Nutrition

for GNM Nursing Students

(As per the INC Syllabus for GNM)

Nursing Knowledge Tree
An Initiative by CBS Nursing Division

Third Edition

Varinder Kaur
PhD (N), MSc (CHN), MA (Pub, Ad.)
Associate Professor
College of Nursing, AIIMS
Bilaspur (Himachal Pradesh)

CBSPD
Dedicated to Education

CBS Publishers & Distributors Pvt Ltd

• New Delhi • Bengaluru • Chennai • Kochi • Kolkata • Lucknow • Mumbai
• Hyderabad • Jharkhand • Nagpur • Patna • Pune • Uttarakhand

Textbook of

Nutrition

for GNM Nursing Students

(As per the INC Syllabus for GNM)

ISBN: 978-93-94525-63-4

Reprint: 2026

Third Edition: 2025

Second Edition: 2022

First Edition: 2018

Published by **Satish Kumar Jain** and produced by **Varun Jain** for

CBS Publishers & Distributors Pvt Ltd

4819/XI Prahlad Street, 24 Ansari Road, Daryaganj, New Delhi 110 002, India.

Ph: +91-11-23289259, 23266861, 23266867 Website: www.cbspd.com

Fax: 011-23243014

e-mail: delhi@cbspd.com; cbspubs@airtelmail.in.

Corporate Office: 204 FIE, Industrial Area, Patparganj, Delhi 110 092

Ph: +91-11-4934 4934 Fax: 4934 4935

e-mail: feedback@cbspd.com

Branches

- **Bengaluru:** Seema House 2975, 17th Cross, K.R. Road, Banashankari 2nd Stage, Bengaluru-560 070, Karnataka
  Ph: +91-80-26771678/79 Fax: +91-80-26771680 e-mail: bangalore@cbspd.com
- **Chennai:** 7, Subbaraya Street, Shenoy Nagar, Chennai-600 030, Tamil Nadu
  Ph: +91-44-26680620, 26681266 Fax: +91-44-42032115 e-mail: chennai@cbspd.com
- **Kochi:** 68/1534, 35, 36-Power House Road, Opp. KSEB, Cochin-682018, Kochi, Kerala
  Ph: +91-484-4059061-65 Fax: +91-484-4059065 e-mail: kochi@cbspd.com
- **Kolkata:** Hind Ceramics Compound, 1st Floor, 147, Nilganj Road, Belghoria, Kolkata-700056, West Bengal
  Ph: +033-2563-3055/56 e-mail: kolkata@cbspd.com
- **Lucknow:** Basement, Khushnuma Complex, 7-Meerabai Marg (Behind Jawahar Bhawan), Lucknow-226001, Uttar Pradesh
  Ph: +0522-4000032 e-mail: tiwari.lucknow@cbspd.com
- **Mumbai:** PWD Shed, Gala No. 25/26, Ramchandra Bhatt Marg, Next to J.J. Hospital Gate No. 2, Opp. Union Bank of India, Noor Baug, Mumbai-400009, Maharashtra
  Ph: +91-22-66661880/89 Fax: +91-22-24902342 e-mail: mumbai@cbspd.com

Representatives

- **Hyderabad** +91-9885175004
- **Jharkhand** +91-9811541605
- **Nagpur** +91-9421945513
- **Patna** +91-9334159340
- **Pune** +91-9623451994
- **Uttarakhand** +91-9716462459

Printed at : Goyal Offset Works Pvt. Ltd. Haryana

CBS Nursing Knowledge Tree

Extends its Tribute to

Florence Nightingale

For glorifying the role of women as nurses,
For holding the title of " The Lady with the Lamp,"
For working tirelessly for humanity–
Florence Nightingale will always be
remembered for her
selfless and memorable services to the
human race.

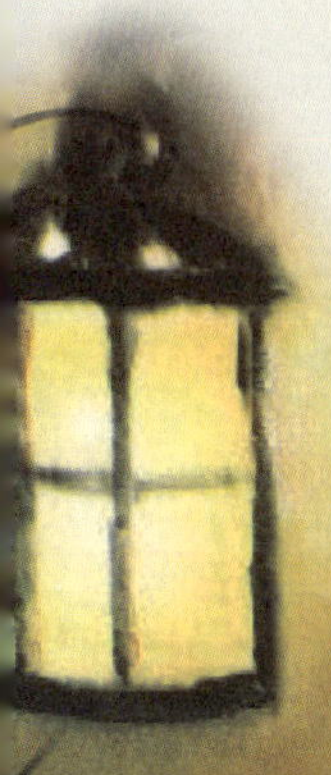

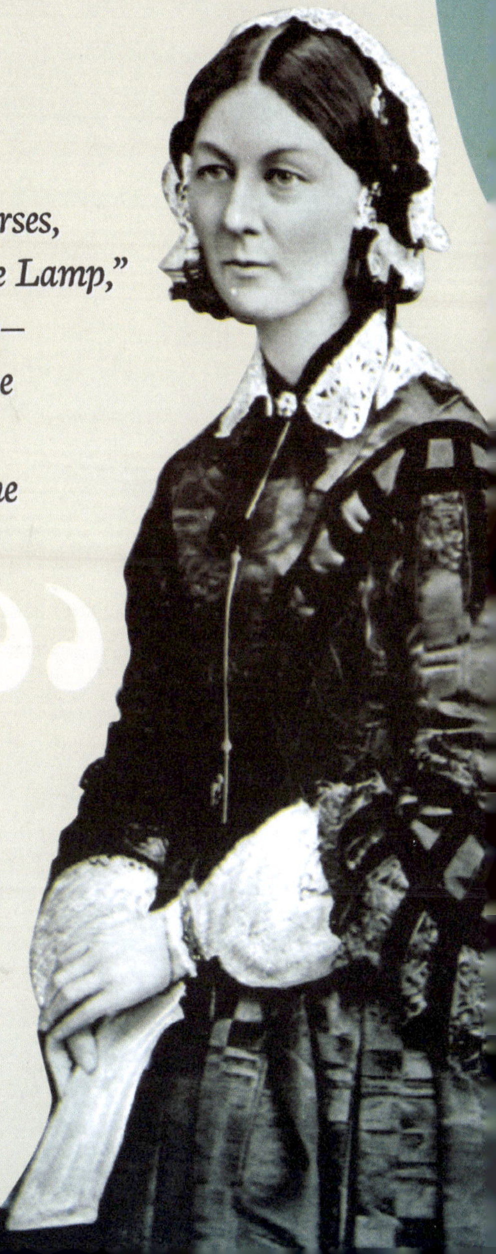

lorence Nightingale
May 1820 – August 1910)

Dedicated to

The Almighty God,

My Family and

Dear Son

Sehaj Preet Singh

Preface to the Third Edition

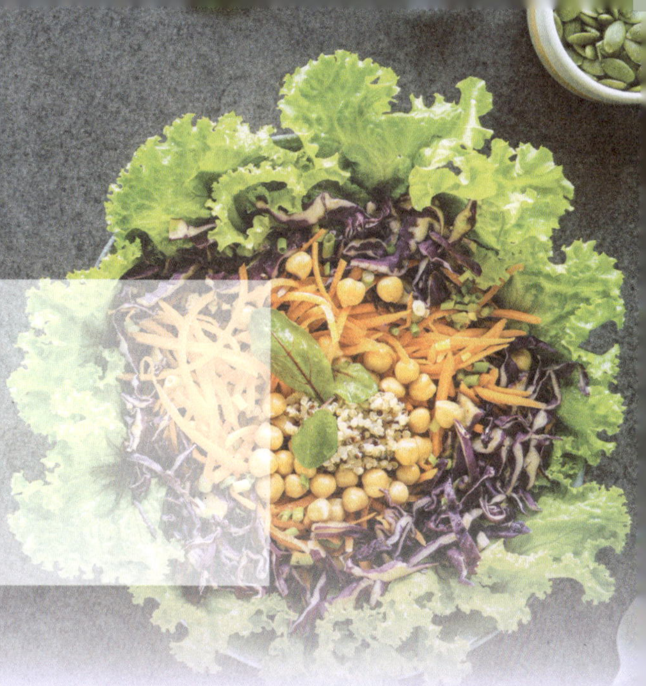

Nutrition plays a vital role in maintaining health and supporting recovery, making it a fundamental aspect of nursing practice. Nurses are not only responsible for promoting healthy eating habits but they also have to spread awareness about the nutritional needs of humans in general and their patients in particular. Therefore, nurses must possess comprehensive knowledge of nutrition to educate patients and their families on the importance of a balanced diet.

Recognizing the critical importance of nutrition in nursing, the third edition of this textbook has been carefully crafted using clear and accessible language, aligned with the updated syllabus prescribed by the Indian Nursing Council (INC). Every topic specified in the INC curriculum has been thoroughly covered. The content has been updated to incorporate recent advancements in health and nutrition with a focus on enhancing comprehension of the subject.

This edition includes detailed dietary plans customized for various health conditions and diseases, aiding nurses in practical application. The inclusion of cooking section aims to support students during hands-on sessions. Each chapter concludes with **Student Assignment** sections containing both subjective and objective questions to assess students' comprehension and learning abilities.

It is my aspiration that this book will assist students in comprehending and retaining the fundamental principles of nutrition. Since nutrition is a vibrant and dynamic field, any suggestions for further enhancing the usefulness of the book are warmly welcomed.

Varinder Kaur

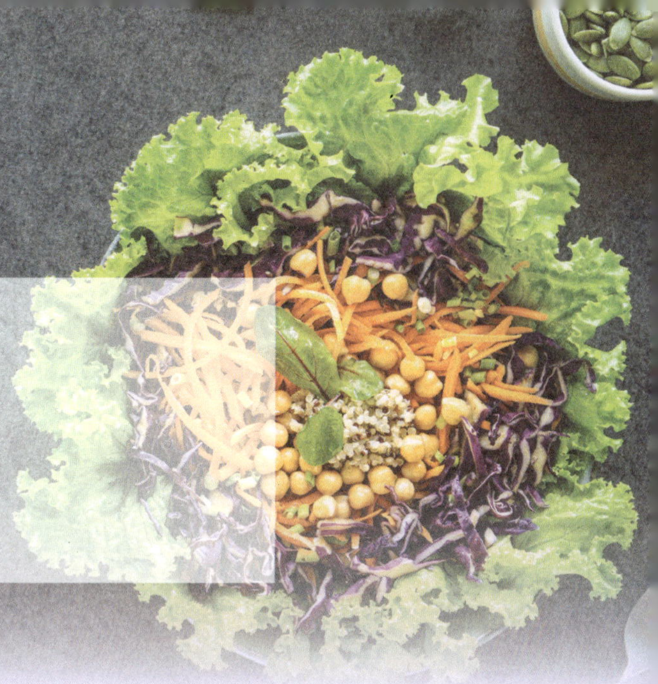

Preface to the Second Edition

Nutrition is a vital component for a healthy life. Nurses play a crucial role in maintaining and restoring nutrition in the individuals. The role of a nurse in nutrition is not only confined to promote healthy dietary habits but also to take care of the nutritional requirements of the people sick or healthy. Therefore, the nurses must be well-versed with all the aspects of nutrition to educate the patients as well as their family members about the importance of a healthy and nutritious diet.

Keeping in view the importance of nutrition in Nursing, this *Textbook of Nutrition for GNM Nursing Students*, 2nd edition has been designed in a very simple and lucid language and as per modified syllabus prescribed by the Indian Nursing Council (INC). Special care has been taken to include each and every topic prescribed in INC curriculum. The whole content of the book is updated keeping in mind the recent advancements in the field of health and nutrition as well as the necessity of immunity-boosting methods. Detailed diet plans related to various conditions and diseases have been included to help the nurses to apply them as and when needed in their profession. The cookery section added in this edition will surely help the students in practicals. Subjective and objective questions under the heading "Assess Yourself" have been included at the end of every chapter to assess students' learning skills.

I hope this book will help the students in memorizing and understanding the basic concepts of nutrition. As nutrition is a vast subject to explore, any suggestions for further improvement of the book will be highly appreciated.

Varinder Kaur

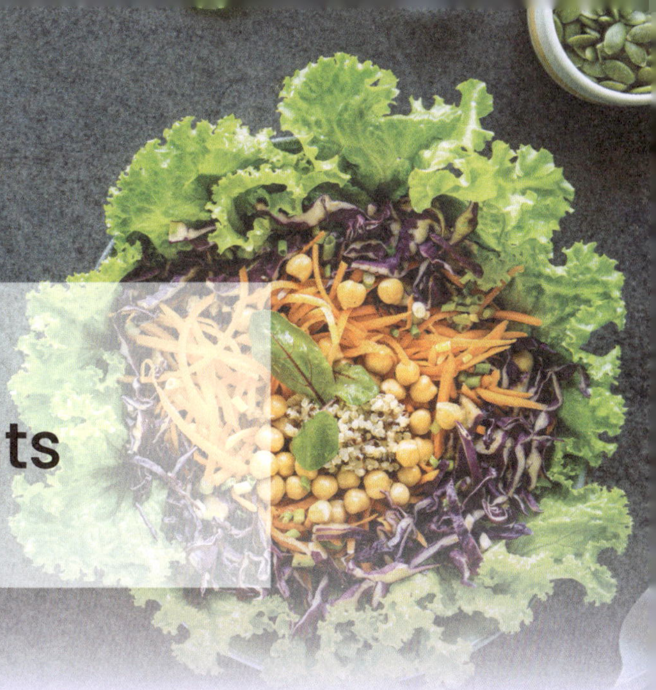

Acknowledgments

Every task demands effort but it cannot reach to its completion without cooperation from all the quarters. I pay my profound gratitude to the **Almighty** to glorify my way that led to the completion of this book. I am extremely grateful to my family, especially my husband, ***Rupinderjit Singh*** and my son ***Sehaj Preet Singh*** for their continued patience, support and encouragement. I express my gratitude and heartfelt thanks to my colleagues ***Ms Kiran*** and ***Ms Jyoti Saini*** for their sincere efforts toward completion of this book.

I extend my special thanks to **Mr Satish Kumar Jain** (Chairman) and **Mr Varun Jain** (Managing Director), M/s CBS Publishers and Distributors Pvt Ltd for their wholehearted support in publication of this book.

I sincerely thank the entire CBS team for bringing out the book with utmost care and attractive presentation. I would like to thank Ms Nitasha Arora (Assistant General Manager – Publishing) and Dr Anju Dhir (Sr. Product Manager cum Commissioning Editor) for their publishing support. I would also like to extend my thanks to Ms Surbhi Gupta (Sr. Editor cum Team Lead), Mr Ashutosh Pathak (Assistant Production Manager cum TL) and all the production team members for devoting laborious hours in editing, designing and typesetting the book.

Special Features of the Book

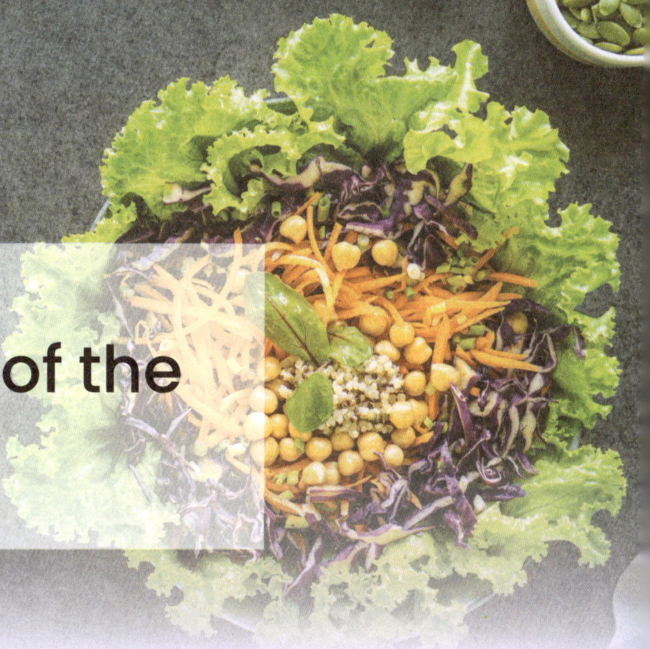

Learning Objectives in the beginning of every Chapter help readers understand the purpose of the chapter.

LEARNING OBJECTIVES

After the completion of the chapter, the readers will be able to:

- Define health, nutrition, nutrients and various other terms.
- Describe factors affecting nutrition.
- Discuss changing concepts of food and nutrition.
- Describe relationship between health and nutrition.

CHAPTER OUTLINE

- Introduction
- History and Changing Concepts of Nutrition
- Nutrition
- Nutrients

Chapter Outline gives a glimpse of the content covered in the chapter.

Key Terms are added in each chapter to help understand difficult scientific terms in easy language.

KEY TERMS

Antioxidants: These are natural or synthetic substances found in food that help in boosting the immunity of body.
Health: According to WHO "health is a state of complete physical, mental, and social well-being and not merely the absence of disease or infirmity."
Imbalance: It is a pathological state resulting from disproportion of the nutrients.
Nutrition: Nutrition is defined as the scientific study of food and its relation to health.

The book is well illustrated with relevant colorful **Figures** to add value to the content.

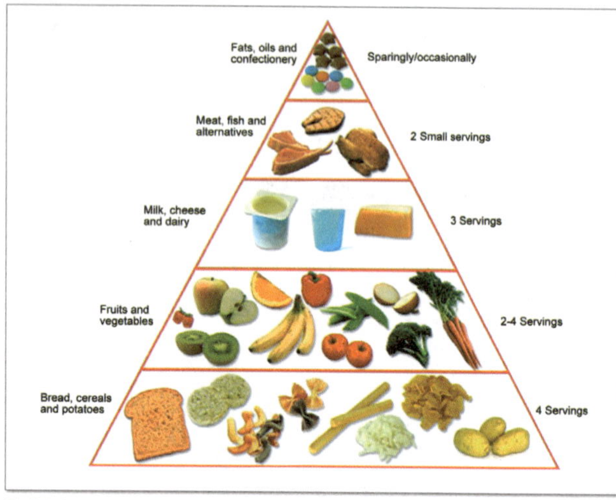

Fig. 3.2: Pyramid showing the amount of food products that should be consumed in form of balanced diet

Table 3.3: Body mass index according to body types

Classification	Body mass index
Underweight	<18.5
Normal range	18.5–24.9
Overweight	≥25.0
Preobese	25.0–29.9

Numerous **Tables** have been used in the chapters to facilitate learning in a quick way.

At the end of chapters, **Student Assignment** section is given which contains subjective and objective questions to help students attain mastery over the subject.

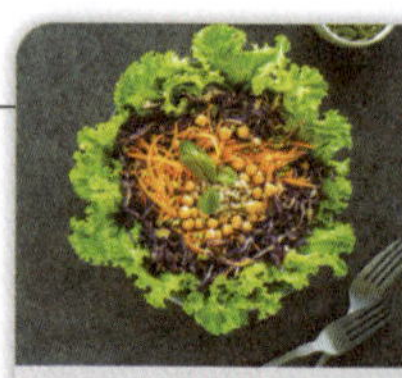

STUDENT ASSIGNMENT

LONG ANSWER QUESTIONS

1. What are the precautions to be taken while preserving the food?
2. How the food can be stored at commercial level?

SHORT ANSWER QUESTIONS

1. Discuss the principles of cooking.
2. Explain the household method of preservation of food.

MULTIPLE CHOICE QUESTIONS

1. **The full form of PFA is:**
   a. Prevention of Food Act
   b. Protection of Food Act
   c. Prevention of Food Adulteration Act
   d. None of these

Studded with a special section on **Cookery Practical** from applied perspective.

Cookery Practical

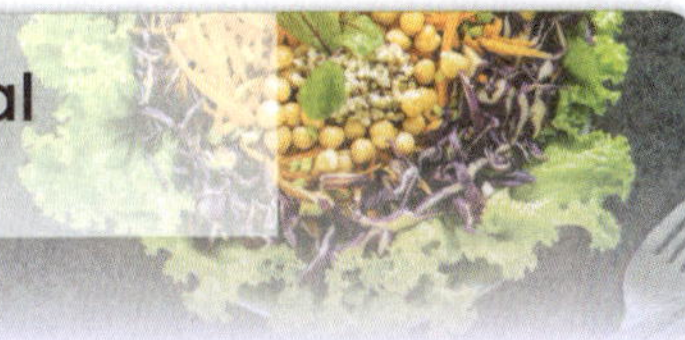

HOUSEHOLD MEASUREMENT

- 1 liter = 1000 milliliter (mL)
- 1 liter = 1 kilograms (kg) = 1000 grams = 1,0000,000 milligrams
- 1 gallon = 4 quarts
- 1 quart = 1 liter
- 1 pint = 500 milliliters (mL)
- 1 cup = 240 milliliters (mL)
- 1 fluid ounce (oz) = 30–32 milliliters (mL)
- 1 ounce = 28 grams
- 1 tbs (tbs) =15 milliliters (mL)
- 1 tsp (tsp) = 5 milliliters (mL)
- 3 tsp (tsp) = 1 tbs (tbs)
- 2.2 pound (lbs) = 1 kilograms (kg)
- 1 quart = 2 pints = 4 cups = 64 tbs (tbs) = 192 tsp
- 1 quart = 16 ounces = 1 pound
- 1 cubic centimeter (cc) = 1 milliliter (mL)

Note: A cubic centimeter (cc) is equal to the volume of a cube with side length of 1 cm.

Annexure

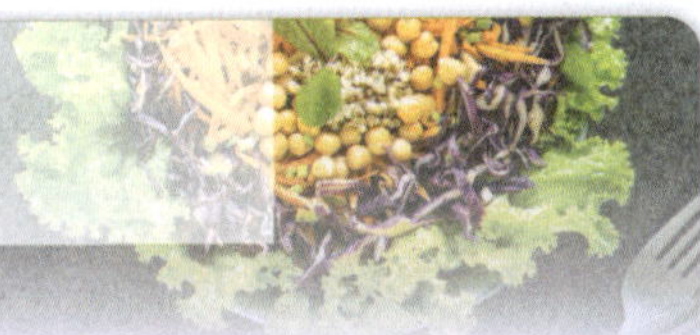

COMMONLY ASKED QUESTIONS IN EXAMINATION

- Explain common nutritional problems in India.
- Discuss dietary sources of proteins.
- Discuss protein deficiency diseases.
- Plan one day diet for toddler.
- Enlist fat soluble vitamins.
- What are the principles of cooking?
- Describe the different factors that help a patient in acceptance of diet.
- Explain different methods of preparation, preservation and cooking of food.
- Write a short note on balanced diet.
- Explain normal dietary requirements.
- Describe factors affecting selection and planning of meal.
- Write about food hygiene and laws related to food.
- Write a short note on classification of food.
- Write down the classification of proteins.
- What are the factors to be kept in mind by the nurse while selection and planning of meal?
- Explain functions of carbohydrates.
- Enlist main vitamin deficiencies.

Annexure provides additional but valuable information related to topics discussed in the book.

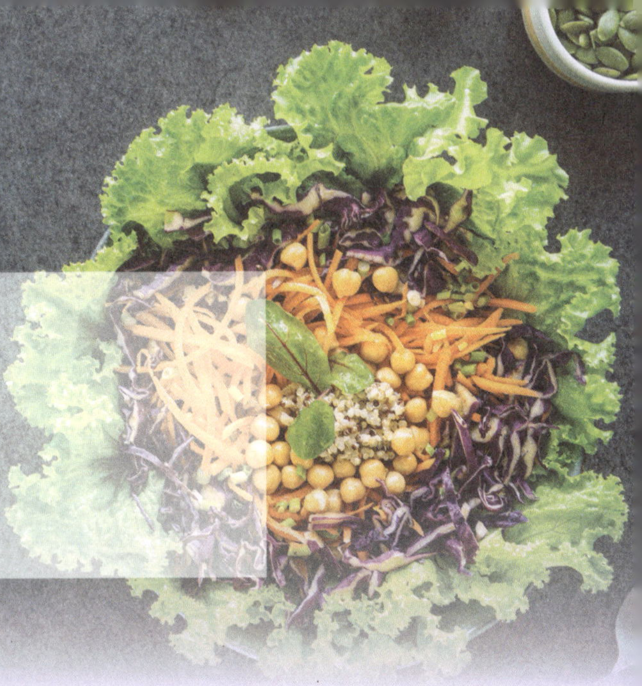

Syllabus

NUTRITION

Course Description

This course is designed to help students understand that nutrition is an integral component of health as nutrients play a vital role in the growth, development and maintenance of the body.

General Objectives

Upon completion of this course, the students will be able to:

- Describe the principles of nutrition and dietetics and their relationship to the human body in health and disease.
- Describe the balanced diet in promotion of health.
- Apply this knowledge in providing therapeutic diet and take care of the sick.
- Demonstrate skills in selection, preparation and preservation of food.

Total Hours: 30

Unit	Learning objectives	Content	Hours	Teaching learning activities	Methods of assessment
I	Describe the relationship between nutrition and health	**Introduction** • Meaning of food, nutrition, nutrients, etc. • Food habits and customs • Factors affecting nutrition • Changing concepts in food and nutrition • Relationship of nutrition and health	2	• Lecture cum discussions • Explain using charts	• Short answer types • Objective type

Contd...

Unit	Learning objectives	Content	Hours	Teaching learning activities	Methods of assessment
II	Describe the classification of food	**Classification of Food** • Classification by origin: ▪ Food of animal origin ▪ Food of plant origin • Classification by chemical composition and sources: ▪ Carbohydrates ▪ Proteins ▪ Fats ▪ Minerals ▪ Vitamins ▪ Water • Classification by predominant functions: ▪ Body building food ▪ Energy giving food ▪ Protective food	2	• Lecture cum discussions • Real food items • Exhibits charts	• Short answer types • Objective type • Essay type
		• Classification by nutritive value: ▪ Cereals and millets ▪ Pulses and legumes ▪ Vegetables ▪ Nuts and oilseeds ▪ Fruits ▪ Animal food ▪ Fats and oils ▪ Sugar and jaggery ▪ Condiments and spices ▪ Miscellaneous food			
III	• Explain normal dietary requirements • Demonstrate skill in calculating normal food requirements	**Normal Dietary Requirements** • **Energy:** Calorie, measurement, body mass index, basal metabolic rate—determination and factors affecting • **Balanced diet:** Nutritive value of foods, calculation for different categories of people, normal food requirement calculation. Menu plan. Combination of food affecting and enhancing the nutritive value of the diet. • Budgeting for food, low cost meals, food substitutes. • Diseases and disorders caused by the imbalance of nutrients. • Food allergy—causes, types, diet modifications in gluten, lactose and protein intolerance, etc. • Food intolerance—inborn errors of metabolism.	4	• Lecture cum discussions • Charts exhibits • Real food • Practical exercise	• Short answer types • Objective type • Essay type

Contd...

Unit	Learning objectives	Content	Hours	Teaching learning activities	Methods of assessment
IV	Describe the principles and various methods of preparation, preservation and storage of food	**Food Preparation, Preservation and Storage** • Principles of cooking, methods of cooking and the effect of cooking on food and various nutrients. Safe food handling, health of food handlers. • Methods of food preservation—household and commercial, precautions. • Food storage—cooked and raw, household and commercial, ill effects of poorly stored food. • Food adulteration and acts related to it.	2	• Lecture cum discussions • Field visit to food processing unit • Demonstration exhibits	• Short answer types • Objective type • Evaluation of exhibit preparation
V	Describe the therapeutic diet	**Therapeutic Diet** • Diet modification in relation to medical and surgical condition of the individual such as Protein Energy Malnutrition (PEM), diabetes, cardiovascular disease, hepatitis, renal, gouts, Irritable Bowel syndrome (IBS), obesity, cholecystectomy, partial gastrectomy, gastrostomy, bariatric surgery and colostomy, etc. • Special diets—low sodium diet, fat free diet, diabetic diet, bland diet, high protein diet, low protein diet, low calorie diet, geriatric diet, iron rich diet, liquid diet, semisolid diet, soft diet and high fiber diet, etc. • Factors affecting diet acceptance, feeding the helpless patient. • Health education on nutrition needs and methods in diet modification.	8	• Lecture cum discussions • Practical of planning therapeutic diet • Demonstration charts • Exhibits	• Short answer types • Objective type • Essay type

Contd...

Unit	Learning objectives	Content	Hours	Teaching learning activities	Methods of assessment
VI	Describe the concept of community nutrition	**Community Nutrition** • Nutritional problems and programs in India • Community food supply, food hygiene and commercially prepared and grown food available locally. • National and international food agencies—Central Food Training Research Institute (CFTRI), Food and Agriculture Organization (FAO), National Institute of Nutrition (NIN), Food Safety and Standards Authority of India (FSSAI), Cooperative for Assistance and Relief Everywhere (CARE), National Institute of Public Cooperation and Child Development (NIPCCD), etc.	4	• Lecture cum discussions • Videos • Government of India nutrition manuals • Visit to the local food preparation/ processing agency.	• Short answer types • Objective type

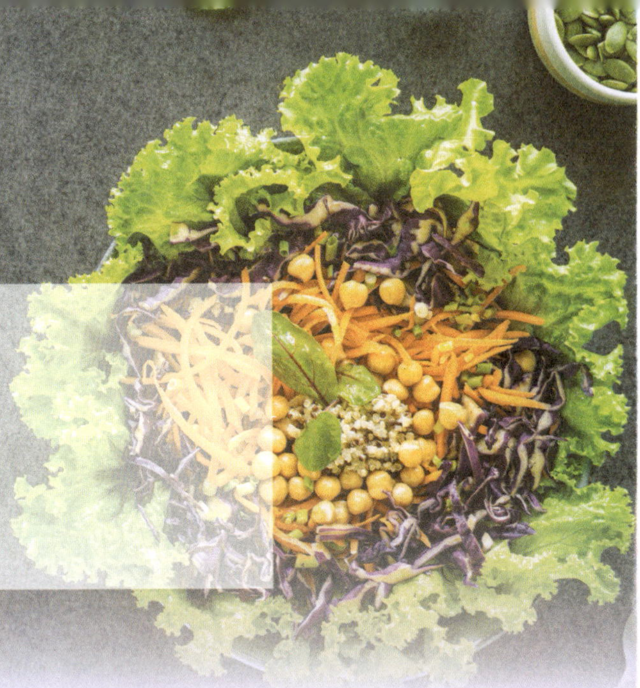

Contents

CHAPTER 3 Normal Dietary Requirements 49–94

CHAPTER 4 Food Preparation, Preservation and Storage 95–116

CHAPTER 5 Therapeutic Diet 117–167

1

Introduction

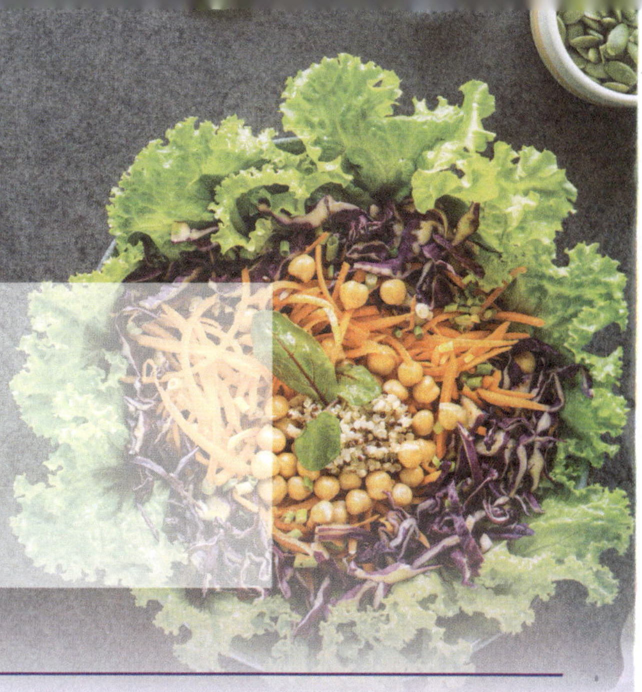

LEARNING OBJECTIVES

After the completion of the chapter, the readers will be able to:

- Define health, nutrition, nutrients and various other terms.
- Describe factors affecting nutrition.
- Discuss changing concepts of food and nutrition.
- Describe relationship between health and nutrition.

CHAPTER OUTLINE

- Introduction
- History and Changing Concepts of Nutrition
- Nutrition
- Nutrients
- Food Habits and Customs
- Factors Affecting Nutrition
- Relationship Between Nutrition and Health

KEY TERMS

Antioxidants: These are natural or synthetic substances found in food that help in boosting the immunity of body.
Health: According to WHO "health is a state of complete physical, mental, and social well-being and not merely the absence of disease or infirmity."
Imbalance: It is a pathological state resulting from disproportion of the nutrients.
Nutrition: Nutrition is defined as the scientific study of food and its relation to health.
Nutritional requirements: It refers to amount of various nutrients needed by an individual to sustain a healthy life.
Nutritional status: It is the state of our body as a result of the food we consume.
Nutritional surveillance: It is defined as the regular collection of information related to nutrition. It is used for making decisions about actions and policies, which affect nutrition.
Nutritionist: A person who advises about various aspects of nutrition is nutritionist.

INTRODUCTION

Food is the basic necessity of life without which survival is not possible. We eat food to live, to grow, to get energy, to work and to keep ourselves healthy. Nurses are important members of the health team. Now in modern era more emphasis is given upon prevention of the diseases and diet plays a key factor to prevent such diseases. Nurses are committed to maintaining good health status of the people, so they must have adequate knowledge regarding food and nutrition.

HISTORY AND CHANGING CONCEPTS OF NUTRITION

History

As nutrition means the process of nourishing or being nourished by the food consumed and using it for growth and development, so knowledge related to nutrition can make a big difference in the life of an organism.

- History of nutrition is as old as the biblical writings in which relationship of health and food was mentioned. In this era, eye diseases were used to treat by putting juices of liver into eyes (liver is very rich source of vitamin A). Hippocrates, known as 'father of medicine', quoted that a wise man should consider health as the greatest blessing.
- The diet of the early humans varied with location and climate as the early human beings were dependent merely upon natural products like food from plants and animals. Gradually, with evolution of time agriculture developed and gifted the world with foods such as rice, wheat, maize, etc. To consume and preserve such food items, process of cooking developed, which further reduced the risk of contamination of food products. Later on with the advancement of technology, milk, dairy products and diversity of vegetables were also available.
- With the beginning of 19th century, **Justus Liebig** from Germany researched chemical composition of carbohydrates, fats and proteins and found that carbohydrates were made of sugars, fats from fatty acids, and proteins were made up of amino acids.
- In the 20th century, role of essential nutrients was identified as a vital factor for various processes in human body. **Dr Casimir Funk** coined the term vitamin as an important factor in the diet. Vitamins and minerals were also considered as important as the macronutrients.
- With the further advancement in research on nutrients, **Linus Pauling and colleagues** recommended that nourishing the body with right nutrients and right concentration can help people to achieve better health and prolonged life, which was considered as a milestone in the history of nutrition.

Changing Concepts

- Significant progress has been achieved during the last 50 years regarding practical application of the new knowledge obtained through various researches.
- Special emphasis was given on the nutritional deficiency diseases like anemia, goiter, nutritional blindness and protein energy malnutrition (PEM).
- The influence of the nutritional science was also extended to other fields like agriculture, animal husbandry, economics, etc. that led to increased food production and helped to achieve **Green revolution** and **White revolution** in India.
- Gradually, nutrition was recognized as a global health issue by international agencies like World Health Organization (WHO), Food and Agriculture Organization (FAO), United Nations Children's Fund (UNICEF). They formulated various strategies to combat with such health and nutritional problems.

- With the further advancement of technology, relationship of nutrition was not only established with the infection, immunity, maternal and child health, family health but also with the noncommunicable diseases such as coronary artery disease, diabetes, etc.
- During the recent years, science of nutrition has moved out of laboratory and has established its link with epidemiology, which is known as nutritional epidemiology. It deals with newer concepts of nutrition such as nutritional assessment, dietary survey, nutritional growth and monitoring, nutritional indicators and nutritional interventions.
- With the newer concepts and newer approaches, nutritional science has become more dynamic and it has proved that nutritional problems are not just a medical problem but are multifactorial in nature as many other factors like education, demography, agriculture, which are equally responsible for nutritional diseases. So a broad intersectoral and integrated approach of all sectors is important to tackle today's nutritional problems.
- By viewing the importance of nutrition, in global campaign of 'Health for All', promotion of proper nutrition is one of the eight elements of primary health care. Many nutritional indicators have been developed to monitor health for all. To achieve the targets many community nutrition programs like Midday Meal Program, Integrated Child Development Services (ICDS) programs, etc. have been implemented.

NUTRITION

The word "nutrition" is derived from a Latin word called '*nūtrīre*', which means to feed, nurse, support, preserve.

Nutrition is defined as the scientific study of food and its relation to health. It also deals with aspects such as what to eat, how much to eat and when to eat.

Definitions

"Nutrition is the intake of food, considered in relation to the body's dietary needs. Good nutrition—an adequate, well-balanced diet combined with regular physical activity—is a cornerstone of good health."

—World Health Organization (WHO)

"Nutrition is the process of taking in nutrients from the foods you eat."

—National Institutes of Health (NIH)

"Nutrition is the science of food and its relationship to health." ***—Academy of Nutrition and Dietetics***

"Nutrition is the study of the nutrients in foods and the body's handling of them."

—American Society for Nutrition

"Nutrition is the process of nourishing or being nourished; specifically: the sum of the processes by which an animal or plant takes in and utilizes food substances." ***—Webster's Dictionary***

- **Food:** Food is any substance consumed to provide nutritional support for the body. It is typically of plant or animal origin and contains essential nutrients such as carbohydrates, proteins, fats, vitamins, minerals, and water. Food is ingested by humans and animals to sustain life, promote growth, and maintain health.

  Or

  Any edible or portable substances (usually of animal or plant origin) consisting of nourishing and nutritive components, which sustain life, generate energy and provide growth, maintenance and health.

- **Dietetics:** It is the practical application of the principles of nutrition or in other words it is the science that deals with the study of nutrition in health and disease.
- **Balanced diet:** It is the selection of right component of food in right proportions for maintaining good health and prevention of disease.

NUTRIENTS

Nutrients are substances that provide nourishment essential for the growth, maintenance, and repair of the body's tissues. They are typically obtained from food and include carbohydrates, proteins, fats, vitamins, minerals, and water. Each nutrient plays a specific role in supporting various bodily functions, from energy production to immune system maintenance and overall health. Nutrients are also known as '**food factors**'. These are the essential substances that are not produced by the body. There are about 40–50 different nutrients that must be supplied through food.

Classification

Depending upon the functions, nutrients can be categorized as:

- **Energy-yielding nutrients:** Carbohydrates and fats
- **Body-building nutrients:** Proteins
- **Protective nutrients:** Minerals and vitamins

Carbohydrates provide 65–80% energy, fats provide 10–30% of energy whereas proteins contribute to 7–15% of total energy to the body.

Depending upon the requirement, nutrients can be categorized as:

- **Macronutrients:** Carbohydrates, fats and proteins
- **Micronutrients:** Minerals and vitamins. The requirement of micronutrients may vary from fraction of milligrams to several grams.

Nutrients play a vital role in the body as human body is made up of proteins (muscles), supported upon minerals (bones), protected by layers (fat), energized by carbohydrates and protected by the vitamins.

Definitions

- **Calorie:** A calorie is defined as the amount of heat required to raise the temperature of one gram of water through 1°C.
- **Calorific value:** It is the amount of heat released by a unit weight or unit volume of a substance during complete combustion.
- **Kilocalorie:** It is 1000 times energy for calorie
  1 kilocalorie = 4.2 kilojoules
- **Calorific values of macronutrients per gram**

Macronutrients	Kilocalorie
Carbohydrates	4
Fats	9
Proteins	4

- **Metabolism:** The complex of physical and chemical processes occurring within a living cell or organism that are necessary for the maintenance of life. In metabolism some substances are broken down to yield energy for vital processes while other substances, necessary for life, are synthesized.
- **Basal metabolic rate (BMR):** It is the amount of energy expressed in calories that a person needs to perform the basic body functions at rest, for example, breathing, blood circulation, cell growth, brain and nerve functions.
- **Malnutrition:** It is a condition resulting from unbalanced diet or insufficient food.

  Or

  It is insufficient, excessive or imbalanced consumption of nutrients.
  - **Overnutrition:** Overnutrition or hyperalimentation is a form of malnutrition in, which intake of nutrients is oversupplied. The amount of nutrients exceeds the amount required for normal growth, development and metabolism.
  - **Undernutrition:** It is defined as the deficient bodily nutrition due to inadequate food intake or faulty assimilation of nutrients. It is also known as hyponutrition.

FOOD HABITS AND CUSTOMS

Food habits are passed from one generation to another and family plays an important role in shaping these food habits. Food habits are also a reflection of the culture or a society. What one society treats normal or highly valuable may be considered inappropriate in another society. Food customs differ widely in regard to likes and dislikes of a society introducing many food taboos. A food taboo is a prohibition against consuming certain foods or is referred to the practices prescribed by the society as improper or unacceptable.

Food habits and customs in India are diverse due to the vast geographical and cultural diversity of the nation.

Some common Indian food habits and customs are:

- **Regional diversity:** India is known for its regional cuisines, each with its own unique flavors, ingredients, and cooking techniques. For example, North Indian cuisine is characterized by dishes like tandoori chicken, naan bread, and rich gravies, while South Indian cuisine features rice-based dishes like dosa, idli, and sambar.
- **Vegetarianism:** Vegetarianism is widespread in India, influenced by religious beliefs such as Hinduism and Jainism, which advocate non-violence toward animals. Many Indians, particularly in North and West India, follow vegetarian diets, and even those who consume meat often have days or periods of vegetarianism.
- **Spices and flavors:** Indian cuisine is known for its use of spices and herbs, which vary by region and dish. Common spices include turmeric, cumin, coriander, cardamom, and mustard seeds, which add depth and complexity to dishes.
- **Traditional eating practices:** Traditional Indian meals typically include a variety of dishes served together, such as rice or bread (roti, naan), dal (lentil curry), vegetable curries, yogurt (raita), and pickles. Meals are often eaten with the right hand, and sharing food with others is a common practice that signifies hospitality.
- **Festive and ritual foods:** Indian festivals and rituals are often associated with specific foods and sweets. For example, during Diwali (the festival of lights), sweets like laddoos and barfis are exchanged, while during Ramadan, Muslims break their fast with special dishes like biryani and kebabs.

- **Ayurvedic influence:** Ayurveda, an ancient system of medicine and wellness, also influences Indian food habits. It emphasizes balancing the body's doshas that is defects (Vata, Pitta and Kapha doshas) through diet, recommending specific foods and spices for different health conditions.
- **Modern influences:** Urbanization and globalization have introduced new foods and culinary influences to India. Fast food chains coexist with traditional food items and fusion cuisines that blend Indian flavors with international dishes are increasingly popular.

Food Taboos

A food taboo is a rule or belief within a culture that says certain foods should not be eaten, often for religious, cultural, or ethical reasons. These taboos can vary widely between different societies and can dictate what foods are considered acceptable or forbidden to eat.

Food taboos, both in India and across the world, are influenced by various factors such as religion, tradition, health beliefs, and superstitions.

Examples of food taboos are:

- **Beef consumption:** In Hindu-majority regions of India, especially among certain communities, the consumption of beef is taboo due to the belief that cows are sacred.
- **Food during religious fasts:** During religious fasts such as Navratri or Janmashtami, followers often avoid specific foods like grains, meat, or even certain vegetables as per religious customs.
- **Eating practices:** Some communities have specific rules about how food should be prepared and consumed. For instance, certain communities may avoid eating onions and garlic, considering them to be tamasic (having negative qualities).
- **Taboos related to pregnancy:** In some regions, pregnant women are advised against consuming certain foods such as papaya, pineapple, or sesame seeds, believed to cause miscarriages or other complications.

Food Taboos Across the World

- **Insects:** While many Western cultures have a taboo against eating insects, they are consumed widely in some Asian, African, and Latin American countries where they are considered a nutritious food.
- **Cultural specificities:** In Western cultures, many people find it wrong to eat cats and dogs. However, in some parts of Asia, it's acceptable to eat these animals.
- **Raw versus cooked food:** Some cultures have taboos against eating raw meat or fish due to health concerns, while others have developed traditions around raw dishes like sushi in Japan.
- **Fasting practices:** Various cultures observe fasting periods where certain foods are restricted or prohibited
- **Superstitions and beliefs:** Some food taboos are related to superstitions or beliefs. For example, in some cultures, eating certain foods during specific times of the year might be believed to bring bad luck or illness.

Healthy Food Habits

- **Hand hygiene:** Always wash hands before eating to prevent the spread of germs and illnesses.
- **Food hygiene:** Ensure that food is covered and prepared in a hygienic manner to avoid contamination.
- **Fresh food:** Consume fresh food whenever possible to maximize nutrient intake and flavor.
- **Proper cooking:** Avoid overcooking or undercooking food to retain nutrients and ensure safety.

- **Limit salt, sugar, and spices:** Reduce excessive intake of salt, sugar, and spices to promote heart health and overall well-being.
- **Balanced diet:** Eat a variety of foods to obtain essential nutrients. Avoid eating the same foods repeatedly (monotonous diet).
- **Timing of fruits and water:** Consume fruits and water half an hour before or after meals to aid digestion and maximize nutrient absorption.
- **Never skip breakfast:** Eat a nutritious breakfast to kickstart metabolism and maintain energy levels throughout the day.
- **Light dinner:** Have a light dinner at least two hours before bedtime to aid digestion and promote better sleep.
- **Regular meals:** Aim to eat regular meals throughout the day to maintain steady energy levels. Skipping meals can lead to overeating later in the day.
- **Mindful eating:** Pay attention to hunger and fullness cues. Eat slowly and enjoy food, avoiding distractions like screens or work during meals.
- **Hydration:** Drink plenty of water throughout the day to stay hydrated. Limit sugary drinks and opt for water or herbal tea.
- **Limit processed foods:** Reduce intake of processed and refined foods that are high in added sugars, unhealthy fats (trans fats and saturated fats).

FACTORS AFFECTING NUTRITION

A number of factors influence the food habits. Nurses are concerned about the nutritional status of the individual. The important role of a nurse is to prevent diseases and to promote health so knowledge of all the factors that influence nutrition and health is very important. The following are the factors that play an important role in the nutritional level of an individual (Fig. 1.1).

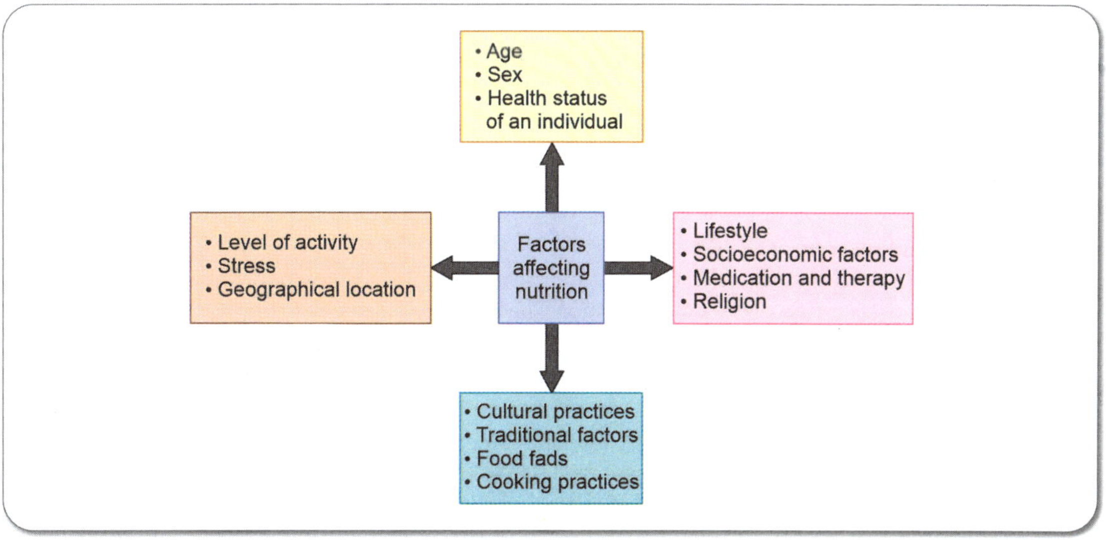

Fig. 1.1: Factors affecting nutrition

- **Age:** Nutritional requirements change as the person gets older. Growing children have different needs, from the adults, for example, they require higher intake of fatty acids than the adults. Similarly, digestion, absorption and utilization of elderly people get affected due to aging process so they have different nutritional requirements.
- **Sex:** Energy requirements are different in men and women. Basal metabolic rate of the women is less than the men. A woman's nutritional requirements also vary through stages like in pregnancy, lactation and in menopause.
- **Health status of an individual:** Health status of an individual greatly affects the eating habits and nutritional status. Lack of teeth, ill-fitting dentures, gastrointestinal and other diseases cause nausea or diarrhea, which adversely affect the appetite and nutritional status of the individual. On the other side, for different diseases, there are different nutritional requirements. Diet has to be modified as per the disease condition, for example, low sodium intake in case of hypertension and low amount of carbohydrates in case of diabetes.
- **Levels of activity:** It also affects the nutritional requirements. An athlete needs different nutrients than that of an office worker. Muscular activity affects the metabolic rate as strenuous activities improve metabolic efficiency in some people and increase the demand of nutrients. Mental activities require only 4 kcal/hr that provides little metabolic stimulation.
- **Stress:** It has also a great impact on the intake of diet. Some people eat less and suffer from nutritional deficient diseases while others can overeat (suffer from coronary artery or obesity) in the same stressful situation.
- **Geographical location:** Consumption of diet also varies according to place of living as people prefer different staple food. Some prefer to take rice whereas others eat wheat or maize depending upon the production of food in the area where they live, for example, wheat is mainly cultivated in regions with high temperature and rice is the main crop in the tropical areas where rainfall is high. This staple food sometimes may lead to certain nutritional deficient diseases, for example, pellagra is prevalent among maize eaters and beriberi spreads among the population consuming highly milled raw rice.
- **Lifestyle:** Lifestyle also has a great impact on eating habits as people who spend enough time at home can prepare healthy meals and take it on proper time. On the other side, people who are always busy and in hurry prefer to buy convenience grocery (fast food) or eat outside, which affects their health. Due to busy schedule fast food has become the first choice of many youngsters.
- **Socioeconomic factors:** What, how much and how often a person eats is frequently affected by the level of income of an individual. Poor people do not have enough resources to buy the food items essential for health and many people in developing countries often sleep without food. Other social factors like level of education, sanitation, family size, knowledge regarding nutritive value of food also affect the nutrition.
- **Medication and therapy:** The effect of drugs on nutrition may alter appetite, disturb taste perception or interfere with nutrient absorption or excretion. Other therapies like chemotherapy, radiation therapy may adversely affect eating pattern and nutrition due to severe side effects like diarrhea, oral ulcers or intestinal bleeding that result from toxicity of antineoplastic agents.
- **Religion:** Some religion does not allow to consume certain foods and drinks. Cow is very sacred for Hindus and those who eat meat are forbidden from consuming beef. Similarly, pork is prohibited in Muslims. Onion and garlic is not eaten by the Jain community and even Hindus during the specified sacred days (Navratri) do not consume these food items. Other religious activities such as fasting (going without food or drink for a specified period) are also believed in many religions, for example, Muslims observe fast during the month of Ramadan that includes abstaining from all foods and drinks from sunrise to sunset. In some religions, strict vegetarian, do not consume even milk or milk products and suffer from severe deficiency diseases.

- **Cultural practices:** Every culture has its own customs and beliefs regarding nutritional practices, for example, papaya is avoided in some societies because it is believed to cause abortion. Similarly, in some parts it is considered that women must eat the leftover food to respect the male members of the family. Another common practice during the menstruation phase of women is they are prohibited to do certain types of activities and have to eat a specified food only. All cultural practices are not bad, some are useful and others have not any effect on health, for example, Jewish taboo against pork was introduced to eliminate prevalence of pork tapeworm, which was causing disease in the Jewish community.
- **Traditional factors:** Traditions also vary from one region to another and these traditions also have a great impact on health. In many parts of country, colostrum (first breast milk rich in antibiotics) is not given to the baby as they consider it impure and hard to digest. Adulteration of milk with water is also very common practice as it is considered that if milk is boiled purely, the milk of the donor animal may dry up. Similarly, certain foods are also categorized as hot and cold food in certain communities such as curd, juices, bananas are considered cold foods and are avoided in case of common flu or in winter season. Pica (craving for unusual substances like clay, chalk) is also considered a very positive symptom of pregnancy that can lead to malnutrition and certain serious health problems.
- **Food fads:** Personal likes and dislikes are called food fads. In the selection of food, these food fads play an important role and may become obstacle in treating certain nutritional problems. Nurses must keep the likes and dislikes of patients in mind related to food while planning diet for them.
- **Cooking practices:** These practices also have a great impact on the nutritive value of food. Excessive boiling of milk, frequently heating of food, cooking food at very high heat (temperature) or draining away the water from rice after cooking are certain practices that can diminish the nutritive value of food.

RELATIONSHIP BETWEEN NUTRITION AND HEALTH

Nutrition and health are the two sides of the same coin. Good health is impossible to maintain without balanced nutrition as adequate nutrition is the foundation of good health. The relationship of health and nutrition is shown in Figure 1.2.

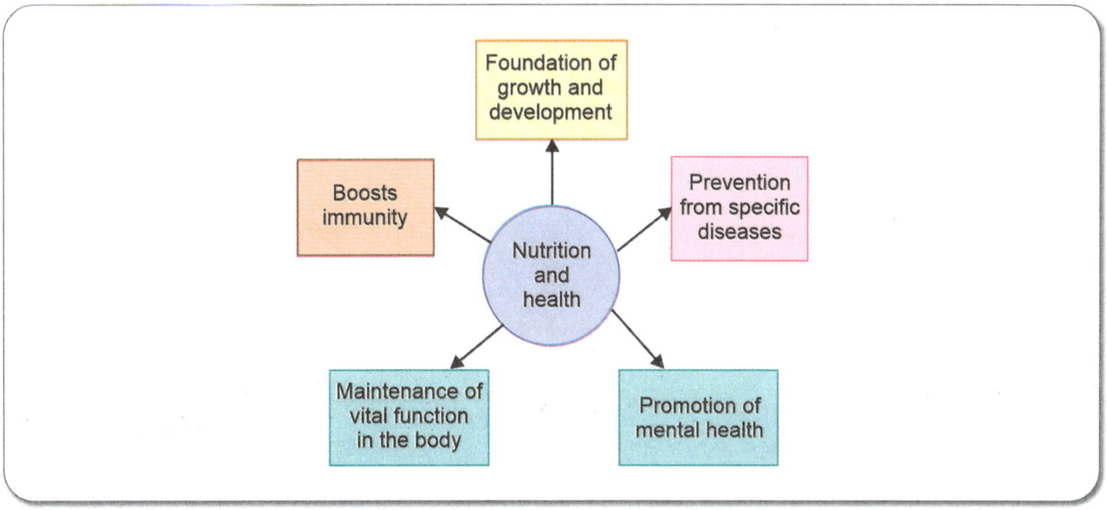

Fig. 1.2: Relationship between nutrition and health

- **Foundation of growth and development**: Balanced nutrition not only promotes fitness but also helps the body to grow and maintain proper functions. A well-balanced diet is important at every stage of life like infancy, childhood, adolescence, pregnancy, lactation and in old age for maintenance of optimum health and efficiency of the body.
- **Immunity booster:** When the body receives enough nutrients, the immune system of the body functions well and protects the body from many infections. A well-balanced diet is required throughout the life to combat with surrounding infections (seasonal allergies). Good nutrition is also mandatory in the disease condition, for example, for early recovery in tuberculosis or for speedy wound healing in case of any surgery and prevention from infections.
- **Prevention from specific diseases:** Recent researches suggest that diet plays an important role in the prevention of certain nutritional deficiency diseases like protein energy malnutrition, goiter, blindness, scurvy, anemia, etc. Malnutrition is also directly responsible for many other associated problems like abortion, premature delivery, stillbirth, low birth-weight babies and death of the mother. Balanced nutrition also reduces the risk of certain chronic diseases like hypertension, obesity, diabetes and heart diseases.
- **Maintenance of vital function in the body:** Carbohydrates and fats give enough energy to the body to function properly throughout the day. Fats also keep the body warm, lubricate joints and keep the muscles movable. The proteins (amino acids) are used by the body to build and repair any muscle tissue. Every tissue in the body is made up of protein so it is important to take good nutrition to replenish and repair the body's tissues.
- **Promotion of mental health:** Recent researches on nutrition have proved that good nutrition not only promotes physical health but also promotes the intellectual ability. Tryptophan is an amino acid that is required to produce chemical called serotonin that promotes sleep and also helps the body to combat with depression. Similarly, omega-3 fatty acids are also found very useful for improving mental health.
- **Bone and muscle health:** Nutrients such as calcium, vitamin D, and protein are essential for maintaining strong bones and muscles. A balanced diet helps prevent conditions like osteoporosis and muscle wasting.
- **Digestive health:** A diet high in fiber, along with adequate hydration, supports healthy digestion and prevents issues like constipation and gastrointestinal disorders.
- **Overall well-being:** Good nutrition contributes to overall well-being and quality of life. It can improve energy levels, promote better sleep, and enhance physical performance.

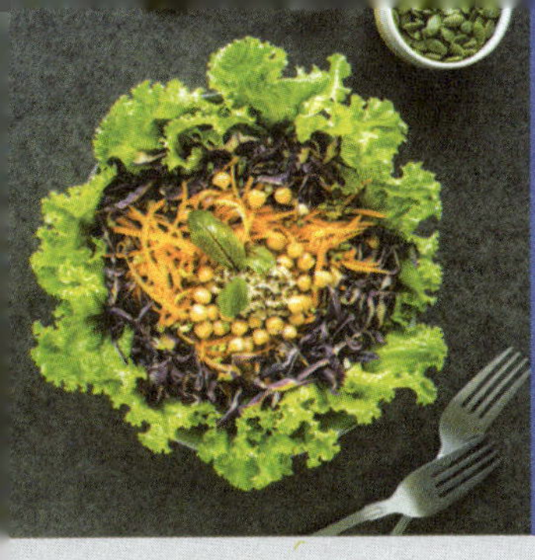

STUDENT ASSIGNMENT

LONG ANSWER QUESTIONS

1. Explain various food habits and customs that can affect the nutritional status of an individual.
2. Define nutrition and enlist the factors affecting nutrition.
3. Explain the relationship of health and nutrition.
4. How has the concept of nutrition changed from past to the present era?

SHORT ANSWER QUESTION

1. **Define the following terms:**
   a. Food
   b. Calorie
   c. Balanced diet
   d. Nutrients
   e. Metabolism

MULTIPLE CHOICE QUESTIONS

1. **A substance needed by the body for growth, energy, repair and maintenance is called:**
   a. Nutrient
   b. Calorie
   c. Vitamins
   d. Folic acid
2. **Nutrients that help the body tissues to repair are:**
   a. Fats
   b. Proteins
   c. Vitamins
   d. None of these
3. **All of the following nutrients are found in food, except:**
   a. Fats
   b. Proteins
   c. Carbohydrates
   d. Plasma
4. **Cereals and breads are good sources of:**
   a. Carbohydrates
   b. Proteins
   c. Vitamin C
   d. Fats
5. **Micronutrients include:**
   a. Carbohydrate
   b. Vitamins and minerals
   c. Proteins
   d. Fat
6. **One kilocalorie is equal to:**
   a. 4.2 Joules
   b. 5 Joules
   c. 8 Joules
   d. None of these

7. **One gram fat provides:**
   a. 7 calorie
   b. 5 calorie
   c. 9 calorie
   d. 12 calorie
8. **Energy-yielding nutrients include:**
   a. Carbohydrate
   b. Fat
   c. Vitamins
   d. Both a and b
9. **Protective nutrients include:**
   a. Fats
   b. Carbohydrates
   c. Vitamins and minerals
   d. None of these
10. **What role do vitamins play in maintaining good health?**
    a. Provide energy
    b. Support immune function
    c. Regulate blood sugar
    d. Build muscle
11. **Which dietary factor is most closely linked to the risk of developing heart disease?**
    a. Sodium intake
    b. Protein consumption
    c. Vitamin D levels
    d. Fiber intake
12. **What mineral is crucial for maintaining strong bones and teeth?**
    a. Iron
    b. Potassium
    c. Magnesium
    d. Calcium
13. **What is the primary function of carbohydrates in the body?**
    a. Build muscle
    b. Provide energy
    c. Support brain function
    d. Strengthen bones
14. **Which nutrient is essential for building and repairing tissues in the body?**
    a. Vitamin C
    b. Protein
    c. Calcium
    d. Iron
15. **What is a food taboo?**
    a. A diet plan for weight loss
    b. A cultural rule against eating certain foods
    c. A recipe for a traditional dish
    d. A list of recommended foods for athletes
16. **In Hindu-majority regions, which animal's meat is often considered taboo due to religious beliefs?**
    a. Chicken
    b. Fish
    c. Cow
    d. Goat
17. **What is a common reason for food taboos related to pregnancy in various cultures?**
    a. To promote weight gain
    b. To prevent allergies
    c. To avoid harming the baby
    d. To reduce food cravings
18. **In some cultures, which type of food is often avoided due to beliefs about its impact on fertility?**
    a. Fruits
    b. Vegetables
    c. Dairy products
    d. Eggs
19. **Which factor often influences the development of food taboos?**
    a. Climate
    b. Language
    c. Religion
    d. Music

20. Which cultural factor can affect dietary habits and food choices?

a. Language spoken
b. Personal preferences
c. Religious beliefs
d. Fashion trends

21. Which is the best source of Iron in the given options?

a. Green vegetables
b. Eggs
c. Milk
d. Carrot

22. Which of the following is responsible for the sweetness of milk?

a. Sucrose
b. Lactose
c. Carotene
d. Microse

ANSWER KEY

1. a	**2.** b	**3.** d	**4.** a	**5.** b	**6.** a	**7.** c	**8.** d	**9.** c
10. b	**11.** a	**12.** d	**13.** b	**14.** b	**15.** b	**16.** c	**17.** c	**18.** d
19. c	**20.** c	**21.** a	**22.** b					

Notes

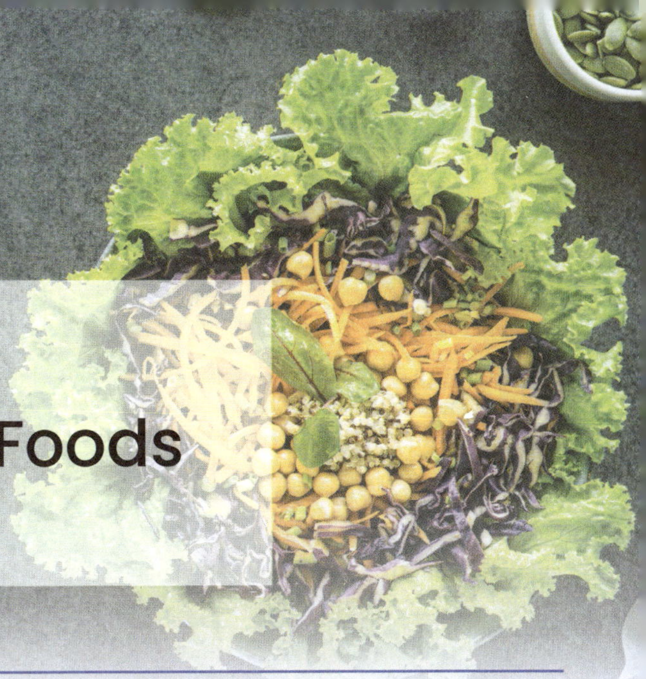

2

Classification of Foods

LEARNING OBJECTIVES

After the completion of the chapter, the readers will be able to:

- Discuss classification of food by plant and animal origin.
- Discuss classification of food by chemical composition.
- Discuss classification of food according to predominant functions.
- Explain classification of food by nutritive value.

CHAPTER OUTLINE

- Classification of Foods
- Classification of Food by Predominant Functions
- Classification of Food by Nutritive Value
- Fats and Oils
- Sugar and Jaggery
- Spices and Condiments
- Miscellaneous Foods

KEY TERMS

Amino acids: They are made up of carbon, nitrogen and oxygen atoms and act as the backbone of protein.
Balanced diet: A diet containing all the essential nutrients in appropriate proportions to meet the requirement of the body effectively.
Carbohydrates (CHO): These are also called saccharides made up of three elements—carbon, hydrogen and oxygen.
Fats: Fats are also known as triglycerides as they are made up of three fatty acids and glycerol. These are generally hydrophobic and are soluble in organic solvents and insoluble in water.
Minerals: A mineral is a naturally occurring substance, represented by a chemical formula, and is usually solid and inorganic and has a crystal-like structure.
Proteins: Proteins are made up of amino acids linked with peptide bonds.
Vitamins: Organic substances, required in small amount but a very essential component of the diet.

CLASSIFICATION OF FOODS

Based on Origin of Food

Animal Origin

Food of animal origin plays an important role in the diet of human being. Nutritionally they are very important sources of good quality of proteins and excellent sources of vitamins and minerals. In addition, animal food in general is more distinctive in flavor and texture. Examples of such food is milk, eggs, cheese, yogurt, honey, meat, etc.

Plant Origin

Food of plant origin contributes major share in the daily diet of every human being. Examples of such foods are various vegetables (potato, tomato, carrot, and cauliflower), cereals (maize, wheat, and barley), nuts, fruits, herbs, etc.

Based on Chemical Composition

Carbohydrates (CHO)

These are also called saccharides made up of three elements—carbon, hydrogen and oxygen. They are further of two types that include monosaccharides (glucose, sucrose small molecules also called sugars) and disaccharides also known as complex sugars (starch). Carbohydrates are found in almost every food, for example, milk, bread, potatoes, cookies and soft drinks. Carbohydrates are very important for the body as chemical reactions in the body requires fuel. During digestion carbohydrates break down into single molecules in the form of glucose or sucrose, which are absorbed by the body through blood supply.

Recommended Dietary Allowances

There is no set recommended dietary allowances (RDA) for carbohydrates as there is for vitamins and minerals. Carbohydrates are mainly used for energy so daily intake will depend on how many calories a person needs. Since the need of basic fuels must be met so required range is **45–65%** of calories that must be provided through carbohydrates to the body. Therefore, if the dietary requirement of calorie is 2000 calories per day then **900–1300** calories must come from carbohydrates that indicate **225–325** grams of carbohydrates per day. Again the recommendations of carbohydrates depend upon the lifestyle and health status of the person, for example, there is restricted need of carbohydrates if the person is suffering from diabetes or obesity.

Functions of Carbohydrates

- **Source and store house of energy:** Carbohydrates are probably the greatest source of energy for humans. The primary role of carbohydrates is to supply energy to all cells in the body. About 70% of the glucose entering the body from digestion is redistributed back into blood for use by other tissues. The brain is highly sensitive to low blood glucose level because it only uses glucose to produce energy and function properly. The primary function of carbohydrates is not only to provide energy but also to store energy in the form of glycogen in the muscles and liver.
- **Build macromolecules:** Glucose is converted to ribose and deoxyribose, which are essential building blocks to prepare RNA, DNA and ATP. Glucose is also used to make the molecule NADPH that is used for other chemical reactions in the body.

- **Help to preserve muscles:** During the period of starvation when carbohydrates are not available, the body can convert amino acids from muscles into glucose to provide energy to the brain. Thus consuming carbohydrates in the diet can prevent muscle breakdown to provide energy to the body.
- **Promote digestive system:** The fiber content in the carbohydrates promotes good digestive health by lowering the risk of digestive tract diseases and reducing the risk of constipation. There are two types of fibers, soluble and insoluble. Soluble fibers when pass through the body draw water and form a gel-like substance that makes the bowel movements easier. On the other hand, insoluble fibers relieve constipation by adding bulk to the stool.
- **Good for healthy heart:** Eating plenty of dietary fibers is good for heart. It helps to lower down the level of cholesterol and keeps the heart healthy.
- **Preserve the fats and proteins:** The presence of adequate glucose spares the breakdown of proteins and fats from being used to make glucose to fulfill the requirements of the body and spares proteins and fats for other uses in the body. Carbohydrates also help in the metabolism of fats; if the body has excessive energy after meeting its daily needs then the extra energy is stored as fats. If the diet is deficient in carbohydrates, the fat metabolism cannot proceed normally and results in the formation of ketones (ketones are acidic molecules formed by partially broken down fats) and leads to the condition called ketosis that makes the blood acidic and hinders the normal functioning of the body.

Sources

Carbohydrates are widely found in almost every food. The best sources are plant foods such as:	
Whole grains (rice, wheat, barley, oats, and cereals, flour) Milk and milk products Breads and other processed foods like fruit juices, snacks, cookies, candies, muffins, squash, syrup Beverages sweetened with sugar	Vegetables (potatoes, beans, and sweet potatoes) Dry fruits (dates, raisins) and nuts Fruits (mango, guava, banana, and grapes)

Digestion

Carbohydrates are broken down to provide glucose for energy. Carbohydrates are consumed in the form of polysaccharides (cellulose or starch fibers) and disaccharides (lactose, sucrose and galactose). They need to be changed into monosaccharide (glucose) for utilization in the body.

The digestion process of the carbohydrates begins in the mouth where it gets hydrolyzed by the salivary enzymes. Food bolus reaches into the stomach and digestion of carbohydrates mainly occur in the small intestine with pancreatic amylase, which converts starch into dextrin and maltose. Other enzymes like glycosidase present in the small intestine break down maltase, lactose and sucrose and convert into monosaccharide.

Absorption and Transportation

Glucose, galactose and fructose (monosaccharide) are transported from the wall of small intestine into the liver by the portal vein. Most of the glucose derived from food is transported via the blood stream to the peripheral tissues. The hormone insulin enables the glucose to be utilized by the cells as an energy source. Glucose is the most important energy source for the body especially for the brain. On the other hand, in the liver galactose and fructose are converted into other metabolites. Most fructose is taken up by the liver and converted into glucose, glycogen and lactate. Galactose is converted into glucose and stored as glycogen.

Storage

Extra glucose is initially stored as glycogen in the liver or muscles. The liver can store approximately 100 g of glycogen, which is used to maintain blood glucose level whereas the muscles store 400–500 g often used during movement. Once these reserves are saturated, excess glucose is converted to fat for long-term storage.

Overconsumption of Carbohydrates

Excess carbohydrates, especially refined sugars and starches, can contribute to weight gain. A diet high in refined carbohydrates can increase blood sugar levels rapidly, leading to insulin spikes. Over time, this can contribute to insulin resistance and increase the risk of type 2 diabetes. Diets high in refined carbohydrates and sugars have been linked to an increased risk of heart disease and other cardiovascular problems.

Underconsumption of Carbohydrates

Carbohydrates are the body's primary source of energy. Inadequate intake can lead to low energy levels, fatigue, and impaired physical performance.

Proteins

Proteins are made up of amino acids linked with peptide bonds. Amino acids are made up of carbon, nitrogen and oxygen atoms and act as the backbone of proteins. Amino acids are building blocks of proteins and play many critical roles inside the body like building of proteins, synthesis of hormones and neurotransmitters. Amino acids sequence is coded by specific genes, which are also known as polypeptide chain. Proteins are the chief body builders of the body; and recommended daily allowance is approximately 45–50 g/day for women and 50–60 g/day for men. Amino acids can be classified as essential and nonessential amino acids.

Essential Amino Acids

Human body needs almost 20 different amino acids to function properly. All amino acids are important for body but 10 are named as essential amino acids as these amino acids cannot be made by the body (Table 2.1).

Table 2.1: List of essential amino acids

Sl. no.	Name of essential amino acids
1.	L-arginine
2.	L-histidine
3.	L-isoleucine
4.	L-leucine
5.	L-lysine
6.	L-methionine
7.	L-phenylalanine
8.	L-threonine
9.	L-tryptophan
10.	L-valine

Nonessential Amino Acids

Nonessential amino acids are those amino acids that can be made by the body (Table 2.2).

Table 2.2: List of nonessential amino acids

Sl. no.	Name of nonessential amino acids
1.	Alanine
2.	Asparagines
3.	Aspartic acid
4.	Cysteine
5.	Glutamic acid
6.	Glutamine
7.	Glycine
8.	Proline
9.	Serine
10.	Tyrosine

Sources

Seafoods are excellent sources of proteins (fish, crabs). Protein is also found in milk and milk products (butter, cheese, yogurt), in animal and poultry products like meat (beef, pork) and eggs. Pulses, legumes, beans, nuts, soya and oats are also very rich sources of proteins (Table 2.3).

Table 2.3: Dietary sources of protein according to National Institute of Nutrition (NIN) per 100 g of food item

Plant source foods	Protein (g)	Animal source foods	Protein (g)
Maize, dry	11.1	Katla fish	19.5
Rice, raw	7.5	Pomfret (white)	17.0
Rice, raw, milled	6.8	Rohu fish	16.6
Wheat, whole	11.8	Sole fish	16.2
Wheat flour (whole)	12.1	Surmai fish	19.9
Wheat flour (refined)	11.0	Egg (hen)	13.3
Wheat bread (brown)	8.8	Goat meat (lean)	21.4
Wheat bread (white)	7.8	Fowl	25.9
Bengal gram	20.8	Milk (buffalo)	4.3
Black gram	24.0	Milk (cow)	3.2
Green gram	24.5	Curd (cow's milk)	3.1
Lentils	25.1	Chenna (cow's milk)	18.3
Dry peas	19.7	Cheese	24.1
Rajma	22.9		
Soybean	43.2		
Almonds	20.8		
Cashewnuts	21.2		
Walnuts	15.6		
Sunflower seeds	19.8		
Safflower seeds	13.5		
Groundnuts	25.3		

Recommended Daily Allowance (RDA) of Protein for Indians

Normally recommended daily allowance (RDA) of protein is approximately 0.8 g/kg of body weight. As per particular groups it is given as in (Table 2.4).

Table 2.4: Recommended daily allowance (RDA) of protein for Indians

Groups	Particulars	Total (g/day)
Infant	0–6 months 6–12 months 1–3 years	1.16 g/kg/day 1.69 g/kg/day 16.7
Children	4–6 years 7–9 years 10–12 years (boys) 10–12 years (girls)	20.1 29.5 39.9 40.4
Adolescents	13–15 years (boys) 13–15 years (girls) 16–18 years (boys) 16–18 years (girls)	54.3 52.0 61.5 55.5
Men (average 60 kg weight)	Sedentary worker Moderate worker Heavy worker	60.0
Women (average 55 kg weight)	Sedentary worker Moderate worker Heavy worker	55.0
	Pregnant	78.0
	Lactating 0–6 months Lactating 7–12 months	79.0 68.0

Functions of Proteins

- **Help in growth, repair and maintenance of body:** Proteins not only play an important role in growth and development of body tissues but also have a vital role in maintenance and repair of these tissues. Proteins are also essential in the growth of fetus in the womb and in the process of lactation after delivery. Therefore, the demand of proteins increases during the period of pregnancy and lactation.
- **Provide stiffness and rigidity to the body:** Some proteins are fibrous in nature that provide stiffness and rigidity to the body. For example, keratin, collagen and elastin. Collagen is the most excessive structural protein found in bones, tendons, ligaments and skin. Similarly, keratin is found in skin, hair and nails. Elastin is hundred times more flexible than collagen and helps many body tissues to return to their original shape after stretching or contracting like uterus, arteries and lungs.
- **Act as messenger:** Some hormones are actually proteins that act as a chemical messenger between cells, tissues and organs. For example, ADH, glucagon and insulin.
- **Maintain pH of the body:** Another important role of proteins is to maintain pH of the body by regulating the concentrations of acids and bases in blood as well as other bodily fluids. For example, hemoglobin that binds small amount of acids to maintain normal pH of blood.

- **Aid in biochemical reactions:** Many enzymes are made up of proteins that help in the biochemical reactions that take place within or outside the cell. Many functions of the body depends upon these enzymes like digestion, blood clotting, etc.
- **Boost the immune system:** Antibodies are actually proteins that help and protect the body to fight with infections when foreign antigens invade the body cells and thus body develops the immunity against the exposed disease.
- **Help in transportation and storage of nutrients:** Many substances are transported by the proteins like vitamins, minerals, blood sugar, cholesterol and oxygen. Hemoglobin helps to carry oxygen from lungs to body tissues and similarly, lipoproteins transport cholesterol and other body fat in the blood. Proteins play a pivotal role in storage like ferritin is a storage protein to store iron.
- **Source of energy:** Proteins provide 4 calories per gram, the same amount of energy that is being provided by carbohydrates.
- **Maintain the body fluids:** Proteins help the body to regulate fluid balance. Albumin and globulins are the proteins that help to maintain body fluid balance by attracting or retaining water.

Digestion

Proteolytic enzymes are not present in the mouth, so there is no digestion of proteins in the mouth. When the proteins enter the stomach, hydrochloric acid and pepsin begin protein digestion in the stomach. Hydrochloric acid makes the stomach very acidic that helps HCl to react with pepsinogen to form pepsin so that it can break the central peptide bond in proteins. In small intestine, trypsin breaks down proteins into single amino acids. Trypsin also activates the enzymes chymotrypsin, carboxypeptidase and elastase that are released into the small intestine for amino acid chain breakdown.

Absorption

Absorption of proteins takes place in the jejunum and ileum portions of the small intestine. Adenosine triphosphate is the energy source that the body utilizes during protein absorption. The sodium and potassium are minerals needed for the amino acids to pass from the intestines through the villi and into the bloodstream. Excessive proteins get converted into fat for storage.

Overconsumption of Proteins

Excessive protein intake can increase uric acid and put a strain on the kidneys, as they are responsible for filtering out waste products from protein metabolism. Some research suggests that very high protein intake, particularly from animal sources, may increase calcium loss through urine and potentially impact bone health over the long term.

Underconsumption of Proteins

Proteins are essential for maintaining and repairing tissues, including muscle tissue. Inadequate protein intake can lead to muscle wasting and weakness over time. Proteins are necessary for the production of antibodies and other components of the immune system. Insufficient protein intake may weaken immune function and impact wound healing.

Fats

Fats are among the three main macronutrients along with carbohydrates and proteins. Fats are also known as triglycerides as they are made up of three fatty acids and glycerol. Fats like other lipids are generally hydrophobic and are soluble in organic solvents and insoluble in water. Fats can also be categorized according to the number and bonding of the carbon atoms in the chain. Fats that are saturated do not have double bonding between the carbon atoms in the chain. Unsaturated fatty acids have one or more double bonded carbons in the chain and some fats have multiple double bonds and thus known as polyunsaturated fats.

Fats not only serve as energy source for the body but also extra fats can be stored in the body to meet the immediate requirement of excessive energy. Fats are broken down in the body to release glycerol and fatty acids. Glycerol itself can be converted to glucose by the liver and used for the energy requirement of the body.

Fats are major source of energy and also aid body in absorbing fat soluble vitamins. Fats are very important for proper growth and development and they also add flavor and taste and give satiety value to the food. Total fat consumption should be 15–30% of the total calorie intake. Saturated fats should be eaten in limited amount compared to unsaturated fats.

Sources

Butter, cream, ghee, fried foods, snacks, chips, oils, whole milk, whole eggs, animal meat like pork, mutton, chicken are the major sources of fat.

Functions of Fats

- **Major source of energy:** Fat provides maximum amount of energy that is 9kcal/grams, more than the energy provided by the same amount of carbohydrates and proteins. Fat can be deposited in adipose tissue to provide energy during starvation. All tissues except central nervous system and brain can utilize fat as a source of energy.
- **Essential for absorption of certain vitamins:** Fat is essential in the body for the absorption of fat soluble vitamins. For example, vitamin A, D, E and K.
- **Retention of body heat:** Fat acts as a thermal insulator in the body and protects the body from cold by retaining body heat.
- **Necessary for synthesis of hormone:** Cholesterol is necessary for the synthesis of hormones like sex hormones.
- **Shock absorber:** Fats not only surround the vital organs to protect them from mechanical shocks and injuries but help them to keep in place.
- **Help in transportation of nutrients:** Fat serves as main component of cell membrane structure and helps in transportation of nutrients, minerals and metabolites across cell membrane.
- **Transmission of nerve impulse:** Fat insulation (myelin) around nerve fibers provides electrical insulation and helps in nerve impulse transmission.
- **Increase satiety value of food:** Fats not only give the feeling of fullness and slow down the emptying of stomach but also add palatability to diet.

Digestion and Absorption of Fats

Digestion of fats (triacylglycerols and phospholipids) begins in the mouth as lipids get mixed with the saliva. The physical action of chewing and the digestive enzymes change the fats into small droplets and water gets separated. Then the fat reaches to the stomach and the enzyme gastric lipase breaks down the triglycerides into diglycerides and fatty acids. Small amount of fat digestion occurs in the stomach. Stomach contents enter the small intestine where it gets mixed with the bile juices, which act as an emulsifier. The act of emulsification increases the surface area of lipids making them more accessible for digestive enzymes. Pancreatic lipase enzyme further breaks the fats into free fatty acids and monoglycerides that can be absorbed directly into the bloodstream from the intestinal microvillus. Long-chain fatty acids form a large lipoprotein structure called a chylomicron and they carry lipids from the digestive tract into circulation. When energy supplies are low the body utilizes its stored fat reserves for energy.

Types of Fatty Acids

- **Saturated fatty acids:** These fatty acid chains have only single bond. They are made up of long chains of carbon atoms and are usually solid at room temperature. They can be derived both from animal and plant sources. For example, butter and fat, meat fat, palm and coconut oils. If taken excessive, they can increase the level of cholesterol and lead to obesity and other heart diseases.
- **Unsaturated fatty acids:** These are fats or fatty acids in which there is one or more double bond in the chain of fatty acids. They are liquid at room temperature.
    - **Monounsaturated fatty acids (MUFA):** These types of fatty acids have only one double bond in their molecular chain. They remain liquid even at extremely low temperature. For example, olive oil and peanut oil. They are helpful in lowering bad cholesterol (LDL) and increasing (HDL) good cholesterol level.
    - **Polyunsaturated fatty acids (PUFA):** These types of fatty acids have two or more double bond in their molecule. Such type of fatty acids are present in fish and soybean oil.

Fats can also be classified as visible and invisible fat:

- Visible fat can be seen like butter or oil.
- Invisible fat is present in the food but cannot be seen, for example, fat in dairy products, fish, etc.

Caloric value: 1 gram of fat gives 9 kcal energy almost 2.5 times more energy per gram as compared to carbohydrates and proteins (Table 2.5).

Table 2.5: According to National Institute of Nutrition, values per 100 g

Foods	Fat	Foods	Fat
Butter	81.0	Curd (cow's milk)	4.0
Ghee (cow)	100.0	Cheese	25.1
Ghee (buffalo)	100.0	Katla fish	2.4
Hydrogenated oil	100.0	Pomfret (white)	1.3
Cooking oils (peanut, mustard, coconut)	100.0	Prawn	1.0
Rohu	1.4	Almonds	58.9
Egg (hen)	13.3	Cashewnuts	46.9
Goat liver	3.0	Coconut (dry)	62.3
Mutton	123.3	Groundnut	40.1
Milk (buffalo)	6.5	Pistachio nut	53.5
Milk (cow)	4.1	Walnuts	64.5
Milk (human)	3.4	Whole wheat flour	1.7
Rice (raw milled)	0.5	Soybean	19.5

Recommended Daily Allowances of Fat (Table 2.6)

Table 2.6: According to ICMR, visible fat (g/day) for different age groups

Group	Particulars	Body weight (kg)	Visible fat (g/day)
Man	Sedentary work	50	20
	Moderate work	50	
	Heavy work	50	
Woman	Sedentary work	50	
	Moderate work	50	
	Heavy work	50	
	Pregnant woman	50	30
	Lactating 0–6 months	50	45
	Lactating 6–12 months	50	
Infant	0–6 months	5.4	—
	6–12 months	8.6	—
Children	1–3 years	12.2	25
	4–6 years	19.0	
	7–9 months	26.9	
Boys	10–12 years	35.4	22
	13–15 years	47.8	
	16–18 years	57.1	
Girls	10–12 years	31.5	
	13–15 years	46.7	
	16–18 years	49.9	

Overconsumption of Fats

Fats are calorie-dense, and excessive consumption can lead to weight gain and obesity, especially if combined with a sedentary lifestyle. Diets high in saturated and trans fats can increase levels of LDL (bad) cholesterol in the blood, which raises the risk of heart disease and stroke. Excessive fat intake, especially saturated fats, can contribute to fatty liver disease and gallstones.

Underconsumption of Fats

Fats are crucial for the absorption of fat-soluble vitamins (A, D, E, K) and for the body's production of essential fatty acids. Inadequate fat intake can lead to deficiencies in these nutrients. Inadequate fat intake can lead to dry, flaky skin, other dermatological issues and inadequate fat intake can disrupt hormonal balance and reproductive health.

Minerals

A mineral is a naturally occurring substance, representable by a chemical formula, is usually solid and inorganic and has a crystal-like structure. It is different from rock as rock can be aggregate of minerals and nonminerals and do not have a specific chemical composition. For example, calcium, phosphorus, and chlorides.

Human body needs many minerals and these are essential for health, growth and development of the body. Minerals can be further divided into major (macro minerals) and trace minerals (micro minerals). These two are equally important but trace minerals are required in smaller amount than the major minerals, for example, iron, zinc, iodine, magnesium, etc. A balanced diet must provide all the essential minerals these are as follows:

Sodium

It is an essential mineral. Sodium is found in most of the things we consume so a supplement of sodium is not much required to a normal healthy individual. We can convert sodium into salt by multiplying it by **2.4**. For example, 1500 mg of sodium is equivalent to 3600 mg of salt.

Functions of sodium: It helps in regulating blood pressure, proper fluid balance, nerve transmission and muscle contraction. It also regulates the acid alkali balance along with other minerals like potassium, calcium and magnesium.

Requirement: It is required in the quantity of approximately **1.5–2.3 g/day**

Overconsumption: Excessive intake of sodium leads to fluid retention, hypertension, put strain on kidney and heart. Hypernatremia is a condition when there is high concentration of sodium in the blood.

Underconsumption: It can lead to hypotension, weakness and muscle cramps. Hyponatremia is a condition when there is low concentration of sodium in the blood.

Sources: Table salt, canned vegetables and juices, pickles, soya, salsa and tomato sauces, processed foods, small amount is also found in breads, vegetables and unprocessed meat, poultry and fish.

Chloride

It is major mineral that works along with sodium and potassium.

Functions of chloride: Chloride is an essential mineral needed for maintaining proper fluid balance, blood volume, blood pressure, transmitting of nerve impulses and pH of our body fluids. The cells in the lining of stomach need chloride to make hydrochloric acid, which is an essential component of digestive juices.

Requirement: It is required approximately 1.5 g/day to 2.3 g/day. Chloride needs are similar for both males and females but slightly vary according to age (Table 2.7).

Table 2.7: Requirement of chloride as per age

Age	Chloride (g/day)
1–3 years	1.5
4–8 years	1.9
9–50 years	2.3
51–70 years	2.0
Above 71 years	1.8

Overconsumption: It can lead to increase in blood pressure, retaining of fluid. **Hyperchloremia** is excessive amount of chlorides in the body.

Underconsumption: Deficiency of chloride may occur in case of heavy fluid loss, like heavy sweating, diarrhea or vomiting. Certain medications like diuretics also cause deficiency of chloride. Deficiency of chlorides can lead to weakness or fatigue, muscle cramps and heart failure. **Hypochloremia** is a condition when there is low amount of chlorides in the body.

Sources: Table salt, vegetables and food with higher amounts of chloride include rye, tomato, celery and olives.

Potassium

Potassium is the third most abundant mineral in the body that acts as an electrolyte. Roughly 80% of the potassium is found in muscle cells and 20% can be found in bones, liver and red cells.

Functions of potassium: Potassium is needed for fluid balance, nerve transmission and muscle contraction.

Requirement: It is required approximately 4–5 g/day.

Sources: Bananas, oranges, apricots, grapefruit, dry fruits, spinach, broccoli, potatoes, sweet potatoes,, mushrooms, cucumber, peas, meat, milk,, whole grains and legumes.

Overconsumption: It can affect the functions of heart muscles leading to irregular heartbeat and may cause heart attack and failure of kidney. **Hyperkalemia** is excessive amount of potassium in the blood.

Underconsumption: Underconsumption of potassium may lead to weakness of muscles, cramp, twitch, or even person may become paralyzed. Low level of potassium can increase blood pressure, depletion of calcium from the bones and increases the risk of kidney stones. Low amount of potassium in the blood is known as **hypokalemia.**

Calcium

Calcium is the most abundant mineral in our body that constitutes about 1.5–2% of total body weight. Calcium is not produced by our body, so we have to depend upon the diet to get the required amount of calcium needed to the body. Vitamin D helps in the absorption of calcium.

Functions of Calcium

- **Growth:** Calcium is essential for growth of children.
- **Formation and maintenance of bones and teeth:** Calcium is required for the formation of healthy bones and teeth.
- **Regulation of heartbeat:** Calcium helps in regulation of heartbeat and functioning of heart muscle.
- **Activation of enzymes:** It activates a number of enzymes such as pancreatic lipase.
- **Helpful in clotting of blood:** Calcium helps in process of blood clotting process by converting prothrombin into thrombin and fibrinogen into fibrin.
- **Contraction and relaxation of muscles:** Free calcium ions act as activators for chemical reaction and large amount of ATP (adenosine triphosphate) gets released that helps in contraction and relaxation of muscles.
- **Transmission of nerve impulse:** Calcium is required for the synthesis of acetylcholine, a neurotransmitter that is necessary for conduction of nerve transmission.
- **Absorption:** It helps in the absorption of essential nutrients such as cobalamin from the ileum.

Sources of Calcium

Milk and milk products, canned fish, tofu, fortified soya milk, dry fruits and green legumes, etc.

Dietary Sources Rich in Calcium (Table 2.8)

Table 2.8: Value of calcium in (mg/100 g) of food item

Food sources	Calcium (mg/100 g)
Milk	300
Spinach, cooked	145

Contd...

Food sources	Calcium (mg/100 g)
Almonds	93
Orange	52
Sesame seeds	51
Mushrooms	18
Cheese	790
Curd	120–210
Broccoli	41

Daily Calcium Requirement (Table 2.9)

Table 2.9: Requirement of calcium as per age

Age	Calcium (mg/day)
0–6 months	210
7–12 months	270
1–3 years	500
4–8 years	800
9–18 years	1300
19–50 years	1000
Above 50 years	1200

Overconsumption of Calcium

Too much calcium in the blood can weaken the bones, create kidney stones and can affect the functioning of heart and brain. Excessive amount of calcium in the blood is known as **hypercalcemia.**

Underconsumption of Calcium

Low level of calcium can cause osteopenia and osteoporosis. This also increases the risk of bone fracture especially in the older individuals. Low amount of calcium in the blood is known as **hypocalcemia.**

Phosphorus

Phosphorus is an essential mineral required for various bodily functions, including bone health, energy production (as part of ATP), and cell membrane structure. The recommended daily intake (RDI) of phosphorus varies by age and gender but generally ranges from 700 mg to 1000 mg per day for adults.

Sources of Phosphorus

- **Food sources:** Phosphorus is found abundantly in many foods, especially protein-rich foods. Good dietary sources include:
  - Meat (especially organ meats like liver and kidney)
  - Poultry
  - Fish and seafood
  - Dairy products (milk, cheese, yogurt)
  - Nuts and seeds

  - Legumes (beans and lentils)
  - Whole grains
- **Phosphorus in beverages:** It is also present in some beverages, particularly carbonated drinks and processed foods due to additives like phosphoric acid.

Overconsumption of Phosphorus

Overconsumption of phosphorus can occur, especially in diets high in processed foods and carbonated drinks containing phosphoric acid. Excessive phosphorus intake, particularly in the form of additives, may disrupt calcium balance in the body, potentially leading to bone loss (osteoporosis) and calcification of soft tissues.

Health concerns: Individuals with chronic kidney disease (CKD) are particularly susceptible to problems related to excess phosphorus because impaired kidney function can lead to difficulty in excreting phosphorus, resulting in high levels in the blood (hyperphosphatemia).

Underconsumption of Phosphorus

Symptoms of phosphorus deficiency (hypophosphatemia) can include muscle weakness, bone pain or fragility, and fatigue. Severe deficiency can lead to conditions like rickets in children or osteomalacia in adults, which are characterized by weakened bones.

Magnesium

Magnesium is found in bones, and is needed for making proteins. It helps in muscle contraction and nerve transmission.

Sources: Nuts, legumes, green leafy vegetables, seafood, bakery products, hard drinking water. Daily requirement of magnesium as per the age given in Table 2.10.

Table 2.10: Requirement of magnesium as per age

Age	Magnesium (mg/day)
0–6 months	30
7–12 months	75
1–3 years	80
4–8 years	130
9–13 years	240
14–18 years	410 (boys), 360 (girls)
19–30 years	400 (men), 310 (women)
Above 30 years	420 (men), 320 (women)

Overconsumption: Overconsumption of magnesium from dietary sources alone is rare because excess magnesium is usually excreted by the kidneys. However, excessive intake from supplements or medications can lead to diarrhea, nausea, and abdominal cramping. In severe cases, very high doses of magnesium supplements can cause irregular heartbeat and dangerously low blood pressure.

Underconsumption: Not getting enough magnesium can lead to symptoms such as muscle cramps and spasms, fatigue, weakness, loss of appetite, nausea, and abnormal heart rhythms.

Sulfur

It is an important part of several amino acids. It helps the body to resist from bacteria, and cleanses the blood. It plays an important role in enzyme reaction and protein synthesis. It is required in quantity of approximately 700–900 mg/day.

Sources: Meat, poultry products, fish, eggs, milk, legumes and nuts.

Trace Minerals

- **Iron:** It is a part of the molecule hemoglobin found in red blood cells that carry oxygen in the body needed for metabolism. It is required approximately 10 mg/day but its requirements vary according to various stages of the body like pregnancy and lactation. Its deficiency may cause anemia.

  Sources: Organ meat, red meat, fish, poultry, egg yolks, legumes, dry fruits, green leafy vegetables and cereals
- **Zinc:** It is an important part of many enzymes needed for making proteins and genetic material, and helps in taste perception, wound healing, normal fetal development, production of sperm, sexual maturation, normal growth and in immune system. It is required approximately 15–20 mg/day.

  Sources: Seafood, oyster, liver, yeast, wheat gram.
- **Iodine:** It is found in thyroid hormone, which helps to regulate growth, development and metabolism. It is required in quantity of approximately 150 µg/day. Deficiency may cause thyroid disorder.

  Sources: Seafoods, iodized salt, bread and dairy products.
- **Copper:** It is an important part of many enzymes and needed for iron metabolism. It is required in quantity of approximately 1–2 mg/day.

  Sources: Legumes, nuts, whole grains, organ meat and drinking water.
- **Fluoride:** It is involved in the formation of bones, teeth and helps to prevent tooth decay. It is required in quantity of approximately 3.8–10 mg/day.

  Sources: Drinking water, fish, poultry products and tea.
- **Chromium:** Chromium works closely with insulin to regulate blood sugar levels. It is required approximately 50–150 mg/day.

  Sources: Unrefined foods, yeast, whole grains, nuts and milk products.

Vitamins

These are the vital amines, which are required by the body for the metabolism. It may be categorized as fat-soluble vitamins, for example, vitamins A, D, E and K and water-soluble vitamins, for example, vitamin B complex and vitamin C. Vitamin deficiency causes many diseases in the body. Vitamin deficiencies occur mainly due to poverty, food fads, faulty food habits, consumption of some drugs or excessive consumption of alcohol.

Water-soluble Vitamins

Vitamin B complex

- **Thiamine (B_1):** Involved in carbohydrates, fats, amino acids and alcohol metabolism. Deficiency causes the disease beriberi and peripheral neuritis. Recommended dietary allowance (RDA) is 1–1.5 mg.

  Sources: Sprouted beans, fortified cereals and green leafy vegetables.
- **Riboflavin (B_2):** Required as a coenzyme for carbohydrates metabolism. Its deficiency causes sore throat, lesions on lips and mouth and dermatitis. RDA varies from 0.5 mg to 1.5 mg depending upon the age.

  Sources: Rich sources are mushroom, yeast, beef, pork and lamb.

- **Niacin (B_3):** It acts as a coenzyme in oxidation reactions vital in cell metabolism. Its deficiency causes Pellagra— a condition characterized by diarrhea, dermatitis, dementia, inflammation of mouth and mental disturbances. RDA is 14–18 mg.

  Sources: Mushrooms, fish, chicken, pork, peanuts, sunflower seeds and green leafy vegetables.
- **Pantothenic Acid (B_5):** Needed in the synthesis of coenzyme that helps in the metabolism of carbohydrates, proteins and fats. RDA for adults is 5 mg /day and varies according to age.

  Sources: Whole grain cereals, legumes, eggs, meat, mushroom, liver.
- **Pyridoxine (B_6):** It helps the body to make several neurotransmitter chemicals that carry signals from one nerve cell to another nerve cell. It is needed for normal brain development and helps the body to make hormones serotonin and norepinephrine, which influence the mood. RDA is 1.3–1.7 mg and increases during the period of pregnancy and lactation.

  Sources: Avocado, banana, legumes, nuts, meat, poultry and whole grains, fortified bread and cereals.
- **Biotin (Vitamin H or B_7):** It acts as a coenzyme for carboxylation reaction essential for fats and carbohydrates metabolism. It also keeps the skin, hair, eyes and nervous system healthy. It is a crucial nutrient during pregnancy as it is important for embryonic growth. RDA is 300 mg.

  Sources: Egg yolk, green leafy vegetables, whole grains, organ meat, nuts, butter and mushroom.
- **Folic acid-(B_9):** It helps in maturation of blood cells and synthesis of purines and pyrimidines required for development of fetal nervous system. Adequate folic acid consumption before conception and during first trimester helps to prevent brain and spinal cord defects in newborn. Its deficiency in old age can also cause dementia. RDA is 400 mg and increases up to 600 mg in pregnancy and lactation.

  Sources: Beans, yeast, green leafy vegetables and fresh fruits.
- **Cyanocobalamin vitamin (B_{12}):** Involved in nucleic acid metabolism, myelin synthesis and repair and necessary for the formation of normal red blood cells. Daily recommended allowance is 2–4 µg. Deficiency can cause megaloblastic anemia, peripheral neuropathy characterized by tingling and numbness in hands and feet, damage to white matter of spinal cord and brain.

  Sources: Seafood, turkey, chicken, beef, pork, green leafy vegetables and dry fruits.

Vitamin C (L-ascorbic acid)

It plays a role in collagen, hormones and amino acid formation. Essential for wound healing, acts as an antioxidant and supports immune system, facilitates absorption of iron. Deficiency can cause scurvy, connective tissue defects, impaired wound healing, fatigue, depression, rashes, gingivitis and internal bleeding. RDA is 75–90 mg.

Sources: Found in citrus fruits (orange, lemon), fresh fruits and green leafy vegetables, amla is the richest source of vitamin C.

Fat-soluble Vitamins

Vitamin A (Retinol, Retinal)

It plays an important role in growth and development, for maintenance of immune system and for good vision. It is needed by the retina of the eye in the form of retinol, which combines with protein opsin to form rhodopsin, the light absorbing molecule necessary for vision. It also serves as growth hormone for epithelial and other cells. Its deficiency is estimated to affect approximately one-third children around the world. It can lead to night blindness, xerophthalmia (dryness of the conjunctiva) and keratomalacia (destruction of cornea). RDA for vitamin A for adults is 900 µg (300 IU) for men and 700 µg (2300 IU) for women, which increases up to 2600 IU in the period of pregnancy and lactation.

Sources: Carrot, cod liver oil, red capsicum, sweet potato, pumpkin, mango, peas, butter, green leafy vegetables, broccoli.

Vitamin D (Calciferol)

It comes into two forms vitamin D3 (cholecalciferol) and D2 (ergocalciferol animal version). It helps in maintenance of blood calcium and phosphorus level and proper mineralization of bones. Vitamin D3 is synthesized in the skin by the exposure to sunlight (ultraviolet rays). Deficiency may result in defective growth in children (rickets) and soft bones in adults (osteomalacia). RDA is 2–30 mg. Daily recommended allowances is given in Table 2.11.

Sources: Fish liver oil, egg yolk, milk and milk products and direct sunlight.

Table 2.11: Recommended daily allowance of vitamin D

Age	Amount of vitamin D required
From birth to 50 years	200 (IU)
51–70 years	400 (IU)
Above 70 years	600 (IU)

Vitamin E (Alpha-Tocopherol)

It works as an antioxidant, protection of polyunsaturated fatty acids, cell membranes. Deficiency may lead to peripheral neuropathy and breakdown of red blood cells. Recommended daily allowance is 20 μg/day.

Sources: Green leafy vegetables, nuts, dry fruits and sun flower oil.

Vitamin K (Menadione)

It helps in synthesis of proteins, involved in blood coagulation and bone metabolism. Recommended daily allowance is 120 μg for men and 90 μg for women.

Sources: Green leafy vegetables such as spinach, broccoli, cauliflower and dry fruits.

Water

Average human body is composed of 50–65% water. Body composition may vary according to gender and fitness level because fatty tissues contain less water than lean tissues. The usual way of adding water in the body is by drinking, through eating foods rich in water such as fresh fruits, vegetables, meat, etc. Loss of water may cause dehydration. A healthy sedentary adult should drink at least 1.5–2 L of water per day. Water plays an essential function in temperature regulation and removal of waste products from the body through urine. Water also plays an important role in chemical and metabolic reaction within the body.

CLASSIFICATION OF FOOD BY PREDOMINANT FUNCTIONS

- **Body building foods:** Foods that are high in proteins and complex carbohydrates such as whole grains. A body building diet generally contains 2500–5500 calories/day for men and 1500–3000 calories/day for women depending upon the type of work and level of exercise. Proteins are important part of body building food. Muscles are composed primarily of proteins and water. If an inadequate amount of proteins is consumed, muscle mass will suffer along with decrease in metabolism. Carbohydrates are also equally important as they not only provide energy to the body but also stimulate the pancreas to release hormone insulin, which helps to regulate glucose. Fats are needed in diet to maintain healthy metabolism.
- **Energy giving foods:** These are the foods that provide humans with energy to carry out the daily routine work. For example, potatoes, rice, and bread, beverages, juices, etc. Some foods give us more energy that can be stored and used later, for example, oil, butter, ghee.

- **Protective foods:** Foods that contain adequate amount of vitamins, minerals, high quality proteins and protect the body against deficiency diseases (scurvy, pellagra, beriberi) are called protective foods. For example, green leafy vegetables, fruits, etc.

CLASSIFICATION OF FOOD BY NUTRITIVE VALUE

Cereals and Millets

Cereals are also known as staple crops (Fig. 2.1). They include rice, brown rice, maize, wheat, barley, sorghum, millet, oats, rye, etc. Most cereals have a huge amount of fiber contents, enriched with a lot of vitamins and minerals (thiamine, niacin and riboflavin, phosphate, sulfate), for example, wheat, oats, barley, etc. They are also abundant in carbohydrates and proteins. Maize, rice and wheat together make up 87% of total grain production all over the world. There are many cereals that are used in specific regions and are not much popular, for example, wild rice is grown moderately in North America.

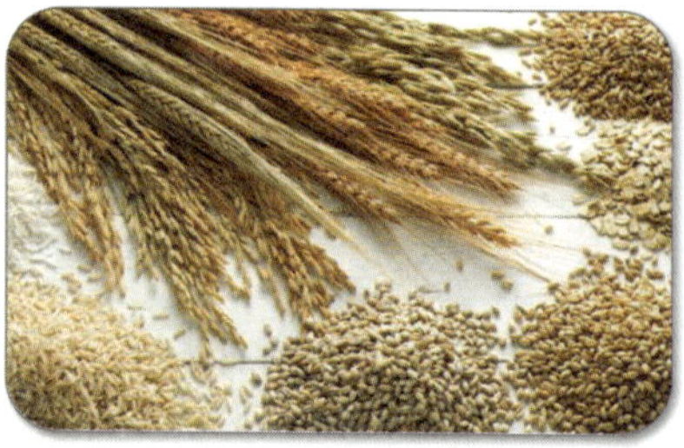

Fig. 2.1: Staple crop

Belonging to the complex carbohydrates food group, cereals are rich sources of minerals, vitamins, carbohydrates, oils, proteins and fats. Whole cereal grains have an outer bran coat, a starchy endosperm, and a germ layer. Bran coat is rich in fiber and minerals and also contains high amounts of thiamine and riboflavin. Endosperm layer gets removed during the process of refining. Endosperm has high percentage of starch and protein and is low in vitamin or mineral content. Germ layer is rich in protein, fat, minerals and vitamins. The germ layer is the storehouse of nutrients for the seed while germinating.

Millets are smaller grains, which are eaten without removing the outer layer, for example, jawar, bajra, etc.

Commonly used Cereals and Millets

Rice

Rice is possibly the most familiar, cultivated kind of cereal in the world. Although consumed in all parts of the world; rice cannot grow especially in cold regions. Most countries use it as their main food.

Types of Rice

Rice is a staple food in many countries. It can be categorized according to size, shape, aroma and color and type of processing.

According to size and shape

It can be long grain, medium grain and short grain.

According to Aroma

- **Basmati rice:** It is grown mainly in India and Pakistan but consumed all over the world. It is expensive and has a wonderful aroma. After cooking, it increases length wise and remains separate and fluffy.
- **Jasmine rice:** It is fragrant, long grained, nonsticky rice. When cooked, its aroma is very delicious and it is mainly used in Thailand.
- **Ambemohar rice:** It is short grain, very soft rice mainly available in Maharashtra, which is also known as mango blossom because of its flavor after cooking.

According to Color

- **Brown rice:** It is unpolished rice. In this type, hull is removed but the bran is retained. It is more nutritious as compared to white rice.
- **White rice:** It is more commonly used all over the world. It is also known as polished rice. While polishing, the nutritious part of rice gets removed, which makes it less nutritious as compared to brown rice. In this type, bran/germ is also removed.
- **Purple/black rice:** It is available in some parts of the world mainly in China and Thailand. It is very nutritious because of antioxidants and iron they contain. It takes longer time to cook as compared to white rice.

According to Processing

- **Unhulled rice:** These cannot be cooked and eaten, for cooking the rice grain chaff is separated.
- **Parboiled rice:** It is very commonly used in Southern part of India. In this type, the rice goes through the steam pressure process while still in the husk. Then the husk is removed and the rice is used in cooking. It cannot be cooked very soft.

Wheat

Wheat is one of the most dominant cereals consumed. Wheat is a significant ingredient in our foods especially in bread, biscuits, pastries, porridge, cakes, crackers, pancakes, pies, cookies, rolls, muffins, doughnuts, and also some breakfast cereals. It is rich in nutrients and has a lot of health benefits in human body. Researches suggest that eating brown bread can benefit health by encouraging growth of beneficial gut bacteria. It is also in a different form and has different species too.

Usage of Wheat

- **Whole wheat flour:** This type of flour is made by grinding or mashing the entire whole grain wheat. The word whole means all the grain (bran, germ and endosperm) is used and nothing is lost in the process of making flour, it has a brownish appearance. It is ideal for making chapatis, a staple food preferred by many Indians. It restores all the nutrients especially fibers, proteins and vitamins. It is also a good source of fibers, calcium, iron and other minerals like selenium. It is also used to make bread, muffins and some other baked items.
- **Refined flour:** It is made from whole wheat grain by peeling off entire husk and bran. Husk and bran are the most nutritious and fiber-rich part of the grain that is lost during the process of refining. Refined flour is also deficit in most of the vitamins and minerals. It is used for making cookies, cakes, white breads, pizza base, garlic breads, chocolates and muffins.
- **Semolina (Suji):** It is made exclusively from the endosperm, the middle part of the wheat. It is a rich source of gluten and is used in preparation of many pastas, cakes, desserts, porridge and dosa, etc. When cooked it has the ability to increase manifold in size but it is also used raw in some recipes to absorb the moisture or liquid, for example, fruit cakes. It is easily digestible, making it suitable food for gastrointestinal (GI) problems and for making the baby foods.
- **All purpose flour (Maida):** It is highly refined wheat flour, it is denatured food where most of the nutrients and fibers are removed and it is deficient in most of the nutrients. It is used to prepare noodles, naan, pooris, biscuits, pastries, sweets and other fast foods.

Other Cereals

- **Brown rice:** Brown rice is another delicious rice that contains a lot of nutrients such as vitamin B group, particularly riboflavin, thiamine, niacin and minerals like potassium, iron, phosphorus, and magnesium.
- **Maize:** This is a vital cereal all over the world. Cornflakes are flaked form of maize and popcorn, a well-known corn product, is one of the best snacks for ages all over the world.
- **Oats:** Oats are types of cereal grains that are especially grown for its seeds. It is grown in the cool and wet region. Oats is a rich source of essential nutrients such as carbohydrates, minerals and dietary fibers. Due to this reason it is considered best food for breakfast especially for the people who are obese and have high cholesterol level. Pure oats are also used as substitute diet for the patient of celiac disease (gluten free diet).
- **Barley:** This is a type of cereal that is not consumed as commonly like wheat or rice but it is very beneficial for the health as it is a rich source of fibers, antioxidants, vitamins and minerals. It is very low in fats and calories. It is very helpful in the improvement of digestion problems, as it not only helps to combat with constipation but also very helpful by providing healthy bacterias in the digestive tract. Antioxidants present in barley lowers the chances of cancer and are beneficial for the healthy heart.
- **Sorghum:** Also known as great millet or Indian millet. In India its local name is jowar or jonna. Sorghum can grow in hot environment where others crops cannot grow. It is high in carbohydrates with small amount of proteins and fats. It also contains some amount of minerals and vitamins like calcium, iron, and vitamin B_1. Its grains can be used as edible oil, dextrose and for some alcoholic beverages.
- **Millets:** This is considered the first grain consumed by the humans for domestic purpose. They can be grown in a short period of time in the areas that are dry and dependent upon rain water. Millets are very rich source of minerals like iron, magnesium, potassium and phosphorus. They are also known as non-gluten food recommended in gluten free diet, for example, ragi. They also have lower level of glucose as compared to rice and wheat.
- **Rye:** This is a type of cereal that can be grown in cold climates. Its grain is longer than the wheat grain and is usually consumed as whole grain because it is difficult to separate the germ and bran layer of the grain and makes it a more nutritious grain. It is used for making breads, beer, whiskeys, vodka and also used as animal feeds. Rye bread is considered better for the diabetic patients as compared to wheat bread.

Health Benefits of Cereals and Millets

Cereals and millets are highly nutritious and have numerous health benefits (Fig. 2.2).

- **Source of energy:** Cereals are the greatest source of energy. It is a rich source of vitamins, minerals, carbohydrates, fats and proteins. Proteins are present in every tissue of the grain. It is also rich in sulfate, phosphate, magnesium, potassium and calcium. Millets carry high amount of fibers. Average composition of cereals and millets is given in Table 2.12.
- **Controls the level of blood sugar:** Cereals, especially, millets are a rich source of magnesium, which is known to increase the efficiency of insulin and glucose receptors in the body and thus prevent from diabetes.
- **Improves digestive health:** Cereals and millets are rich in fibers so they prevent many problems of digestive system like constipation, gas and bloating, etc. They also regulate the digestive process and prevent gastric ulcers and reduce the chance of colon cancer.
- **Boosts the immune system:** Many of the antioxidants present in the cereals and millets not only boost the immunity but also detoxify the body by eliminating the waste products and neutralize the free radicals that can cause many diseases.

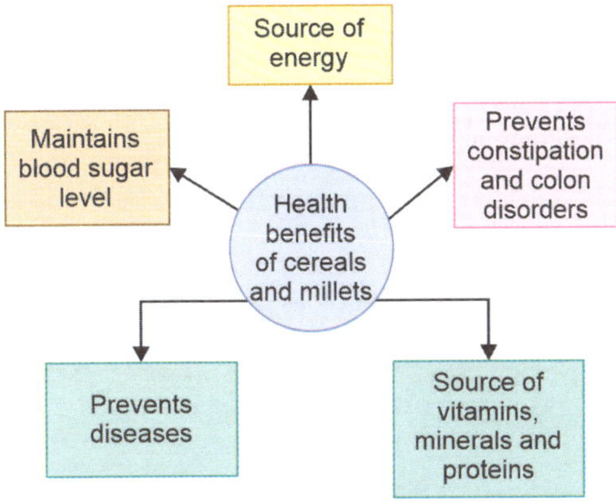

Fig. 2.2: Health benefits of cereals and millets

Table 2.12: Average composition of cereals and millets

Components	Wheat	Rye	Corn	Barley	Oats	Rice
Fat (%)	1.9	1.8	4.3	2.1	5.1	1.3
Fiber (%)	3.4	2.2	2.3	5.6	12.4	2.2
Thiamine mg/kg	5.4	4.4	4.6	5.7	7.0	3.2
Niacin mg/kg	63.6	1.3	26.6	64.5	17.8	40.0
Riboflavin mg/kg	1.3	1.8	1.3	2.2	1.8	0.7
Pantothenic acid mg/kg	13.6	7.7	5.9	7.3	14.5	7.0

- **Important for healthy heart:** Cereals and millets are rich sources of magnesium, and are very important agents to reduce blood pressure and minimize the risk of stroke and other heart diseases. Potassium present in millets act as a vasodilator and controls the blood pressure and optimize the circulatory system. High level of fibers in cereals and millets also control the level of cholesterol and keep the heart healthy.

Pulses and Legumes

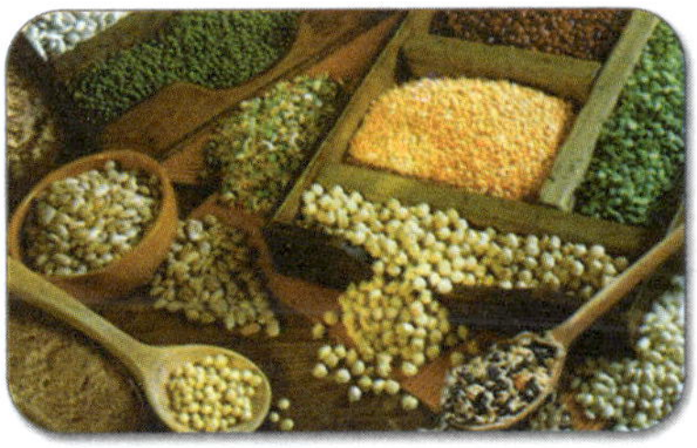

Fig. 2.3: Pulses and legumes

Pulses are part of legume family that includes fresh peas, soy and peanuts but the term pulse refers to dried seeds like edible beans, lentils (Fig. 2.3). Pulses are an important part of healthy balanced diet. Pulses are very high in fiber content that helps to decrease blood cholesterol level and controls blood glucose level. Pulses are rich source of proteins almost double the amount as found in cereals. In most of the developing countries like India, pulses are the main source of proteins for majority of the population. Pulses provide good amounts of vitamins and minerals. Pulses are rich in vitamin B complex and in minerals like potassium, magnesium and zinc. World Health Organization (WHO) estimates that 80% of noncommunicable diseases (Diabetes mellitus, stroke and cancer) could be prevented by eliminating risk factors, such as unhealthy diet and promoting better eating habits, of, which pulses are an essential component (Table 2.13). The World Food Program (WFP) includes 60 grams of pulses in its daily food basket alongside cereals, oil, sugar and salt.

Soybeans are a type of legume that has become incredibly popular worldwide because of their many health benefits. They are often used by strict vegetarians as a protein substitute for meat. Along with being high in protein, soybeans also contain saturated fats, fiber, antioxidants and Omega-3 fatty acids., which are important nutrients for the body. Recently, soybean derivatives like tofu and soy milk have gained popularity as well.

Table 2.13: Nutritive value of common pulses and legumes per 100 g

Nutritive value	Chickpeas	Lentils	Dry peas	White beans
Calories (Kcal)	341	116	302	92
Total fat	6 g	1.7 g	1.44 g	1.6 g
Cholesterol	0 mg	0 mg	0 mg	0 mg
Carbohydrate	44.3 g	40.6 g	41.2 g	34.7 g
Dietary fiber	17 g	17 g	16.7 g	23.2 g
Total sugar	11 g	1.8 g	3.11 g	3.47 g
Protein	20.8 g	23.18 g	22.9 g	21.1 g
Magnesium	115 mg	125 mg	118 mg	140 mg
Calcium	143 mg	70 mg	72 mg	15 mg
Sodium	25 mg	2 mg	26 mg	13 mg
Potassium	875 mg	837 mg	941 mg	1137 mg
Iron	6.8 mg	8.2 mg	5 mg	6.2 mg
Zinc	3.43 mg	3.1 mg	3.3 mg	2.6 mg
Vitamin C	4 mg	1.5 mg	2 mg	2.5 mg
Vitamin A	33 IU	8 IU	42 IU	4 IU
Vitamin D	0 IU	0 IU	0 IU	0 IU
Vitamin B12	0 IU	0 IU	0 IU	0 IU
Vitamin B6	0.5 mg	0.7 mg	0.12 mg	0.41 mg
Vitamin B3	4.57 mg	6.58 mg	10.33 mg	5.28 mg
Vitamin B9	185 IU	168 IU	151 IU	388 IU
Vitamin K	264 IU	123 IU	81 IU	19 IU

Source: The U.S. Department of Agriculture (USDA)

Vegetables

Vegetables have a rich content of nutrients like protein, vitamins, potassium, phosphorus, and magnesium, calcium, selenium, iron, manganese, copper and zinc (Fig. 2.4). A diet rich in vegetables definitely assures a relief from the deficiency diseases of the body so they are also classified as protective foods. They help in protecting our body against cancers,

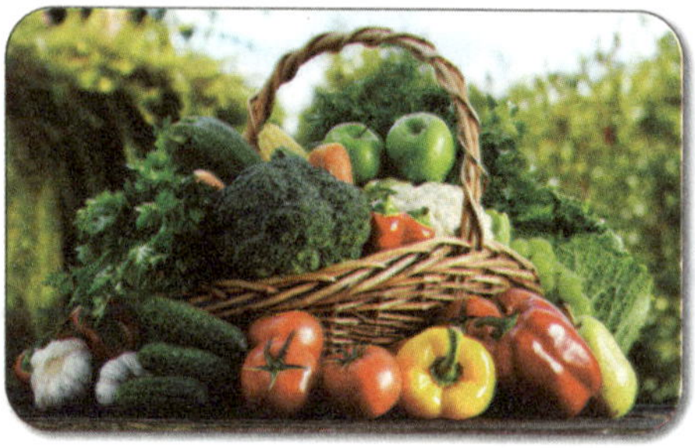

Fig. 2.4: Vegetables

diabetes and heart diseases. Almost all the vegetables are low in fat and calories, none have cholesterol and many of them are great sources of fiber. In order to stay healthy, it is essential for human beings to eat lot of vegetables. As per nutritionists, people must eat at least a couple of vegetables in a day. Vegetables can be divided into green leafy vegetables, vegetables with roots and other vegetables. Green leafy vegetables are rich in iron, potassium, folic acid, vitamin B complex and vitamin C, for example, spinach, cabbage, and amaranth (Table 2.14).

Vegetables with roots are rich in fibers, low in fat and good source of carbohydrates, for example, potato, sweet potato, reddish, onion, etc. Other vegetables are brinjal, cauliflower, etc. that are rich in minerals and vitamins.

Table 2.14: Nutritive values of vegetables per 100 g

Vegetable	Protein (g)	Fiber (g)	Vitamin A (IU)	Vitamin C (mg)	Calcium (mg)	Iron (mg)
Spinach	2.9	2.2	4693	28.1	99	2.7
Broccoli	2.8	2.6	623	89.2	47	0.7
Carrots	0.9	2.8	17033	9.3	33	0.6
Capsicum	0.9	2.1	1577	128.0	10	0.6
Sweet Potatoes	1.6	3.0	19218	2.4	26	0.8

Sources: USDA National Nutrient Database

Nuts and Oilseeds

Nuts and seeds are rich in energy and nutrients (Fig. 2.5). Nuts are excellent source of monounsaturated-fatty acids (MUFA) such as oleic acid, which help to lower LDL or bad cholesterol and increase HDL or good cholesterol. They are rich source of all important omega-3 essential fatty acids like Linoleic acid. Nuts and seeds have been found to offer protection against cancers, heart disease, degenerative nerve disease, Alzheimer's disease, and viral/fungal infections. Nuts not only provide calories, but they are also rich source of vitamins and minerals like manganese, potassium, calcium, iron, magnesium, zinc, fluoride and selenium. They contain very good levels of vitamin E, a powerful lipid soluble antioxidant. (Vitamin E is required for maintaining the integrity of cell membrane of mucus membranes and skin; thus, protecting it from harmful oxygen-free radicals). Nuts, nutrition provides many vital B-complex groups of vitamins such as riboflavin, niacin, thiamin, pantothenic acid, vitamin B_6, and folates. These vitamins are essential for optimum health and well-being (Table 2.15).

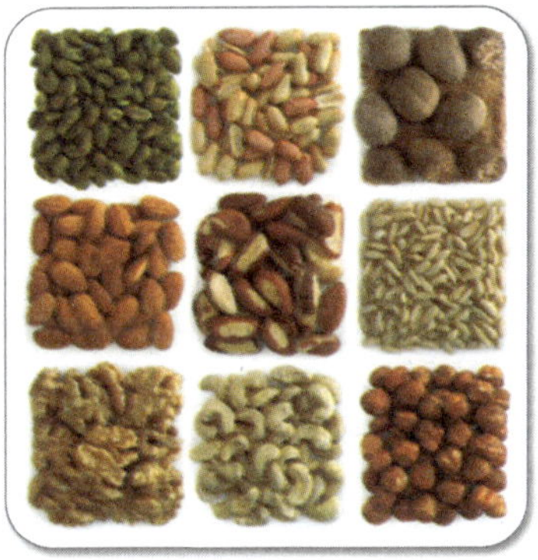

Fig. 2.5: Nuts and oilseeds

Table 2.15: Nutritive values of various nuts and seeds per 100 g

Nut/seed	Protein (g)	Fiber (g)	Vitamin E (mg)	Magnesium (mg)	Zinc (mg)	Iron (mg)
Almonds	21.2	12.2	25.6	270	3.3	3.7
Walnuts	15.2	6.7	0.7	158	3.1	2.9
Pistachios	20.3	10.3	2.9	121	2.2	3.2

Contd...

Nut/seed	Protein (g)	Fiber (g)	Vitamin E (mg)	Magnesium (mg)	Zinc (mg)	Iron (mg)
Cashews	18.2	3.3	0.9	292	5.8	6.7
Pumpkin Seeds	29.8	18.4	2.6	535	7.8	8.8
Chia Seeds	16.5	34.4	0.5	335	4.6	7.7

Sources: USDA National Nutrient Database

Fruits

Fruits are an important source of vitamins, minerals, and enzymes (Fig. 2.6). Fructose is the principal sugar in most fruits, whereas sucrose is present in fruits such as oranges, melons, and peaches. Fructose is absorbed slowly into the bloodstream, so fruit gives you energy without triggering the insulin cycle. Fruits, their nutrients and calorific values are given in Table 2.16.

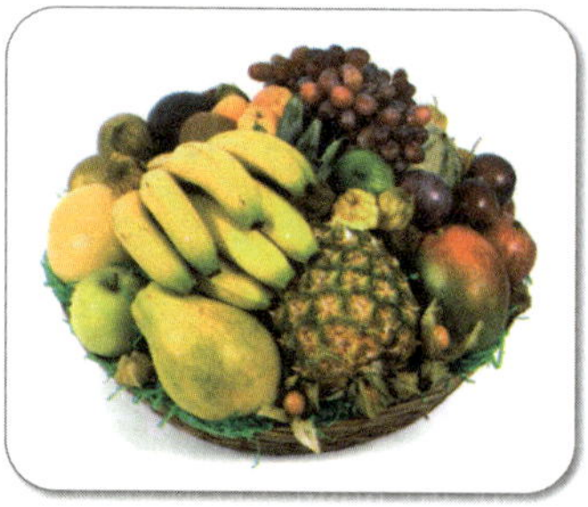

Fig. 2.6: Fruits

- **Apple:** An apple is a rich source of fibers, vitamins, minerals and antioxidants. It is very low in saturated fats, cholesterol and sodium and calories. It is one of the healthiest foods to eat and also known as nutritional powerhouse. It not only promotes the digestion but also boosts the immunity.
- **Bananas:** This fruit is also a good source of energy, fibers, vitamins and minerals, especially potassium. It is very helpful when immediate energy is required, for example, in case of athletes.
- **Apricot:** Apricots are rich source of vitamin A, C, fibers, copper, zinc and potassium, folic acid and antioxidants.
- **Cherries:** Cherries are good source of vitamin C, A, calcium, potassium, proteins and iron. They have low level of calorie, fats and cholesterol.
- **Dates and figs:** Dates are good source of fiber, iron, and niacin. Dried figs are not only high in calories and carbohydrates but also contain abundant amounts of other nutrients, such as calcium, fiber, protein, and potassium.
- **Grapes:** Grapes contain cancer-fighting anthocyanin pigments, vitamin C, carbohydrates and vitamins.
- **Guava:** Rich source of fiber, vitamin E and minerals.
- **Melon:** Melon is rich source of proteins, fiber, calcium, and beta carotene.
- **Mango:** Mangoes are rich in fiber, beta carotene and vitamin C and A along with the calories as compared to other fruits.
- **Orange:** Oranges are known for their vitamin C content, but they are also a good source of foliate and fiber. They even contain some calcium.
- **Papaya:** High in calcium, folic acid, vitamin C, fiber and carotenoids.
- **Peach:** They are low in calorie, moderate source of antioxidants and vitamin C. They also contain small source of vitamin A and carotene. These are rich in minerals like potassium, fluoride and iron.
- **Pear:** High in fibers, makes it ideal for persons suffering from constipation. Most of the vitamin C in pears is concentrated in the skin so peeled, canned pears are less nutritious than fresh.
- **Pineapple:** This fruit is highest in the essential nutrient, manganese, and it has digestive enzymes.

- **Plum:** These are low in calories and saturated fats, rich in dietary fibers, antioxidants and flavonoids. They are also helpful in regulating digestive system functioning and relieving constipation. They are also a modest source of vitamin B complex.
- **Strawberries:** Strawberries are higher in vitamin C per calorie than any other fruit and they are high in fiber.
- **Watermelon:** Watermelon is the top fruit source of the carotenoid and antioxidant.
- **California Avocado:** Avocados are usually thought of as a vegetable, but they are really a fruit, with a great amount of nutrition. They also contain nearly 20 vitamins, minerals, and beneficial plant compounds—such as B vitamins, vitamin A, vitamin E, potassium, folate, and fiber.

Table 2.16: Nutrient and calorific values of fruits

Fruits	Energy	Water	Fiber	Fat	Protein	Sugar	Vit. A	Vit. C	Vit. B_1	Vit. B_2	Vit. B_6	Vit. E
Substance = 100 g	kJ/kcal	%	g	g	g	g	ug	mg	mg	mg	mg	mg
Apple	207/49	84	2.3	0	0.4	11.8	2	15	0.02	0.01	0.05	0.5
Apricot	153/36	87	2.1	0	1.0	8.0	420	5	0.06	0.05	0.06	0.5
Avocado	523/126	81	0.2	10	2.0	7.0	20	17	0.06	0.12	0.36	3.2
Blueberry	204/48	80	8.4	0	1.0	11.0	0	10	0.02	0.03	0.05	1.9
Blackberry	170/40	85	8.7	0	2.0	8.0	30	150	0.08	0.04	0.07	1.0
Banana	375/88	76	2.7	0	1.2	20.4	3	10	0.04	0.03	0.36	0.3
Carrots	48 /11	92	3.3	0	0.6	2.2	312	2	0.03	0.04	0.08	0.2
Cranberry	68 /16	89	4.2	0	0.0	4.0	0	15	0.00	0.01	0.07	0.0
Cherry	221/52	86	1.2	0	0.0	13.0	40	10	0.02	0.02	0.04	0.1
Date	1275/300	20	7.5	0	2.0	73.0	0	0	0.05	0.10	0.10	0.7
Fig	340/80	80	2.0	0	1.0	19.0	10	3	0.06	0.05	0.11	—
Grapefruit	128/30	90	1.4	0	0.9	6.6	0	40	0.07	0.02	0.03	0.5
Red grapes	274/64	83	2.2	0	0.6	15.5	0	3	0.03	0.01	0.08	0.6
Guava	306/72	81	5.3	0	1.0	17.0	30	218	0.04	0.04	0.14	—
Gooseberry	170/40	88	3.2	0	1.0	9.0	0	30	0.02	0.01	0.08	0.4
Kiwi fruit	168/40	84	2.1	0	1.1	8.8	5	70	0.01	0.02	0.12	1.9
Kumquat	289/68	82	1.5	0	1.0	16.0	160	55	0.14	0.06	—	—
Lemon	51/12	96	1.8	0	0.0	3.0	0	40	0.06	0.02	0.04	0.8
Lime	156/37	91	0.3	0	0.0	7.0	0	40	0.03	0.02	0.08	—
Lychee	323/76	82	1.5	0	1.0	18.0	0	39	0.05	0.05	—	—
Mandarin/ tangerine	177/42	88	1.9	0	0.9	9.5	12	30	0.08	0.03	0.084	0.4
Mango	255/60	84	1.0	0	0.0	15.0	210	53	0.05	0.06	0.13	1.0
Melon	153/36	93	0.6	0	1.0	8.0	30	6	0.04	0.05	0.07	—
Red water melon, cantaloupe	122/29	89	0.6	0	0.9	6.3	7	32	0.05	0.02	0.10	0.2

Contd...

Fruits	Energy	Water	Fiber	Fat	Protein	Sugar	Vit. A	Vit. C	Vit. B_1	Vit. B_2	Vit. B_6	Vit. E
Substance = 100 g	kJ/kcal	%	g	g	g	g	ug	mg	mg	mg	mg	mg
Olive	586/142	75	4.4	14	1.0	3.0	50	0	0.03	0.08	0.00	2.0
Orange	198/47	87	1.8	0	1.0	10.6	2	49	0.07	0.03	0.06	0.1
Papaya	136/32	91	0.6	0	0.0	8.0	40	46	0.03	0.04	0.04	—
Passion fruit	158/37	88	3.3	0.4	2.6	5.8	125	23	0.03	0.12	—	0.5
Peach	151/36	89	1.4	0	1.0	7.9	15	7	0.01	0.02	0.02	0.0
Pear	201/47	86	2.1	0	0.3	11.5	0.0	4	0.01	0.01	0.02	0.1
Red bell pepper	119/28	91	2.2	0	1.0	6.0	172	80	0.04	0.14	0.43	6.4
Persimmon	325/76	81	0.5	0	0.5	18.6	260	16	0.02	0.03	—	—
Pineapple	211/50	84	1.2	0	0.4	12.0	20	25	0.07	0.02	0.09	0.1
Pomegranate	343/81	82	3.4	0	1.0	17.0	10	7	0.05	0.02	0.31	—
Plum	177/42	84	2.2	0	0.8	9.6	18	5	0.02	0.03	0.10	0.7
Strawberry	99/23	91	2.2	0	0.7	5.1	10	60	0.02	0.03	0.06	0.4
Tomato	48/11	97	1.4	0	0.9	1.9	140	15	0.05	0.02	0.08	0.7

Animal Food

Milk

Milk is the complete diet in itself. Milk is the primary source of nutrition for infants until they are ready to digest other foods. However, some people are unable to digest the milk due to lack of an enzyme known as lactase. Milk is considered as the healthiest drink as it is full of nutrients. It provides all the elements necessary for proper growth and development. It is not only important for infants but also serves as an essential component of diet for all the age groups. Nutritional elements in a cup of milk are listed in Table 2.17.

Milk-derived Products

They are the food products that are derived from milk. They can be produced by coagulation of the milk protein known as casein in many different flavors, texture and forms. So their composition and nutritional elements are almost same as milk. They not only add flavor in the diet but also provide essential nutrients like calcium, potassium, vitamin D, fats and proteins. Examples of such products are yogurt, hard white cheese, and creamy cheese, cream, butter and ice cream.

Health benefits

- Building and maintaining bone and teeth
- Keeping the blood pressure at a normal rate
- Improving the digestion process

- Boosting the immunity
- Maintaining the skin, hair, and delicate membranes
- Treating the dehydration
- Providing the body with energy
- Preventing cardiac diseases

Table 2.17: Breaking down the nutritional elements in a cup of milk

Nutrients	Low-fat milk	Fat-free milk	Full-fat milk
Calories	102	86	146
Fats	2 mg	0 mg	8 mg
Cholesterol	12 mg	5 mg	24 mg
Sodium	107 mg	128 mg	98 mg
Carbohydrates	13 mg	12 mg	13 mg
Sugar	13 mg	12 mg	13 mg
Proteins	8 mg	8 mg	8 mg

Eggs

Eggs are an important source of protein, essential vitamins and minerals and can make a significant contribution to a healthy diet. Nutritional requirements can vary considerably between men, women and children and can also vary in individuals from time to time. Nutritional value of egg is listed in Table 2.18.

Table 2.18: Nutritional value of egg without its shell

Constituents of egg	Amount per 100 g egg
Energy	151 kcal
Protein	12.5 g
Carbohydrate	trace
Fat	11.2 g
Saturated fatty acid	3.2 g
Monounsaturated fatty acid	4.4 g
Polyunsaturated fatty acid	1.7 g
Dietary fiber	None
Minerals and trace elements	
Sodium	140 mg
Potassium	130 mg
Calcium	57 mg
Phosphorus	200 mg
Magnesium	12 mg
Iron	1.9 mg
Zinc	1.3 mg
Copper	0.08 mg

Contd...

Constituents of egg	Amount per 100 g egg
Iodine	53 mg
Chlorine	160 mg
Sulfur	180 mg
Selenium	11 mg
Vitamins	
Vitamin A	190 mg
Vitamin D	1.8 mg
Vitamin E	1.11 mg
Vitamin C	None
Thiamin (B_1)	0.09 mg
Riboflavin (B_2)	0.47 mg
Niacin	0.1 mg
Vitamin B_6	0.12 mg
Folate	50 mg
Vitamin B_{12}	2.5 mg
Biotin	20 mg
Pantothenic acid	1.77 mg

- **Protein:** Eggs are an excellent source of protein. Egg protein is of high biological value as it contains all the essential amino acids needed by the human body. Eggs, therefore, complement other food proteins of lower biological value by providing the amino acids that are in short supply in those foods. 12.5% of the weight of the egg is due to proteins and it is found in both the yolk and the albumen.
- **Vitamins:** Eggs contain most of the vitamins with the exception of vitamin C. The egg is a good source of all the B vitamins, plus the fat-soluble vitamin A. It also provides useful amounts of vitamin D, as well as some vitamin E.
- **Minerals:** Eggs contain most of the minerals that the human body requires for health. In particular, eggs are an excellent source of iodine, required to make the thyroid hormone, and phosphorus, required for bone health. The egg provides significant amounts of zinc, important for wound healing, growth and fighting infection; selenium, an important antioxidant; and calcium, needed for bone and growth structure and nervous functions. Eggs also contain significant amounts of iron.
- **Carbohydrate and dietary fibers:** Eggs contain only traces of carbohydrate and no dietary fiber.
- **Fat:** Approximately 17% of an egg's fatty acids are polyunsaturated, 44% monounsaturated and only 32% saturated.

Fish

Fish is a food that provides high quality proteins and a wide variety of vitamins and minerals. It is rich source of vitamin A, D and many minerals like phosphorus, magnesium, selenium and iodine. Proteins of fish are easily digestible and provide all the essential amino acids that are low in quantities in vegetable diet. Fish oil is very useful as it provides essential fatty acids required for the normal brain development.

Meat

Meat is animal flesh that is eaten as food. Meat products contain several vitamins that include vitamin B_1, B_2, B_3 and B_6. Meat products are also rich in mineral content that include magnesium, iron and zinc. Meat products are an excellent source of complete proteins that contain all the amino acids that body needs to function properly. Meat products are rich source of unsaturated fats like omega-3 fatty acids. These fatty acids play an important part in lowering the level of LDL, cholesterol, blood pressure and triglycerides and also decrease the risk of cardiovascular diseases.

Poultry

Poultry are domesticated birds kept by humans for the production of eggs or meat. They are rich source of nutrients like proteins, vitamin B, including thiamine, riboflavin, niacin, pyridoxine, vitamin E, zinc, iron and magnesium. Poultry meat is second most widely eaten type of meat in the world. It is available as fresh or frozen, bone in or deboned, raw or ready to cook.

FATS AND OILS

Dietary fats and oils are the most concentrated form of energy. Besides rich in energy, fats are also rich source of essential fatty acids, vitamin E and transport vehicle for fat soluble vitamins and hormones. Essential fatty acids (linolenic acid) as their name suggests must be present in the diet as their deficiency may result in impaired brain growth, mental retardation, poor wound healing, hair loss and learning difficulties. The fat soluble vitamins A, D, E and K require fats and oils in the food to be absorbed through the gut. Inadequate intake of fats and oils may result in deficiency of these vitamins. Fats and oils can be categorized as visible fats, which are present in oil, butter, ghee, etc. and invisible fat (not visible with naked eyes) such as present in food items like in cereals, pulses in small amount.

SUGAR AND JAGGERY

Sugar

Sugar is derived from sugarcane or sugar beets. It is a highly refined carbohydrate. It consists of sucrose, a disaccharide made up of glucose and fructose molecules.

Nutritional Value

- It is primarily composed of carbohydrates, with almost 100% of its weight as sugars (sucrose).
- Provides quick energy due to its high glycemic index.
- Contains minimal amounts of other nutrients such as calcium, iron, and potassium.

Jaggery (Gur)

Jaggery is an unrefined sugar product made from sugarcane juice. Sugar undergoes extensive refining, while jaggery is less processed and retains more nutrients. Jaggery contains minerals like iron, calcium, and potassium, which are absent in refined sugar.

Nutritional Value

- Contains sucrose, but also retains significant amounts of other nutrients from the cane juice, including iron, calcium, and potassium.
- It has a lower glycemic index compared to refined sugar, meaning it raises blood sugar levels more slowly.
- Also contains trace amounts of vitamins and minerals.

SPICES AND CONDIMENTS

Spices are heart and soul of Indian cuisine. It is impossible to cook Indian dishes without spices. Spices are an ingredient used to season a dish in the meal during its preparation and condiments are for using at the table to enhance the flavor of dish as preferred by an individual.

Commonly used spices with their common names in India and medicinal properties

- **Turmeric (*haldi*):** It is effective as an antibiotic. It has anti-inflammatory properties. It is also used as a remedy for common cold, cough, asthma and throat infection.
- **Tamarind (*imli*):** It is a good source of iron, potassium and magnesium.
- **Fennel seeds (*moti saunf*):** It is used in reducing gastritis and aids in digestion.
- **Fenugreek seeds (*methi dana*):** It improves sense of taste and smell and is also considered good to reduce blood sugar levels.
- **Cumin seeds (*jeera*):** It is very useful in morning sickness, flatulence and indigestion.
- **Coriander (*dhaniya*):** It is useful in digestion also known to lower blood cholesterol level.
- **Cloves (*laung*):** Cloves or laung have anesthetic properties especially used for toothache. When used with other spices clove also acts as effective treatment for common cold and cough.
- **Cinnamon (*dalchini*):** It is used in sore throat and dysmenorrhea.
- **Onion seeds (*kalonji*):** Onion seeds help to treat indigestion and treat migraine pain.
- **Curry leaves (*kadhi patta*):** These leaves help in digestion, anti-inflammatory properties and are considered useful in treating gout, and quite useful in lowering blood cholesterol and blood sugar level.
- **Carom seeds (*ajwain*):** Also known as thymol or omum these seeds are useful in colic pain, indigestion and relieve diarrhea and flatulence.
- **Cardamoms (*elaichi*):** Elaichi helps to relieve morning sickness, relieves gas and removes foul smell from mouth.
- **Black peppercorns (*sabut kali mirch*):** Black peppercorns help to reduce inflammation and pain, also used as a treatment for common cold and cough.
- **Poppy seeds (*khuskhus*):** These seeds help to relieve insomnia and colic pain.
- **Chilli and chilli powder (*mirchi*):** Chilli is a good source of vitamin C.
- **Ginger (*adrak*):** It is very useful in treating colic, vomiting, spasm, relieves common cold and cough.
- **Garlic (*lahsan*):** Garlic is considered effective treatment for arthritis, controlling blood pressure and treating asthma.
- **Pomegranate seeds (*anar dana*):** These seeds are useful to treat indigestion, colic, heartburn and vomiting and morning sickness.
- **Nutmeg (*jaiphal*):** It is used to treat hiccups, morning sickness and colic pain.
- **Saffron (*kesar*):** It helps to improve memory and treat inflammation.

MISCELLANEOUS FOODS

These are the types of foods that include frozen prepared meals, canned and packaged foods. Examples of such foods are soups, potato chips, nuts, snacks; condiments, pickles, relishes, sauces and gravies, salads, desserts, baby foods, and vitamin supplements.

Miscellaneous foods can be categorized in the following manner:

- **Meat products:** Poultry slaughtering and processing, sausages and other meat products
- **Dairy products:** Dry, condensed, evaporated dairy products and frozen desserts
- **Fruits and vegetables:** Canned, frozen and preserved fruits and vegetables
- **Flour and other grain mill products:** Consist of wide range of food items derived from grains. For instance, rice flour, barley flour, sorghum flour, oat meal, etc.
- **Bakery products:** Bread, cookies and crackers and fast foods
- **Beverages:** Soft drinks, carbonated water, mineral water, wines, brandy, distilled and blended liquors
- **Sugar and confectionery products:** Cane sugar, beet sugar, chocolate, coca products and chewing gums
- **Fats and oils:** Cotton seed, soybean, margarine, animal and other edible fats and oils.

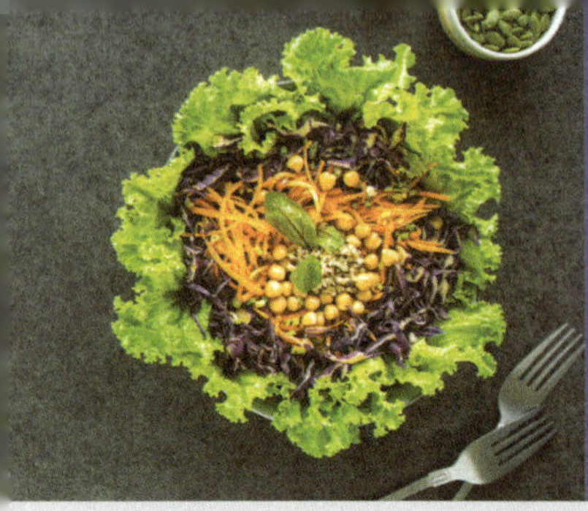

STUDENT ASSIGNMENT

LONG ANSWER QUESTIONS

1. Classify the food on basis of its origin.
2. **Explain the sources of following nutrients:**
   a. Carbohydrates
   b. Fats
   c. Proteins

SHORT ANSWER QUESTIONS

1. Classify Vitamins.
2. How can food be classified on the basis of its functions?
3. Enlist the macro and microminerals.

MULTIPLE CHOICE QUESTIONS

1. **Milk is a poor source of:**
   a. Iron
   b. Protein
   c. Calcium
   d. Phosphorus
2. **The richest natural source of vitamin A is:**
   a. Peas
   b. Green leafy vegetables
   c. Fresh fruits
   d. Cod liver oil
3. **Amino acids help in the formation of:**
   a. Proteins
   b. Carbohydrates
   c. Fats
   d. Minerals
4. **Rich source of vitamin C is:**
   a. Banana
   b. Citrus fruits
   c. Milk
   d. Grapes
5. **The amount of proteins in daily energy intake should be:**
   a. 15–25%
   b. 10–15%
   c. 20–25%
   d. 25–30%
6. **Following nutrient requirement is more in females than males:**
   a. Phosphorus
   b. Sulfur
   c. Fluoride
   d. Iron

7. **Tryptophan is present in all, except:**
   a. Maize
   b. Cheese
   c. Fish
   d. Chicken

8. **Amino acid deficient in wheat is:**
   a. Leucine
   b. Methionine
   c. Lysine
   d. Cysteine

9. **Which of the following is not an energy yielding food?**
   a. Carbohydrates
   b. Vitamins and minerals
   c. Fats
   d. Proteins

10. **Which of the following vegetable is known for its high vitamin A and vitamin C content per 100 grams?**
    a. Spinach
    b. Carrots
    c. Bell Peppers
    d. Broccoli

11. **Which nut is highest in protein content per 100 g?**
    a. Almonds
    b. Walnuts
    c. Cashews
    d. Pistachios

12. **Which oil is highest in polyunsaturated fats per 100 g?**
    a. Olive oil
    b. Coconut oil
    c. Flaxseed oil
    d. Canola oil

13. **Among these spices, which one is known for its anti-inflammatory properties?**
    a. Cumin
    b. Turmeric
    c. Coriander
    d. Cardamom

14. **Which of these grains is highest in fiber content per 100 g?**
    a. Wheat flour
    b. Rice flour
    c. Oatmeal
    d. Cornmeal

15. **Which fruit is highest in vitamin C content per 100 g?**
    a. Apples
    b. Bananas
    c. Oranges
    d. Grapes

16. **Which one of these dairy products is highest in calcium content per 100 g?**
    a. Greek Yogurt
    b. Milk
    c. Cheese
    d. Butter

17. **Which legume is highest in iron content per 100 g?**
    a. Lentils
    b. Chickpeas
    c. Black beans
    d. Kidney beans

18. **Which seafood is highest in omega-3 fatty acids per 100 g?**
    a. Shrimp
    b. Salmon
    c. Tuna
    d. Cod

19. **Which sweetener is highest in antioxidants and minerals like iron and calcium per 100 g?**
    a. Sugar
    b. Honey
    c. Jaggery
    d. Maple syrup

20. Which food is known for its high antioxidant content, supporting heart health and immune function?

a. White bread
b. Blueberries
c. Potato chips
d. Ice cream

21. Which nut is known for its heart-healthy fats and ability to lower LDL cholesterol levels?

a. Almonds
b. Cashews
c. Peanuts
d. Walnuts

22. Which grain is known for its high fiber content, aiding digestion and promoting satiety?

a. White rice
b. Quinoa
c. Couscous
d. Buckwheat

23. Which vegetable is rich in vitamin K and calcium, supporting bone health and blood clotting?

a. Spinach
b. Bell peppers
c. Onions
d. Cauliflower

24. Which fruit is rich in vitamin C, supporting immune function and collagen production?

a. Watermelon
b. Pineapple
c. Oranges
d. Kiwi

25. Which dairy product is high in probiotics, promoting gut health and digestion?

a. Cheese
b. Butter
c. Yogurt
d. Milk

26. Which legume is high in protein and fiber, beneficial for muscle repair and blood sugar regulation?

a. Lentils
b. Kidney beans
c. Chickpeas
d. Black beans

27. Which oil is known for its heart-healthy monounsaturated fats and antioxidants?

a. Coconut oil
b. Olive oil
c. Canola oil
d. Palm oil

ANSWER KEY

1. a	**2.** d	**3.** a	**4.** b	**5.** a	**6.** d	**7.** a	**8.** c	**9.** b
10. b	**11.** a	**12.** c	**13.** b	**14.** c	**15.** c	**16.** a	**17.** c	**18.** b
19. c	**20.** b	**21.** d	**22.** b	**23.** a	**24.** c	**25.** c	**26.** a	**27.** b

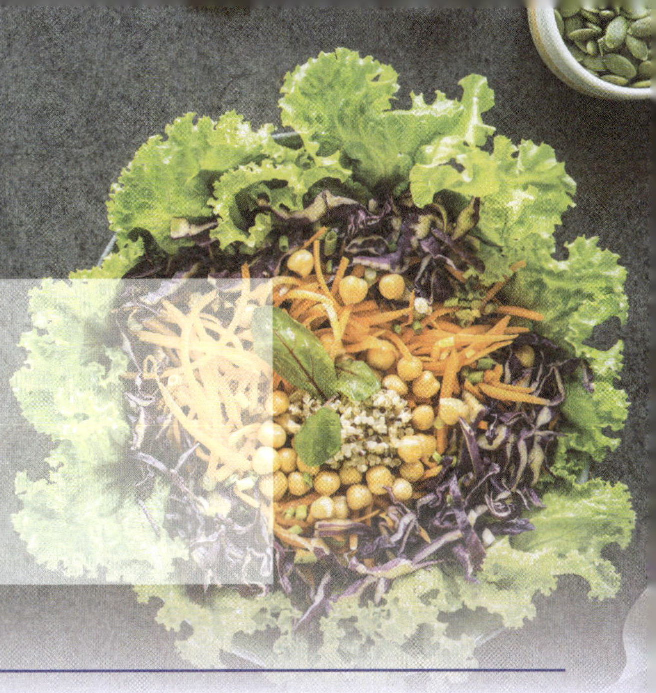

3

Normal Dietary Requirements

LEARNING OBJECTIVES

After the completion of the chapter, the readers will be able to:

- Define various terms like energy, basal metabolism, body mass index.
- Discuss balanced diet and nutritive value of foods.
- Describe budgeting of food and plan food for all categories of people.
- Explain diseases and disorders caused by imbalance of nutrients.
- Discuss diet modification in various types of diseases.

CHAPTER OUTLINE

- Energy
- Basal Metabolism
- Body Mass Index
- Balanced Diet
- Food Groups
- Menu Planning/Meal Planning
- Balanced Diet for Adults
- Diet in Pregnancy
- Diet for Lactating Woman
- Diet for Elderly or Old Age People
- Combination of Food Enhancing the Nutritive Value of Food
- Budgeting for Food
- Food Substitutes
- Food Exchange
- Low Cost Meals
- Diseases and Disorders caused by Imbalance of Nutrients
- Food Allergies
- Food Intolerance
- Inborn Errors of Metabolism

KEY TERMS

Balanced diet: A diet that contains all the nutrients in appropriate proportions.
Basal metabolic rate (BMR): The amount of energy, which is required to carry out involuntary (not in our control) activities of body.
Calorie: It is a unit of energy.
Food allergy: It is a hypersensitive reaction as a result of exposure to a particular allergen.
Food intolerance: It is the digestive problem that occurs after a certain food is eaten.
Metabolism: It is a complex process that converts fat molecule into energy.
Recommended dietary allowance (RDA): RDA is the level of intake of essential nutrients on the basis of scientific knowledge. The level of nutrients is judged by the food and nutrition board and must be adequate to meet the known nutrient needs of healthy people.

ENERGY

Body requires energy for its proper functioning. Energy is required for the optimum growth and development of body. Main sources of energy are fats, carbohydrates and proteins.

Definition

It is defined as strength and vitality required for the sustained physical and mental activity.

Measurements of Energy

Kilocalorie is the unit of energy, which was used for long time but recently the international union of science and international union of nutritional sciences have replaced kcal with joule. Now Joule is internationally accepted unit of energy.

- 1 kcal = 4.184 KJ (kilo joule)
- 1000 kcal = 4.84 MJ (mega joule)
- 1 KJ = 0.239 kcal
- 239 kcal = 1 mega joule

Energy Value of Foods

Calorimetry is used to measure the energy. It is the measurement of heat loss. The instrument known as Bomb calorimeter is used to measure the energy value of food. Energy value of food is listed in Table 3.1.

Table 3.1: Food ingredients and its energy value

Food ingredients	Value (kcal/g)
Carbohydrates	4
Fats	9
Proteins	4

Energy Requirement

Energy requirement refers to the amount of energy (calories) that an individual needs to consume daily to maintain his or her body weight, support bodily functions, and fuel physical activity. This requirement can vary widely depending on factors such as age, sex, weight, height, metabolism, and level of physical activity.

Components about energy requirements include:

- **Basal metabolic rate (BMR):** This is the minimum amount of energy required to sustain basic physiological functions at rest, such as breathing, circulation, and cell production.
- **Physical activity level (PAL):** This factor accounts for the additional energy needed for physical activity beyond basic metabolic needs. Sedentary individuals have lower physical activity level (PAL) compared to those who are more physically active.
- **Total daily energy expenditure (TDEE):** This is the sum of basal metabolic rate (BMR) and energy expended through physical activity. It represents the total amount of energy a person needs per day to maintain his or her current weight.

Factors Affecting Energy Requirement

Weight

Weight is an important factor that affects the energy requirement of the body. Weight is directly proportional to the energy requirement. It means with increase in body weight energy requirement of body also increases.

Age

With age energy requirement also changes. Adolescents require more energy than the old age people.

Physical Activity

Higher is the physical activity, more is the calorie requirement. Heavy workers require more calorie as compared to moderate and light worker.

Climate

On cold days, energy requirement of a person increases as a person requires more energy to conserve heat in the body and vice versa.

Sex

Males require more energy as compared to females.

Specific Groups

Pregnancy/lactation

During pregnancy and lactation, energy requirement of women increases. It is increased during pregnancy (+300 kcal daily). During first 6 months of lactation, it increases + 550 kcal/day and for next 6 months it increases + 400 kcal/day.

Children

Children require more energy because of their rapid growth. Children above 13 years of age require as much energy as adult because of puberty changes.

Elderly People

In elderly people, energy requirement decreases due to decreased activity and decreased basal metabolic rate. The FAO and WHO committee suggested that after the age of 40 years requirement should be reduced by 5% each decade until the age of 60 and by 10% for each decade thereafter.

BASAL METABOLISM

Basal metabolism is the amount of energy used while at rest in a warm environment, in the postabsorptive state (means person has not had a meal for 12 hours). In this state, the amount of energy that is released is sufficient only for the functioning of vital organs such as heart, lungs, kidneys, liver, nervous system, skin, muscles, etc.

Basal Metabolic Rate (BMR)

Definition

It is defined as the amount of energy, which is required to carry out involuntary (not in our control) activities of body such as pumping action of heart, filtration of blood by kidneys, etc.

Factors Affecting Basal Metabolic Rate

There are many factors that affect the BMR (Fig. 3.1):

- **Age:** The BMR is the highest during first few years of life. It decreases gradually as the baby grows. The FAO and WHO committee suggested that after the age of 40 years requirement should be reduced by 5% each decade until the age 60 and by 10% for each decade thereafter.
- **Sex:** It has been found that females have 2–12% less BMR as compared to males. The difference is more clearly visible in older age groups. The BMR of women is also affected by the hormones as seen during menstrual cycle (BMR increases before menstruation and decreases after the menstruation).
- **Climate:** BMR increases in cold months because more energy is required to conserve the body heat. Likewise, it also increases in summer days because work and temperature increase heat loss.
- **Body temperature:** BMR increases by 7%, with a rise in body temperature by each degree Fahrenheit, Thus, a patient with temperature of 105°F would have about 50% more BMR as compared to the person with normal temperature of 98°F.
- **Diet:** Non-vegetarians have 11% more BMR as compared to the vegetarians. BMR decreases after prolonged starvation. Thus, any illness that decreases food intake results in a decrease in BMR.
- **Hormones:** Hormones also affect BMR. BMR increases with the increased secretion of thyroid hormone and vice versa. BMR also increases in response to release of adrenaline and noradrenaline.
- **Sleep:** The more relaxation of muscles during sleep compared to walking decreases BMR by about 10%.
- **Pregnancy/Lactation:** BMR is increased in pregnancy and lactation.
- **Physical activity:** Individuals with more physical activity have more BMR as compared to the sedentary workers, e.g., laborers have higher BMR than sedentary workers.
- **Drugs:** Certain drugs are also responsible for increase in BMR. For example, caffeine, nicotine, etc.

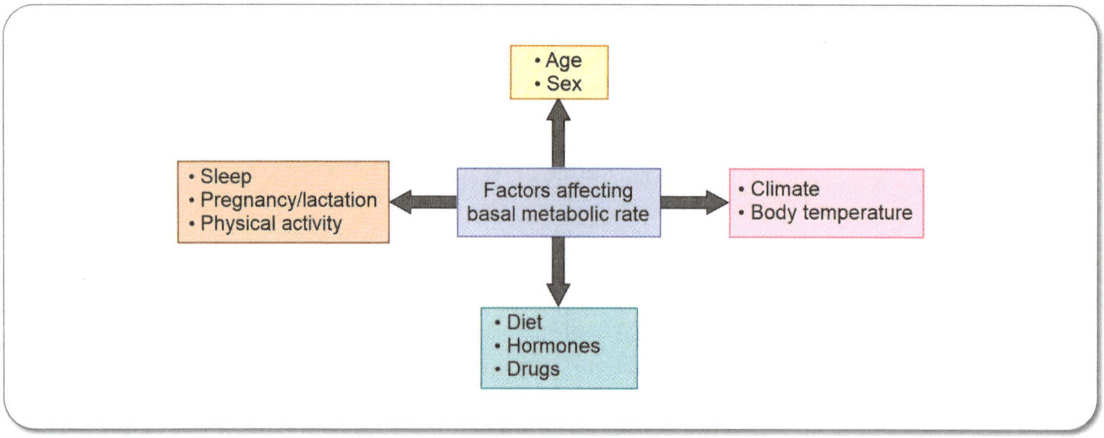

Fig. 3.1: Factors affecting basal metabolic rate

- **Diseases:** Diseases affect BMR in two ways:
  (i) **Increased BMR:** Diseases such as hyperthyroidism, Cushing's syndrome, and diabetes insipidus, Leukemias and polycythemia increase BMR because of cells of body.
  (ii) **Decreased BMR:** Diseases such as hypothyroidism, Addison's disease and hypopituitarism and shock decrease BMR.

Determination of Basal Metabolic Rate

- The amount of energy that is required by the body to support vital functions while the body is at rest. BMR is the single largest component of total energy burnt each day.
- For the assessment of energy requirement, several methods are available. These can be categorized as assessment of energy requirement by direct or indirect calorimetry or an empirical approximate equation.
- **Direct calorimetry:** The human body requires 45% of the energy content of the food intake for work and 55% for heat. Work can be further categorized as internal work (respiration, pumping) and external work (muscular movements). So in this method body's energy requirement is measured by measuring the heat production by the temperature change produced in a medium. This is a complicated method as equipment required is very large, immobile and expensive.
- **Indirect calorimetry:** It measures gas exchange via oxygen consumption and carbon dioxide production. In this method, the expired air is collected and is analyzed for its oxygen and carbon dioxide content. A person is isolated from outside air and is made to breathe from a reservoir that contains pure oxygen. When gas is expired by the patient, carbon dioxide is removed. The decrease in gas volume is directly related to the rate of oxygen consumption and thus it can be used to calculate metabolic rate. It is a simple method than direct calorimetry. In other words, heat production is calculated from oxygen consumption and carbon dioxide production. When related during a given time period, this factor is known as respiratory coefficient (RQ). Table 3.2 shows the respiratory coefficient of food items.
  - RQ = VCO_2/VO_2
  - VCO_2 = Is expired CO_2 volume per unit per time
  - VO_2 = Is consumed O_2 volume per unit per time
  - Value of RQ, VCO_2 and VO_2 varies from food to food

Table 3.2: Value of respiratory quotient (RQ)

Food item	VO_2	VCO_2	RQ
Protein	0.94	0.75	0.80
Carbohydrates	0.81	0.81	1.00
Fats	1.96	1.39	0.71

- **Empirical approximate equation**
  It can be calculated using the following formula:
  - BMR (male) = $66 + (13.7 \times BW) + 5(H) - (6.8 \times A)$
  - BMR (female) = $65 + (9.6 \times BW) + 1.73(H) - (4.7 \times A)$
  Where, BW = body weight in kg, H = height in cm, A = age in years

BODY MASS INDEX

The body mass index (BMI) is defined as the body mass divided by the square of the body height. It is used for the determination of overweight and underweight in adults.

Body mass index = Weight in kilograms/ (height in meters)^2

For example, if you want to calculate body mass index of an adult women who weighs 55 kg and height is 5′5″ feet

1 ft = 30.48 cm

5′5″ × 30.48 = 1.67 m

Body mass index = $55/(1.67)^2 = 19.7$

Classification of obesity on the basis of body mass index is given in Table 3.3.

Table 3.3: Body mass index according to body types

Classification	Body mass index
Underweight	<18.5
Normal range	18.5–24.9
Overweight	≥25.0
Preobese	25.0–29.9
Obese	≥30.0
Obese Grade I	30.0–34.9
Obese Grade II	35.0–39.9
Obese Grade III	≥40.0

BALANCED DIET

Definition

Balanced diet is defined as a diet that contains all the nutrients such as energy, protein, carbohydrates, vitamins, minerals, fats in right proportion adequate to maintain normal functioning and health of a human being (Fig. 3.2).

A balanced diet needs to contain foods from all the main food groups in the correct proportion to provide the body with optimum nutrition. It should be made up of correct number of calories to maintain healthy weight and should not contain processed food. Every person is different and hence the energy requirement also varies from person to person. However, the diet that covers all foods groups and is low in undesirable nutrients such as sodium, saturated fats and sugar is considered healthy for the body.

A balanced diet not only provides essential nutrients but also helps maintain a healthy weight, supports overall well-being, and reduces the risk of chronic diseases such as heart disease, diabetes, and certain cancers.

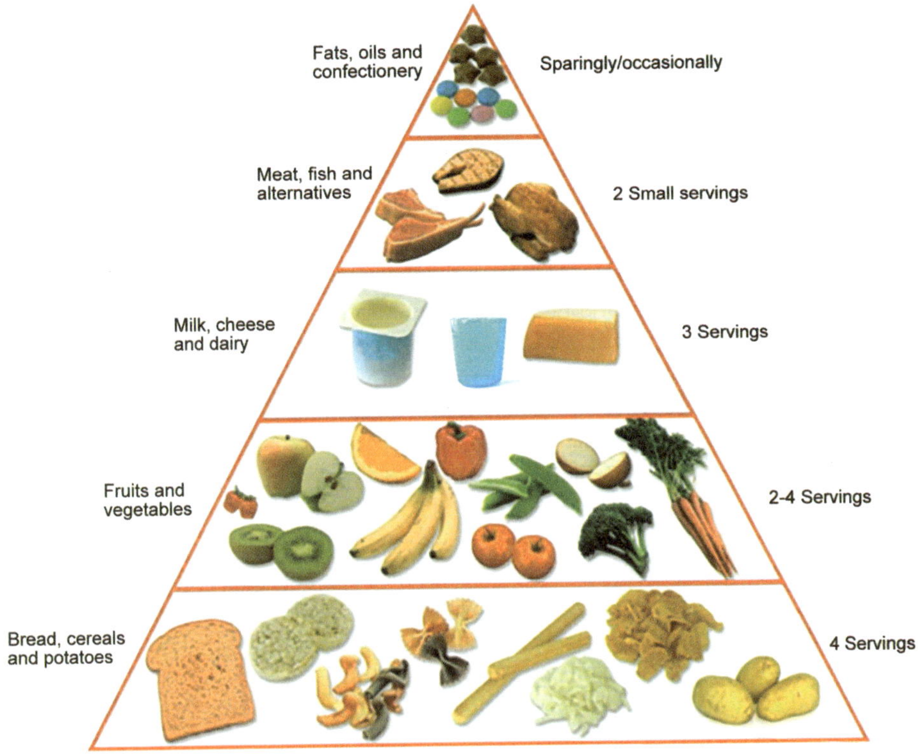

Fig. 3.2: Pyramid showing the amount of food products that should be consumed in form of balanced diet

Instructions for Balanced Diet

- **Regular meal patterns:** Establishing consistent meal times is beneficial for maintaining energy levels throughout the day. It's advisable to eat meals at regular intervals, placing particular importance on breakfast. Skipping breakfast can lower energy levels and potentially lead to overeating later in the day.
- **Carbohydrate intake:** Guidelines recommend that 45–60% of a person's daily calories should come from carbohydrates, or carbs. That's equal to about 225–325 g of carbs if person consumes 2,000 calories a day. Choose complex carbohydrates such as oats, chapati (whole wheat flatbread), brown rice, whole grain bread, and potatoes. These provide sustained energy and fiber.
- **Protein sources:** Proteins should contribute to 25–30% of daily calories. Include sources like milk, legumes (beans and lentils), nuts, poultry (chicken, turkey), lean meats, eggs, and fish. Proteins are essential for muscle repair, immune function, and overall body maintenance.
- **Fat consumption:** Fat intake should not exceed 20–25% of daily calories. Emphasize sources of healthy fats, such as polyunsaturated and monounsaturated fats found in nuts, seeds, avocados, and olive oil. Limit saturated fats to less than 7% of daily calories and avoid trans fats altogether.

- **Cholesterol limit:** Limit cholesterol intake to <300 mg/day. Cholesterol is found in animal products like meat, eggs, and dairy. Choose lean cuts of meat and low-fat dairy options to help manage cholesterol levels.
- **Oil consumption:** Consume no >5–7 teaspoons of oil per day, depending on age and sex. Be mindful of hidden oils in foods such as olives, nuts, and processed snacks. Opt for cooking methods that use less oil, such as baking, grilling, or steaming.
- **Portion control and eating habits:** Eat until 75% full to prevent overeating and promote digestion. Avoid lying down immediately after eating to aid digestion and prevent discomfort.
- **Light dinner:** Dinner should be lighter than lunch, comprising about 3/4th the quantity of lunch. This helps prevent overloading the digestive system before bedtime and promotes better sleep quality.
- **Inclusion of raw vegetables:** Incorporate at least two servings of raw vegetables daily. Raw vegetables provide essential vitamins, minerals, and fiber that may be lost during cooking.
- **Hydration:** Drink an adequate amount of water throughout the day to stay hydrated. Water is essential for digestion, nutrient absorption, circulation, and temperature regulation. Aim for at least 8 glasses (about 2 liters) of water daily, adjusting based on individual needs and activity levels.
- **Fiber-rich foods:** Include fiber-rich foods such as whole grains (oats, whole wheat), legumes (beans, lentils), fruits, and vegetables. Fiber promotes digestive health, helps maintain healthy cholesterol levels, and contributes to feelings of fullness.
- **Limit added sugars and sodium:** Reduce intake of foods and beverages high in added sugars, such as sugary drinks, candies, and desserts. Choose naturally sweet alternatives like fruits. Limit consumption of high-sodium foods like processed meats, canned soups, and salty snacks. Choose low-sodium options and season foods with herbs and spices instead of salt.
- Recommended dietary allowances for various categories are given in Table 3.4.

Elements of Balanced Diet

- **Macronutrients:** Macronutrients are the nutrients, which are required in large quantities for the normal functioning of the body, e.g., carbohydrates, proteins, and lipids.
- **Micronutrients:** These are required in small quantities, for example, vitamins and minerals.

FOOD GROUPS

Indian Council of Medical Research (ICMR) has given five food groups. This five food group system helps to plan the menu, which further helps to meet nutrient requirements as recommended. Five food group systems given by ICMR are shown in Table 3.5.

Table 3.4: Recommended dietary allowances for various categories

Group	Particulars	Body wt. (kg)	Net energy kcal/day	Protein g/day	Visible fat g/day	Calcium mg/day	Iron mg/day	Vitamin-A retinol	Vitamin-A β-carotene	Thiamine mg/day	Riboflavin mg/day	Niacin equivalent	Pyridoxine mg/day	Ascorbic acid mg/day	Dietary folate µg/day	Vit-B_{12} µg/day	Magnesium mg/day	Zinc mg/day
Man	Sedentary work		2320		25					1.2	1.4	16						
	Moderate work	60	2730	60.0	30	600	17	600	4800	1.4	1.6	18	2.0	40	200	1.0	340	12
	Heavy work		3490		40					1.7	2.1	21						
Woman	Sedentary work		1900		20					1.0	1.1	12						
	Moderate work		2230	55.0	25	600	21	600	4800	1.1	1.3	14	2.0	40	200	1.0		10
	Heavy work		2850		30					1.4	1.7	16						
	Pregnant	55	+350	82.2	30	1200	35	800	6400	+0.2	+0.3	+2	2.5	60	500	1.2	310	
	Lactation 0–6 m		+600	77.9	30			950	7600	+0.3	+0.4	+4	2.5	80	500	1.5		12
	6–12 m		+520	70.2	30	1200	25			+0.2	+0.3	+3	2.5					
Infants	0–6 m	5.4	92 kcal/kg/day	1.16 g/kg/day	—	500	46 µg/kg/d	350	—	0.2	0.3	710 µg/kg	0.1	25	25	0.2	30	—
	6–12 m	8.4	80 kcal/kg/day	1.69 g/kg/day	19		05		2800	0.3	0.4	650 µg/kg	0.4				45	—
Children	1–3 years	12.9	1060	16.7	27		09	400	3200	0.5	0.6	8	0.9		80		50	5
	4–6 years	18.0	1350	20.1	25	600	13			0.7	0.8	11	0.9	40	100	0.2-1.0	70	7
	7–9 years	25.1	1690	29.5	30		16	600	4800	0.8	1.0	13	1.6		120		100	8
Boys	10–12 years	34.3	2190	39.9	35	800	21	600	4800	1.1	1.3	15	1.6	40	140	0.2-1.0	120	9
Girls	10–12 years	35.0	2010	40.4	35	800	27			1.0	1.2	13	1.6	40	140	0.2-1.0	160	9
Boys	13–15 years	47.6	2750	54.3	45	800	32			1.4	1.6	16	2.0	40			165	11
Girls	13–15 years	46.6	2330	51.9	40	800	27			1.2	1.4	14	2.0	40	150	0.2-1.0	210	11
Boys	16–17 years	55.4	3020	61.5	50	800	28	600	4800	1.5	1.8	17	2.0	40			195	12
Girls	16–17 years	52.1	2440	55.5	35	800	26			1.0	1.2	14	2.0	40	200	0.2-1.0	235	12

Source: *Indian Council of Medical Research, 2010*

Table 3.5: Five food group systems given by ICMR

Sl. no.	Food groups	Main nutrients
1.	**Cereals, grains and products** Wheat, rice, ragi, jowar, bajra, maize, barley, rice flakes, wheat flour.	Energy, protein, invisible fat, vitamin B_1, vitamin B_2, folic acid, iron, fiber.
2.	**Pulses and legumes** Bengal gram, black gram, green gram, red gram, lentil, cow pea, peas, rajmah, soybeans, beans.	Energy, protein, invisible fat, vitamin B_1, vitamin B_2, folic acid, iron, fiber, calcium
3.	**Milk and meat products** **Milk and milk products:** Milk, skimmed milk, curd, cheese. **Meat:** Chicken, liver, fish, egg, meat.	Protein, vitamin B_{12}, calcium, fat. Protein, vitamin B_2, fat.
4.	**Fruits** Mango, papaya, orange, guava, sweet lime, watermelon, etc.	Carotenoids, fiber, vitamin C
5.	**Vegetables** **Green leafy:** Spinach, amaranth, coriander leaves, drumstick leaves, mustard leaves, fenugreek leaves. **Other vegetables:** Radish, carrots, brinjal, beans, onions, carrots, gourds, drumsticks, lady finger, capsicum **Fats and sugars:** **Fats:** Butter, ghee, cooking oils like mustard oil, coconut oil, sunflower oil, etc. **Sugars:** Sugar and jaggery	Carotenoids, invisible fat, vitamin B_2, iron, calcium, folic acid, fiber. Carotenoids, folic acid, calcium, fiber Energy, fat, essential fatty acids Energy

MENU PLANNING/MEAL PLANNING

Meal planning is defined as a simple process that involves application of the knowledge of food, nutrients, food habits and likes and dislikes to plan wholesome and attractive meals.

Aims

- To provide well balanced diet
- To save time and money
- To promote healing and recovery of patient
- To plan meal according to family budget

Principles

- **Meal pattern must suit the family:** Menu planning should be done according to the family distribution such as age, sex, height, weight, and special conditions such as pregnancy and lactation.
- **Disease condition of the patient:** Menu planning should be done according to the disease condition of the patient, e.g., low sodium diet for the patient with hypertension, sugar free diet for diabetic patient, etc.
- **Save time and money:** Menu planning should be in such a way that it saves time and money.
- **Meal planning should induce variety:** Meal planning should provide variety of foods so as to avoid monotony of foods.

- **Food habits and food customs:** Menu planning should be done according to likes and dislikes and food customs of the family.
- **Individual preferences:** Menu planning must be done according to an individual's preferences like preference of vegetarian and nonvegetarian food.
- **Meals should provide satiable value:** Proteins and fats should be included in one's food as they have higher satiety value as compared to that of carbohydrates. There should be an interval between two meals.
- **Budgetary considerations:** Menu planning should be done according to the family budget. Menu planning can be made cost effective by including seasonal foods.
- **Provide maximum nutrients:** Menu planning should be done in such a way so that it provides all the required nutrients in diet.

Different Categories for Calculating Nutritional Requirement

Nutritional requirement changes in every stage of life of a human being. Calculation for the different category is necessary to ensure the availability of all nutrients to different categories. Different categories are as follows:

- Infant (0–6 months)
- Infant (6–12 months)
- Toddler (1–3 years)
- Preschooler (3–6 years)
- Young school age (6–13 years)
- Adolescent (13–18 years)
- Young adulthood (18–40 years)
- Middle adulthood (40–60 years)
- Late adulthood (60–80 years)

Steps for Calculating

- **Step I: Collection of information**—Collect basic information of person with reference to age, sex, lifestyle, religion, habits, likes and dislikes, socioeconomic status.
- **Step II: Identify recommended dietary allowances (RDA)**—Second step involves identification of RDA. It depends upon many factors such as age, gender, activity, etc.
- **Step III: Prepare food lists**—Third step involves the preparation of food lists along with their quantities so that it meets the recommended dietary allowances. It can be prepared by using ICMR five food group systems.
- **Step IV: Menu plan**—Last step is planning menu. It involves planning of meals beforehand. List of foods that was prepared earlier is converted into recipes and is distributed to various meals such as breakfast, lunch and dinner.

Calculation of Nutritional Requirements for Different Categories

Infant (0–6 months)

Nutritional requirement during this age is more because of rapid growth during this period. Energy and protein requirement during this period is more, i.e., 92 kcal/kg of body weight/day and 1.16 g of body weight/day respectively. During this period nutritional requirement is fulfilled by either breast milk or formula feeding.

Advantages of Breastfeed over Bottle Feed

- It contains all the nutrients, which are sufficient to meet the requirement of infants.
- Breast milk is easy to digest.
- It contains immunoglobulins IgA, IgM, lymphocytes, macrophages and lysozyme, which protects the baby from infection.
- It contains large amounts of lactose and galactose, which is essential for brain growth.

Infant (6–12 months)

At this time, requirement of infant is increased due to rapid growth. Breast milk is not sufficient to fulfil the nutritional requirement of infants so weaning is started to meet the nutritional requirement of infants.

Weaning

Weaning is the introduction of foods other than the breast milk. The infant is put off from breastfeeding and complementary feeding is given. It is the process of gradually introducing foods other than breast milk in the child's feeding schedule.

Principles

- One food is given at one time.
- Weaning is started at the age of 6 months.
- Consistency of food is such that it suits the age of the child. At first liquid diet is given to the infant and gradually semisolid foods are introduced.
- Spicy and fried foods are avoided.
- In the beginning, small amounts of foods are given and then slowly the amount of food is increased.
- If the child dislikes any food substance then the food is changed with other food item. The child should not be forced to eat the food that he/she dislikes.
- Variety of food should be introduced to the child's diet.
- Nuts, eggs or fish, etc. should not be given as they may trigger allergy to the infant.

WHO Recommendations for Weaning

WHO recommends that infants start receiving complementary foods at 6 months of age in addition to breast milk. Initially 2–3 times a day, between 6 and 8 months and increasing to 3–4 times daily between 9 and 11 months and during 12–24 months additional nutritious snacks are offered 1–2 times per day, as desired. Table 3.6 shows list of weaning foods for infants.

Table 3.6: Weaning foods for infants

Infant's age	6 months	7–8 months	9–12 months
Food items	Vegetable soup Dal soup Fruit juice Cow's milk	Mashed banana Cerelac	Suji kheer Custard Boiled potato Khichdi Dalia

Toddler (1–3 years)

During this time-period, child starts exploring his environment, which affects the food behavior and eating patterns. Dietary requirement of toddler is different from infants. As the child grows, his/her dietary requirements also change. Balanced diet for the toddler is essential for the maintenance of his/her optimum level of growth and development. Recommended dietary allowances of calories for children (1–3 years) are 900–1100 kcal. A sample menu plan for toddler is given in Table 3.7.

Table 3.7: Sample menu plan for toddler

Meal timing	Food items	Serving	Amount (kcal)
Early morning	Milk	1 glass	120
	Biscuits	2	36
Breakfast	Dalia	1 bowl	87
Midmorning	Fruit (banana medium)	1	105
Lunch	Chapati (medium)	1	102
	Mix vegetable	1 bowl	102
	Curd	½ bowl	65
Evening	Fruit custard	1 bowl	144
Dinner	Rice	½ bowl	69
	Dal (moong)	½ bowl	70
Bed time	Milk with almonds	1 glass	153
Total			**1053**

Preschooler (3–6 years)

Preschooler period is a period during which growth occur in spurts, therefore the child needs more nutrients. At this stages, the child has to learn eating habits of the family. Preschooler child eats in less quantity so small frequent meals should be provided to the child. As the child has less interest in food, so likes and dislikes of the child should be kept in mind. Provide colorful and attractive meal to stimulate eating. Recommended dietary allowances of calories for children (3–6 years) are 1300–1400 kcal. Sample menu plan for preschooler is given in Table 3.8.

Table 3.8: Sample menu plan for preschooler

Meal timings	Food items	Serving	Calories
Early morning	Milk	1 glass	120
Breakfast	Stuffed potato paratha Curd	1 1 small bowl	178 60
Midmorning	Banana (medium sized)	1	105
Lunch	Rice Chapati (small) Vegetables (ladyfinger) Dal (Bengal gram)	½ bowl 1 1 bowl 1 bowl	69 85 50 180
Evening	Vegetable soup	½ bowl	64

Contd...

Meal timings	Food items	Serving	Calories
Dinner	Chapati (small) Mixed vegetable Dal (washed urad)	1 1 bowl 1 bowl	85 102 156
Bed time	Milk	1 glass	120
Total			**1374**
Note: 1 bowl = 150 mL			

School Going Children (6–13) Years

At this stage, children enjoy company of their friends and spend most of the time with them. They are curious and also learn to think in more compound way. During this age, it is essential to give variety of healthy food to the children. The parents need to pay more attention to diet of children because sedentary habits in the school age can lead to obesity. Recommended dietary allowances of calories for children (6–13 years) is 1600–2000 kcal and is listed in Table 3.9.

Table 3.9: Sample menu plan for children of age 6–13 years

Meal timings	Food items	Amount	Calories (kcal)
Early morning	Milk with Biscuits	1 glass 2	120 36
Breakfast	Bread toast	2	128
Midmorning	Fruit chat (apple, guava, banana)	1 fruit (banana)	113
Lunch	Chapati Rice Dal (rajmah) Vegetable Curd	1 big sized 1 bowl 1 bowl 1 small bowl 1 bowl	136 138 121 57 120
Evening	Dalia with coconut	1 bowl	132
Dinner	Chapati Dal (malka masoor) Salad	2 (big) 1 bowl 1 bowl	272 137 56
Bed time	Milk	1 glass	120
Total			**1686**

Adolescents

This is the most vulnerable period because many biological changes take place during this period like increase in height, development of secondary sexual characteristics, etc. During adolescent years girls become more figure conscious and are at risk for developing anorexia nervosa, which leads to malnutrition and anemia. It is mandatory to provide well-balanced diet to the adolescents.

Recommended dietary allowances of calories for adolescent are given in Table 3.10:

- Boys (13–15 years) — 2750 kcal
- Girls (13–15 years) — 2330 kcal
- Boys (16–17 years) — 3020 kcal
- Girls (16–17 years) — 2440 kcal

Table 3.10: Sample menu plan for adolescent boys and girls (13–15 years)

Meal timings	Food items	Amount for boys	Calories	Amount for girls	Calories
Early morning	Milk Biscuits	1 glass 2	120 36	1 glass 2	120 36
Breakfast	Paratha Curd	3 1 bowl	533 120	2 1 bowl	356 120
Midmorning	Fruit chat (banana, grapes, apple)	1	181	1	181
Lunch	Chapati Rice Dal (urad chana) Vegetable Curd	2 1 bowl 1 bowl 1 bowl 1 bowl	272 138 123 118 120	1 medium sized 1 bowl 1 bowl 1 bowl 1 bowl	136 138 123 118 120
Evening	Dalia	1 bowl	87	1 bowl	87
Dinner	Chapati Dal (washed moong) Vegetable (beans and potato) Salad	3 big 1 bowl 1 bowl 1 bowl	408 139 195 56	3 medium sized 1 bowl 1 bowl 1 bowl	306 139 195 56
Bed time	Milk	1 glass	120	1 glass	120
Total			**2766**		**2351**

BALANCED DIET FOR ADULTS

Activity is one of the most important factors, which influences the requirement of nutrients for the adults. In adults, body growth such as increase in height stops to certain extent but the bodily processes like tissue repair and breakdown go on continuously. Nutritional requirement of adults are influenced by various factors such as age, sex, body weight, height. Nutritional requirements for males and females are also different because of difference in body composition and body weight.

A recommended dietary allowance of calories for sedentary, moderate and heavy male and female worker is given in Tables 3.11 to 3.15:

- **For males:**
  - For sedentary male worker: 2320 kcal
  - For moderate male worker: 2730 kcal
  - For heavy male worker: 3490 kcal
- **For females:**
  - For sedentary female worker: 1900 kcal
  - For moderate female worker: 2230 kcal
  - For heavy female worker: 2850 kcal

Classification of work based on occupation (Indian Council of Medical Research 1990)

Sedentary work: It involves very limited physical activities. For example, teacher, shoemaker, priest, tailor, executive, driver, receptionist, etc.

Moderate work: It involves moderate or average amount of physical activities. Examples are fisherman, potter, carpenter, goldsmith, welder, basket maker, weaver, nurse, agricultural laborer, etc.

Heavy worker: It involves extensive physical activities. For example, stone-cutter, mine worker, wood cutter, dance teachers, fire fighters, construction workers, etc.

Table 3.11: Sample menu plan for adult male-sedentary/moderate activities

Meal timings	Food items	Amount for sedentary worker	Calories (kcal)	Amount for moderate worker	Calories (kcal)
Early morning Breakfast	Tea	1 cup - 53	53	1 cup	53
Midmorning	Stuffed paratha Curd Fruit juice	2 1 bowl 1 glass	356 120 207	2 and half 1 bowl 1 glass	445 120 207
Lunch	Chapati Salad Rice Moong dal Palak paneer	2 big 1 bowl 1 bowl 1 bowl 1 bowl	272 56 138 83 427	3 big sized 1 bowl 1 bowl 1 bowl 1 bowl	408 56 138 83 427
Evening	Tea Biscuit	1 cup 2	53 36	1 cup 2	53 36
Dinner	Chapati Rice Dal (arhar) Capsicum potato vegetable	1 1 bowl 1 bowl 1 bowl	136 138 117 81	2 big sized 1 bowl 1 bowl 1 bowl	272 138 117 81
Bed time	Milk	1 glass	120	1 glass	120
Total			**2393**		**2754**

Table 3.12: Sample menu plan for adult male—heavy worker

Meal timings	Food items	Amount for heavy worker	Calories (kcal)
Early morning	Tea Biscuit	1 cup 4	53 72
Breakfast	Stuffed paratha Curd	3 1 bowl	543 120
Mid morning	Fruit juice	1 glass	207
Lunch	Chapati Curd Rice Moong dal Palak paneer	4 big sized 1 bowl 1 bowl 1 bowl 1 bowl	544 120 138 83 427
Evening	Tea Roasted groundnuts	1 cup 2 tbs	53 180

Contd...

Meal timings	Food items	Amount for heavy worker	Calories (kcal)
Dinner	Chapati Rice Dal (arhar) Capsicum potato vegetable Salad	3 big sized 1 bowl 1 bowl 1 bowl 1 bowl	408 138 117 81 56
Bed time	Milk with almonds	1 glass	153
Total			3493

Abbreviation: tbs, tablespoon

Table 3.13: Sample menu plan for the adult female—sedentary worker

Meal timings	Food items	Amount for sedentary worker	Calories (kcal)
Early morning	Tea	1 cup	53
Breakfast	Methi paratha Curd	2 1 bowl	395 120
Mid morning	Banana	1	116
Lunch	Chapati Rice Dal (rajmah) Vegetable (brinjal potato) Curd	1 big sized 1 bowl 1 bowl 1 bowl 1 bowl	136 138 121 81 120
Evening	Tea Biscuits	1 cup 2	53 36
Dinner	Chapati Dal (malka masoor) Vegetable (pumpkin) Salad	2 small sized 1 bowl 1 bowl 1 bowl	170 137 78 56
Bed time	Milk	1 glass	120
Total			1930

Table 3.14: Sample menu plan for the adult female—moderate worker

Meal timings	Food items	Amount for moderate worker	Calories (kcal)
Early morning	Tea Biscuit	1 cup 2	53 36
Breakfast	Methi paratha Curd	2 1 bowl	395 120
Midmorning	Fruit juice	1 glass	207

Contd...

Meal timings	Food items	Amount for moderate worker	Calories (kcal)
Lunch	Chapati Rice Dal (rajmah) Vegetable (brinjal potato) Curd	3 medium sized 1 bowl 1 bowl 1 bowl 1 bowl	306 138 121 81 120
Evening	Tea Biscuits	1 cup 2	53 36
Dinner	Chapati Dal (malka masoor) Vegetable (pumpkin) Salad	3 medium sized 1 bowl 1 bowl 1 bowl	306 137 78 56
Bed time	Milk	1 glass	120
Total			**2363**

Table 3.15: Sample menu plan for the adult female—heavy worker

Meal timings	Food items	Amount for heavy worker	Calories (kcal)
Early morning	Tea	1 cup	53
Breakfast	Methi paratha Curd	3 1 bowl	590 120
Mid morning	Fruit juice	1 glass	207
Lunch	Chapati Rice Dal (rajmah) Vegetable (brinjal potato) Curd	3 big sized 1 bowl 1 bowl 1 bowl 1 bowl	408 138 121 81 120
Evening	Tea Roasted groundnuts	1 cup 2 tbs	53 180
Dinner	Chapati Dal (malka masoor) Vegetable (pumpkin) Salad	3 big sized 1 bowl 1 bowl 1 bowl	408 137 78 56
Bed time	Milk	1 glass	120
Total			**2870**

DIET IN PREGNANCY

During pregnancy, marked physiological, biochemical and hormonal changes occur in the body of female. Nutritious diet during pregnancy is essential as she carries fetus in her womb and it affects the growth and development of fetus. If any nutrient is lacking in the diet of pregnant lady it can lead to serious birth defects, e.g., deficiency of folic acid can lead to neural tube defects. Poor nutrition of mother is directly proportional to the intrauterine growth retardation (IUGR). Poor nutrition can also increase complications during labor and lactation. Recommended dietary allowances of calories for pregnant lady is 1900 + 350 kcal (Table 3.16).

Table 3.16: Sample menu plan for the pregnant woman

Meal timings	Food items	Amount	Calories (kcal)
Early morning	Tea Biscuits	1 cup 2	53 36
Breakfast	Palak paratha Curd Milk	2 1 bowl I glass	391 120 120
Mid morning	Mixed fruit juice	1 glass	207
Lunch	Chapati Dal (moong washed) Rice Vegetable (capsicum potato) Salad Curd	2 medium sized 1 bowl 1 bowl 1 bowl 1 bowl 1 bowl	204 139 138 81 56 120
Evening	Dalia	1 bowl	87
Dinner	Chapati Dal (arhar) Vegetable (mixed)	2 big sized 1 bowl 1 bowl	272 117 102
Bed time	Milk with almonds	1 glass	153
Total			**2396**

DIET FOR LACTATING WOMAN

Lactation is the process of milk secretion through the mammary glands. In the first few months of the life, infant derives all the nutrients from the breast milk. A well-nourished mother secretes an average of about 850 mL of milk per day. Nutrition of lactating mother has effect on both quantity and quality of milk production. In a poorly nourished lactating mother, quantity of milk decreases about 400 mL/day. Therefore, it is essential to provide well-balanced diet to the lactating women. Recommended dietary allowances for lactating women during first 6 months of lactation is + 600 kcal (1900 + 600) and for the next 6 months it is + 520 kcal (1900+520). Menu plan for the lactating woman is given in Table 3.17.

Table 3.17: Sample menu plan for the lactating woman

Meal timings	Food items	Amount	Calories (kcal)
Early morning	Tea Biscuits	1 cup 2	53 36
Breakfast	Methi paratha Curd	2 1 bowl	395 120
Midmorning	Mixed fruit juice	1 glass	207

Contd...

Meal timings	Food items	Amount	Calories (kcal)
Lunch	Chapati Rice Chana dal Vegetable (palak paneer) Salad	2 medium sized 1 bowl 1 bowl 1 bowl 1 bowl	272 136 117 427 56
Evening	Tea Biscuits	1 cup 2	53 36
Dinner	Chapati Dal (moong washed) Vegetable (brinjal potato)	2 medium sized 1 bowl 1 bowl	272 139 81
Bed time	Milk	1 glass	120
Total			**2520**

DIET FOR ELDERLY OR OLD AGE PEOPLE

As the process of aging greatly affects the nutritional needs of the old age people so older people are vulnerable to malnutrition. Old age people are at the risk of developing diabetes mellitus, obesity, cardiovascular diseases and osteoporosis. Well-balanced diet is important during aging because many degenerative changes are taking place in the body of the older people. They have difficulty in digesting and utilizing the food. The recommended dietary allowances for the old age people are given in Tables 3.18 and 3.19.

Table 3.18: Recommended dietary allowances for the old age people

Sex	Body weight (kg)	Age >60 years	
		Sedentary	Moderate
Males	45	1590	1870
	50	1688	1985
	55	1786	2101
	60	1883	2216
	65	1981	2331
	70	2079	2446
	75	2177	2565
Females	40	1477	1737
	45	1553	1627
	50	1630	1917
	55	1706	2007
	60	1782	2097
	65	1860	2187
	70	1936	2277

Source: Indian Council of Medical Research, 2010

Table 3.19: Sample menu plan for the old age sedentary female worker

Meals	Food items	Amount	Calories (kcal)
Early morning	Tea Fiber biscuits	1 cup 2	53 50
Breakfast	Vegetable upma	1 big bowl	71
Mid morning	Banana	1	116
Lunch	Chapati Rice Rajmah Curd Vegetable (carrot, pea, potato) Salad	1 big sized 1 bowl 1 bowl 1 bowl 1 bowl	136 138 121 120 55
Evening	Tea	1 cup	53
Dinner	Chapati Dal (malka masoor) Pumpkin	2 big sized 1 bowl 1 bowl	272 137 78
Bed time	Milk	1 glass	120
Total			**1520**

COMBINATION OF FOOD ENHANCING THE NUTRITIVE VALUE OF FOOD

New researches show that some food that taste great together are also more nutritious when eaten in combination. According to Ayurveda and other alternative medicine, if we combine the wrong foods, the body will become acidic and unbalanced and actually will secrete enzymes that can lead to impaired digestion resulting in bloating, gas, etc. Proper food combination not only enhances the taste but also increases the nutritive value of the food and boosts the immunity, for example, lemon and green tea.

The following are the proper food combinations:

- **Whole grains and legumes:** Rice and beans, whole grain bread with lentil soup.

  Nutritive value: Combining whole grains (such as rice or bread) with legumes (like beans or lentils) enhances protein value by providing all essential amino acids. This combination also offers a good balance of carbohydrates, fiber, vitamins, and minerals.
- **Greens leafy with vitamin C-rich foods:** Spinach salad with strawberries or oranges.

  Nutritive value: Vitamin C enhances the absorption of iron from green leafy vegetables (like spinach or kale).
- **Yogurt with nuts or seeds:** Yogurt with almonds or chia seeds.

  Nutritive value: Yogurt provides probiotics and calcium, while nuts or seeds offer healthy fats, protein, and additional vitamins and minerals. This combination supports gut health, bone health, and provides sustained energy.
- **Eggs with whole grain toast:** Scrambled eggs with whole grain toast.

  Nutritive value: Eggs are a source of high-quality protein, vitamins, and minerals, while whole grain toast provides fiber and sustained energy. This combination supports muscle repair, satiety, and overall nutrient intake.

In India, people usually consume their diet in combination, which compensate the requirement of nutrients like in South India people take sambar, rasam or idli/dosa in combination similarly North Indians combine dal-chawal or khichdi, curd and butter milk. Such combinations make the diet healthy, tasty and more nutritive.

BUDGETING FOR FOOD

Budget is a financial plan that helps people make the best possible use of their money. It identifies source of income and assists in planning expenditures. Largest part of a family's income is spent in buying food. Family's budget is influenced by size of family, number of children in family, age of family members, activity and special needs during pregnancy, lactation or sick individuals with modified dietary needs. The choice of food for family depends upon family income. It is necessary to plan the expenditure of food so that one can achieve maximum nutrients from spent money. For example, the main source of protein is meat, fish, egg and pulses but pulses are available at cheaper price as compared to animal foods. Seasonal fruits and vegetables are cheaper. One should buy seasonal fruits and vegetables to cut down the expense on food purchase. Economy in food purchasing can be exercised by having small kitchen gardens.

The following points must be considered while planning the budget:

- **Socioeconomic status of the family:** The amount of money spent on food depends upon the basic income of the family. Budget for food increases with increase in family income similarly, it decreases when family income decreases. Poor people focus on buying basic and cheaper food products whereas people with higher income do not bother for calculations. Socioeconomic status of the family has great impact on budget planning.
- **Size of the family:** Expenditure on food depends upon family size, age, sex and special requirement in the family, for example, in case of pregnancy, lactation or in sickness more attention must be paid on nutritional requirement of the individual. Nuclear families can plan their budget according to their convenience but in joint families everyone's choice has to be considered.
- **Availability of resources:** Food is available at low costs in local markets where seasonal fruits and vegetables are available but transportation charges may put additional burden for poor people. Other resources like ration stores and wholesale markets sells food items at cheaper prices. Foods available in these stores, sometimes are not good in quality but has good nutritive value.
- **Preference of the family members:** While planning the budget, preferences of the food items must be kept in mind. Buying the food items that nobody likes in the family is the wastage of money.

Points to be kept in mind before purchasing food items are:

- It is necessary to plan budget for a month or at least for a week.
- Make a list and stick with it. Do not buy too much items that are not necessary, for example, pies, cakes, chips, soda, donuts, etc.
- Buy seasonal fruits and vegetables because they are cheaper and easily available.
- Before purchasing, compare the cost and nutritive value of two similar food items.
- Buy low priced brands because they are similar in nutritive value as compared to more expensive one.
- Avoid pre-packed foods because they are expensive, for example, frozen vegetables are more expensive as compared to fresh vegetables.
- Make kitchen gardens to grow fruits and vegetables to reduce expenditure on food if possible.
- Try to avoid shopping of the food items when you are hungry, late at night or in hurry.

- Always check the ingredients, nutritive value, cost, manufacturing and expiry date of the packaged food items.
- Buy the things without any pressure. Do not buy looking at others if you are shopping in a group, always keep in mind the needs of your family.

FOOD SUBSTITUTES

Food substitutes are the food products, which provide same or nearly same amounts of nutrients as provided by other food products. Food substitutes provide variety to the meal along with fulfilling the nutritional requirement. Food substitutes can also be given to the person who is allergic to that particular food product.

Nutritional Food Substitutes

Food substitution for food items is given in Table 3.20.

Table 3.20: Food items and their substitutes

Food items	Food substitutes
Milk	Milk powder, soy milk
Almonds	Peanuts
Sugar	Jaggery
Jelly/jam	Fresh fruits
White rice	Brown rice
French fries	Baked potatoes
Canned fruits, vegetable	Fresh fruits and vegetables
Fried fish	Chicken/baked fish
Canned soups	Fresh juice/soups

Food Substitutes for Allergy

Food substitution for the allergic food is given in Table 3.21.

Table 3.21: Food items and their substitutes in case of allergy

Food items	Food substitutes
Milk	Soya milk, rice milk
Wheat	Maize, ragi
Meat	Seitan
Butter	Margarine
Dairy cheese	Soya cheese/tofu

FOOD EXCHANGE

The word exchange refers to the fact that each item on a particular list in the portion listed may be interchanged with any other food item on the same list. An exchange can be explained as a substitution, choice, or serving. Each list is a group of measured or weighed foods of approximately the same nutritional value. Within each food list, one exchange is approximately equal to another in calories, carbohydrate, protein, and fat. To use the exchange lists, an individual needs an individualized meal plan that outlines the number of exchanges from each list for each meal and for snacks. The meal plan is developed in cooperation with the person and is based on an assessment of diet changes that would assist the individual in achieving his or her target metabolic goals. Because of the accuracy and convenience of the exchange system, the exchange lists are used for weight management as well for other diseases, for example, diabetes management.

Food Exchange List

Cereal Exchange (Table 3.22)

- **30 g provide:** Carbohydrate 20 g, protein 2 g

Table 3.22: List of cereals that can be interchanged with any other food items on the same list

Cereals	Household measures	Wt./Vol.	Calories
Rice		30 g uncooked	100
Wheat flour		30 g uncooked	100
Dalia	½ bowl cooked	30 g uncooked	100
Sago		30 g uncooked	100
White flour		30 g uncooked	100
Bread	2 slices	40 g	100
Chapati	1.5 (approx. 5-6" diameter)	44 g	100
Jowar roti	0.5	55 g	100
Ragi		30 g	100
Rice flakes	1 bowl	30 g	100
Oat meal		30 g	100
Vermicelli	½ bowl cooked	30 g	100
Corn flakes		30 g	100
Maize dry		30 g	100
Marie biscuit	8 No.		100
Monaco biscuit	4 No.		100
Idlis	2 No.		100
Poha	½ bowl		100
Upma	½ bowl		100
Dosa ordinary			120
Note: 1 bowl-volume is 150 mL.			

Fat Exchange (Table 3.23)

- 50 g calories; fat 5.5 g

Table 3.23: List of fats that can be interchanged with any other food items on the same list

Fats	Household measures	Wt. (g)	Calories
Butter	1.5 tsp	7.5	50
Ghee	1 tsp	5.5	50
Hydrogenated fat (vanaspati)	1 tsp	5.5	50
Oil (coconut, mustard, sunflower, corn, groundnut, cotton seed, til, palm)	1 tsp	5.5	50
Cashewnuts		10	50
Groundnuts roasted		10	50
Walnuts		7.5	50
Pistachio		7.5	50
Almonds		7.5	50

Abbreviation: tsp, teaspoon

Milk and Milk Products (Table 3.24)

- 50 calories; protein 2.5 g

Table 3.24: Milk and milk products that can be interchanged with any other food products on the same list

Milk and milk products	Household measures	Wt./Vol.	Calories
Curd	⅔ glass	105 g	50
Butter milk	3 glasses	375 mL	50
Cheese	1 ice cube	15 g	50
Milk (buffalo)	⅓ glass	45 mL	50
Milk (cow)	⅔ glass	90 mL	50
Milk, skimmed*	1 glass	130 mL	50
Milk skimmed powder*		15 g	50
Coffee Nescafe + 75 mL milk (without sugar)			50
Tea + 75 mL milk			50
Khoya		15 g	50

1 medium glass 150 mL provides 5 g protein*

Vegetable Exchange (Table 3.25)

- 50 calories; carbohydrate 10 g

Table 3.25: List of vegetables that can be interchanged with any other vegetable on the same list

Vegetables	Household measures	Wt. (g)	Calories
Beetroot (chukander)		75	50
Carrot	1–2 No.	105	50
Colocasia (arbi)		45	50
Onion (big)	1 No.	90	50
Onion (small)	2 No.	75	50
Potato	½ No.	45	50
Sweet potato		30	50
Tapioca		30	50
Yam (zimikand)		45	50
Broad beans		90	50
Cluster beans		90	50
Double beans		50	50
Jackfruit, tender		105	50
Jackfruit seeds		30	50
Leeks		60	50
Peas		45	50
Singhara		45	50
Sambar	¼ bowl	35 mL	50
Cooked vegetable	½ bowl		50
Note: *1* bowl*: Volume 150 mL*			

Fruit Exchange (Table 3.26)

- 50 calories; carbohydrate 10 g

Table 3.26: List of fruits that can be interchanged with any other fruits on the same list

Fruits	Size/no.	Wt. (g)	Calories
Apple	1 small	75	50
Amla	20 medium	90	50
Banana	¼ medium	30	50
Cashew fruit	2 medium	90	50
Custard apple	¼	50	50
Dates	3	30	50

Contd...

Fruits	Size/no.	Wt. (g)	Calories
Figs	6 medium	135	50
Grapes	20	105	50
Grapefruit	½ big	150	50
Jackfruit	3 medium pieces	60	50
Mango	1 small	90	50
Melon	¼ medium	270	50
Orange	1 small	90	50
Lemon	1 medium	90	50
Papaya	2 medium	120	50
Peach	1 medium	135	50
Pear	1 medium	90	50
Plums	4 medium	120	50
Pineapple	1½ slices (round)	90	50
Strawberry	40	105	50
Sweet lime	1 medium	150	50
Tomato	4 medium	240	50
Watermelon	¼ small	175	50

Legume and Pulse Exchange (Table 3.27)

- 30 g provides: carbohydrate 15 g, protein 6 g

Table 3.27: Legumes and pulses that can be interchanged with any other items on the same list

Pulse (uncooked)	Household measures	Wt. (g)	Calories
Bengal gram	3/4 bowl cooked	30	100
Bengal gram roasted		30	100
Bengal gram-flour (besan)		30	100
Cow gram	1 bowl cooked	30	100
Horse gram		30	100
Kabuli Chana (white gram)		30	100
Lentils	¾ bowl cooked	30	100
Moth beans		30	100
Peas, dried	1 bowl cooked	30	100
Rajmah (kidney beans)	¾ bowl cooked	60	100
Red gram	¾ bowl cooked	30	100
1 bowl-volume is 150 mL			

Flesh Food Exchange (Table 3.28)

- 70 calories; protein 10 g

Table 3.28: Flesh food that can be interchanged with the flesh on the same list

Flesh foods	Household measures	Wt. (g)	Calories
Egg Hen	2 No.		100
Fish	1 piece	60	70
Liver (sheep)		60	70
Mutton (muscle)	3 piece	60	100
Pork	1 slice	60	70
Prawn	5–7 pieces	60	70
Chicken	1 breast	60	70
Crab	120 g		70
Beef	1 slice	60	70

Drinks (Table 3.29)

Table 3.29: Drinks that can be interchanged with the drink on the same list

	Household measures	Vol. (mL)	Calories
Orange juice	1 big glass	200	30
Tomato juice	1 big glass	200	30
Apple juice	1 big glass	200	100
Grape juice	1 big glass	200	80
Mango juice	1 big glass	200	150

Fast Food (Table 3.30)

Table 3.30: Fast food that can be interchanged with items on the same list

	Household measures	Vol.	Calories
Soft drink	1 bottle	300 mL	120–135
Potato wafers		50 g	430
Samosa	1	40 g	130
Vegetable cutlet	1	100 g	140
Vada	1		150

Cakes and Pastries (Table 3.31)

Table 3.31: Cakes and pastries that can be interchanged with items on the same list

	Wt. (g)	Calories
Cake plain	50	150
Chocolate cake	50	250
Sponge cake	50	150
Pastry	50	250–400

Desserts (Table 3.32)

Table 3.32: Desserts that can be interchanged within the group

	Household measures	Wt. (g)	Calories
Custard		150	360
Fruit salad		150	150
Fruit salad with cream		150	300
Icecream		150	380
Carrot halwa	1 medium bowl	100	600
Badami halwa		100	570

Sweets (Table 3.33)

Table 3.33: Sweets that can be interchanged with item on the same list

	Household measures	Wt. (g)	Calories
Coconut burfi		25	110
Gulab Jamun		25	200
Ladoo		30	160
Rasgulla		150	140
Jam	2 tbs		80
Honey	2 tbs		48

Beverages (Table 3.34)

Table 3.34: Beverages that can be interchanged with items on the same list

	Vol. (mL)	Calories
Beer	150	65
Wine dry	30	30
Wine dessert	30	40
Whisky, brandy, gin, rum	30	65
Vodka	30	65
Ginger ale	30	9

Source: Based on American Dietetic Association Exchange Lists

LOW COST MEALS

A low cost meal is one, which is easily available and cost effective. It is difficult most of the time to fulfil all nutrient requirements with low cost meals but proper planning can satisfy most of the nutritional requirement. Low cost meals include seasonal fruits and vegetables, cereals having low cost such as wheat and maize. List of low cost Indian food items is given in Table 3.35.

Table 3.35: Low cost Indian vegetarian diet

Food composition	Amount g/day	Protein content (g)	Other nutrients	
Cereals and millets	460	46.0	Calories (kcal)	2736
Pulses (legumes)	40	9.5	Protein (g)[b]	65
Green leafy vegetables	50	4.0	Calcium (mg)	781
Other vegetables	60		Iron (mg)	17
Roots and tubers	50		Vitamin A (mg)	715
Fruits[a]	30		Riboflavin (mg)	1.15
Milk	150	5.7	Thiamine (mg)	2.45
Fats and oils	40		Vitamin C (mg)	74.8
Sugar and jaggery	30		Niacin (mg)	15.7
			Total fat (g)	67

Source: Indian Council of Medical Research, 2010

[a]*Additionally included*

[b]*Protein content depends on the type of protein containing foods*

Points to be considered while planning low cost meals are:

- Avoid packed food as they are expensive.
- Add seasonal fruits and vegetables in the diet.
- Making small kitchen gardens can cut off expense on food.
- Look for bargains.
- Two food items may be similar in nutritive value but they are different in cost so one must avoid high cost food.

DISEASES AND DISORDERS CAUSED BY IMBALANCE OF NUTRIENTS

Intake of adequate amount of nutrients is essential for maintaining optimum level of health. Inadequate intake of nutrients can cause various disorders.

Carbohydrates

Deficiency

- **Hypoglycemia:** Starvation and lack of carbohydrates in diet causes drop in blood sugar level, which is known as hypoglycemia. It occurs when blood glucose level falls below its normal value, i.e., 70 mg/dL. Symptoms include fatigue, giddiness, delirium and distress.
- **Muscle wasting:** Deficiency of carbohydrates leads to muscle wasting because during deficiency of carbohydrates, body utilizes stored fats and proteins for energy production.
- **Acidosis:** Depletion of carbohydrates in diet results in breakdown of glucose and lipids, which leads to production of ketone bodies, which in turn increases acidity in the blood.

Overconsumption

- **Type-2 diabetes:** Breakdown product of carbohydrates releases glucose, which is absorbed from small intestine. Insulin is necessary for controlling blood sugar level. When pancreas is unable to secrete adequate insulin, blood sugar level rises, which leads to diabetes mellitus.
- **Obesity:** All carbohydrates do not cause obesity. Only refined carbohydrates without fibers lead to weight gain. Carbohydrates increase blood sugar levels, which in turn stimulate release of insulin. The insulin moves excess glucose into adipose tissue from blood.

Fats

Deficiency

- **Stunted growth:** Deficiency of fat in the diet causes the deficiency of essential fatty acids, which leads to cessation of growth.
- **Poor vitamin absorption:** Low intake of fat leads to poor absorption of fat soluble vitamins, i.e., A, D, E and K. Vitamins are essential for maintaining good vision, absorption of calcium, blood clotting, growth and immunity. Poor absorption of fat soluble vitamins may lead to vitamin deficiency diseases.

Overconsumption

- **Cardiovascular diseases:** Excess intake of low density lipoproteins and triglycerides can cause cardiovascular diseases, e.g., atherosclerosis, coronary artery diseases.
- **Risk of obesity:** Excess intake of fats leads to obesity.
- **Risk for cancer:** Researchers revealed that men and women who consume more fat especially animal fats had a higher incidence of pancreatic cancer as compared to those who consume low fat. Large intake of fats is related with increased incidence of cancer, e.g., colon cancer.

Proteins

Deficiency

Deficiency of proteins includes protein energy malnutrition (PEM). Protein energy malnutrition is caused by deficiency of protein and energy. It mainly occurs in pre-school children.

Risk Factors

- Poor socioeconomic condition
- Inadequate intake of protein and energy in diet
- Unhygienic living conditions
- Maternal malnutrition
- Infection

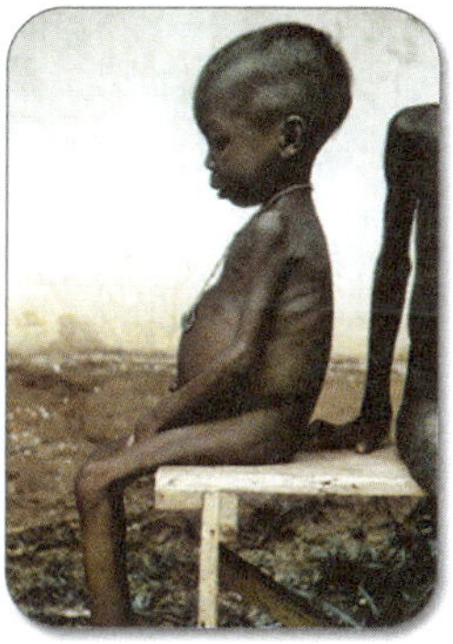

Fig. 3.3: Kwashiorkor

Types

It includes:

- **Kwashiorkor:** Deficiency of proteins in diet leads to kwashiorkor (Fig. 3.3).

  Clinical features:

  - Muscle wasting

- Pitting edema of feet, ankles, which eventually spreads to rest of the body due to reduced plasma proteins
- Moon-shaped face
- Hair are sparse, silky and easily pulled out
- Hyperpigmentation of the skin
- Dermatitis
- Stunt growth
- Weight loss
- Delayed puberty
- Poor appetite
- Impaired immunity

- **Marasmus:** It is a severe form of protein energy malnutrition. It is caused by deficiency of both protein and calories (Fig. 3.4).

Clinical features:

- Skin is thin, flaccid, dry and wrinkled
- Face looks like little old man or monkey
- Bitot's spot (spots in the conjunctiva)
- Weight loss
- Dizziness
- Fatigue
- Chronic diarrhea
- Distended abdomen
- Growth retardation
- Lethargy
- Hypotonic (decreased muscle tone)

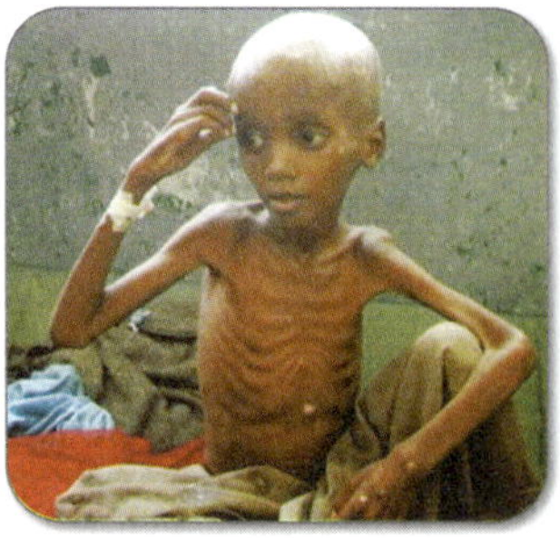

Fig. 3.4: Marasmus

The differences between kwashiorkor and marasmus is given in Table 3.36.

Table 3.36: Differences between kwashiorkor and marasmus

Kwashiorkor	Marasmus
It is caused due to deficiency of proteins only	It is caused due to deficiency of both proteins and calories
Pitting edema is present	Edema is absent
Face is moon-like	Face is monkey-like
Distended abdomen is not present	Distended abdomen is present
Skin is hyperpigmented	Skin is thin, flaccid, dry and wrinkled
Child with kwashiorkor has poor appetite	Child with marasmus has good appetite
Child is irritable and apathetic	Child is alert

- **Marasmic Kwashiorkor:** It is a mixed form of both kwashiorkor and marasmus. It is characterized by the presence of both kwashiorkor and marasmic symptoms.

Overconsumption

Overconsumption of proteins leads to weight gain.

Treatment

In the beginning, more calories in the form of carbohydrates, sugars, and fats are given. Once these calories provide energy, give foods rich in proteins.

Vitamins

Vitamin A

Deficiency

- **Night blindness or nyctalopia:** It is first manifestation of vitamin A deficiency. It is a condition in which a person is unable to see properly in darkness or dim light. In this condition a person is unable to adapt to the dark area when he/she comes from bright area due to delayed formation of rhodopsin because of decreased quantity of vitamin A.
- **Xerophthalmia:** It is manifested by dryness of conjunctiva and cornea.
- **Keratomalacia:** It is characterized by drying and clouding of cornea.
- **Phrynoderma:** It is characterized by hyperkeratinization of epithelial lining of the hair follicles.
- **Bitot's spots:** It is named after a French physician Pierre Bitot who firstly described these spots. These spots are oval, triangular or irregular in shape, are made up of keratin and are located superficially on the conjunctiva.

Overconsumption

Hypervitaminosis: Excess intake of vitamin A in children leads to toxic effects. Symptoms include nausea, vomiting, abdominal pain, loss of hair, itching. Severe toxicity leads to hepatomegaly (enlargement of liver) and papillary edema.

Treatment

The consumption of vitamin A-rich foods, such as liver, beef, chicken, eggs, fortified milk, carrots, mangoes, sweet potatoes, and leafy green vegetables.

Vitamin D

Deficiency

- **Deficiency of vitamin D:** Vitamin D is essential for the absorption of calcium. Deficiency of vitamin D results in inadequate absorption of calcium, rickets and osteomalacia.
- **Rickets:** It mainly occurs in children in the age group of 6 months to 2 years. It is more common in dark skinned children. It is caused due to reduced calcification and mineralization of soft bones. Signs and symptoms include bone tenderness, dental problems, and muscle weakness, increased risk for fracture, skeletal deformities and growth disturbances (Fig. 3.5).

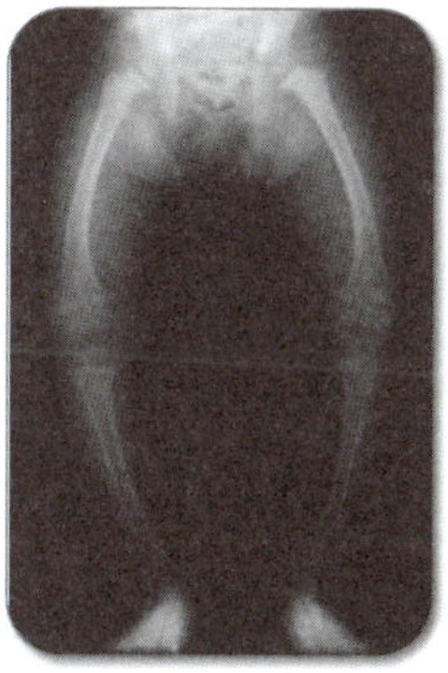

Fig. 3.5: Rickets

- **Osteomalacia:** It is a disease of adults, which occurs mainly in women especially during pregnancy and lactation. In this disease, there is softening of bones. It is characterized by bone pain and muscle weakness. The most common symptom is bone fracture (Fig. 3.6).

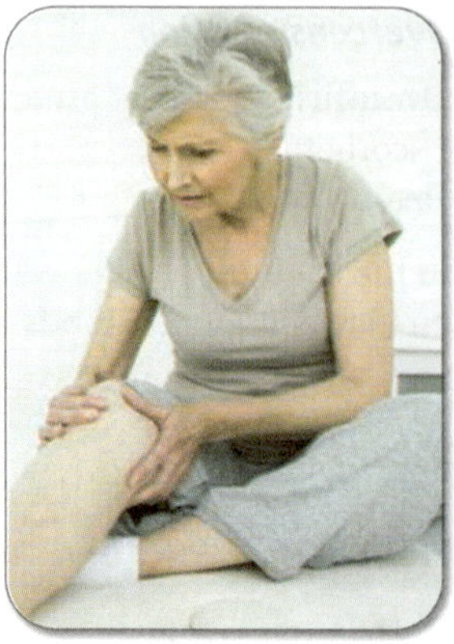

Fig. 3.6: Osteomalacia

Overconsumption

Hypervitaminosis D: This occurs when vitamin D exceeds from its normal concentration, i.e., 30–70 ng/mL (nanogram/mL). Signs and symptoms include nausea, vomiting, confusion, fatigue, irritability, ringing in the ear (tinnitus).

Treatment

Treatment includes vitamin D supplementation, i.e., 1000–5000 IU daily for month followed by 800 IU daily for the next six months.

Prevention

- Educating the parents and family members to expose their children routinely to the sunlight.
- Educating the people to include vitamin D fortified food such as milk in the diet.
- Provide vitamin D supplementation.

Vitamin E

Deficiency

Hypovitaminosis E: It occurs due to deficiency of vitamin E. Signs and symptoms include neurological problems, impairment of immune response, sterility (reproductive failure), anemia and muscular dystrophy.

Treatment

Supplements may cause complications, so it's best to eat a healthy diet that includes many foods rich in vitamin E.

Vitamin K

Deficiency

It can occur at any age but most commonly faced during infancy. Signs and symptoms include uncontrolled bleeding, hematomas, bruising, petechiae (purple spots caused by the bleeding under the skin).Vitamin K plays important role in blood clotting. Deficiency of vitamin K leads to prolonged clotting time and decreased clotting tendency.

Treatment

Drug phytonadione, which is vitamin K_1 is given as an oral medication or may also be injected under the skin.

Vitamin C

Vitamin C is also known as ascorbic acid. Vitamin C is helpful to make a subspace collagen, which is required for repair of various body tissues of skin, bone, teeth, etc.

Deficiency

Insufficient amount of vitamin C in the body causes scurvy. The word scurvy is derived from Latin word 'scorbutus'.

Types of scurvy:

- **Infantile scurvy:** In early stages, symptoms are listlessness, loss of appetite; infant cries when arms and legs are moved. As the disease progresses, there is bleeding and swollen gums, bleeding under the skin.
- **Scurvy in adults:** At the beginning of disease, there is loss of appetite, poor weight gain, weakness. As the disease progresses, there are spongy bleeding gums, swollen tender joints and hemorrhages under the skin.

Treatment

Taking vitamin C supplements and by eating a diet rich in vitamin C.

Vitamin B_1

Deficiency

Another name of vitamin B_1 is thiamine. Thiamine deficiency causes two diseases, i.e., beriberi, wryneck's encephalopathy.

Beriberi is also known as "rice eater's disease" because it mainly occurs in people whose major part of diet is rice.

Types of beriberi:

- **Wet beriberi:** It affects cardiovascular system and other systems. Signs and symptoms include vasodilatation, tachycardia, dyspnea, peripheral edema and elevated jugular venous pressure.
- **Dry beriberi:** It affects the neuromuscular system causing paralysis, numbness and poor coordination.

Treatment

Food rich in vitamin B such as meat, salmon and cod, milk and other dairy products, eggs and yeast extract.

FOOD ALLERGIES

Allergy is a hypersensitive reaction as a result of exposure to a particular allergen. Food allergy is an immune system reaction that occurs soon after eating a certain food. Even tiny amount of allergy causing food can trigger signs and symptoms such as redness, digestive problems and swollen airways.

Allergy causing foods include milk, eggs, peanuts, soy, wheat, fish, shellfish (shrimp, lobster, crab), mushrooms, wheat, tree nuts like walnuts and almonds.

Signs and Symptoms

Specific signs and symptoms that usually develop after consumption of food, within few minutes or 2–3 hours are:

- Tingling or itching in the mouth
- Swelling of lips, face, tongue or throat

- Nasal congestion
- Rapid pulse
- Abdominal cramps
- Bloating

The following are the general signs and symptoms of food allergy:

- Urticaria
- Eczema
- Purpura
- Hay fever
- Bronchial asthma
- Sinusitis
- Dyspepsia
- Nausea and vomiting
- Tingling in the hands, feet, lips or scalp

FOOD INTOLERANCE

It may be defined as digestive problems that occur after a certain food is eaten. It may be defined as detrimental reaction, often related to a food item or beverage, food additives or compounds found in food that produce symptoms in one or more body organs but generally are different from food allergies.

Gluten Allergy/Wheat Intolerance

Gluten allergy is defined as ingestion of gluten, which leads to appearance of intestinal symptoms. Gluten is a protein found in wheat, barley, rye and sometimes in oats. The inflammation and destruction of the inner lining of the small intestine in **celiac disease** is caused by an allergic reaction in the diet. There is no cure for celiac disease; the only effective treatment for this disorder is gluten-free diet.

Common Signs and Symptoms

- Abdominal cramps, gas and bloating
- Bone and joint pain
- Diarrhea
- Failure to thrive in children
- Foul smelling stool
- General weakness and fatigue
- Fluid retention
- Easy bruising
- Gastritis
- Depression

Food Items

Food items made from grains that do not contain harmful gluten and can be consumed in gluten intolerance include:

- Corn in all forms, for example, corn flour, corn meal
- Plain rice in all forms like white, brown, basmati, etc.
- Amaranth, arrowroot, buckwheat, flax, millet, sorghum, soy
- Flours made from gluten free grains, nuts, beans and coconut
- Milk, butter, margarine, real cheese, plain yogurt and most of the ice creams
- Plain fruits, vegetables, meat, sea food, potatoes, eggs, nuts, nut butter, beans and legumes
- Distilled vinegar, distilled alcoholic beverages are gluten free
- Mono- and diglycerides fats, and spices are also gluten-free

Food items that must be avoided in gluten intolerance:

- Wheat in all forms that is in bread, cake flour, cereals, cookies, pasta, pizza crusts, burger, crackers, etc.
- Barley and malt that include malt syrup, malt extract, malt vinegar
- Breaded or floured meat and foods that are fried in the same oil as breaded products are not considered to be safe
- Processed cheese, soy sauce and beer fermented from wheat is also considered harmful

Dietary Management

- **People with gluten intolerance should take gluten free foods. Gluten free foods are given as follows:**
  - Rice
  - Sorghum
  - Soy
  - Nuts
  - Maize
  - Potatoes
  - Beans
- **Dietary modifications:**
  - Wheat can be substituted by maize and ragi.
- **People with gluten allergy should avoid following food items:**
  - Wheat
  - Barley
  - Rye
  - Pasta
  - Bread
  - Wheat germ

Lactose Intolerance

Lactose intolerance is a condition in which persons are unable to digest sugar. Lactose is present in the milk and milk products. It occurs due to the lack of enzyme lactase in small intestine, which is indispensable for the breakdown of sugar lactose into glucose and galactose. Symptoms appear within half to two hours after drinking milk.

Types

- **Primary lactose intolerance:** It is the most common type of lactose intolerance. It occurs due to decrease in enzyme lactase, for example, in old age.
- **Secondary lactose intolerance:** It occurs due to injury, infection or any disease of small intestine, e.g., inflammatory bowel disorder, celiac disease, Crohn's disease and ulcerative colitis, etc. It can also occur due to surgery involving small intestine.
- **Developmental lactose intolerance:** It occurs for short time period in premature babies because they have insufficient levels of enzyme lactase.
- **Congenital lactose intolerance:** It is very rare genetic disorder, which is characterized by presence of little or absence of enzyme lactase from birth.

Signs and Symptoms

Signs and symptoms depend upon amount of lactose consumed and amount of enzyme lactase. Some people can tolerate little amounts of lactose without the appearance of symptoms.

Most common symptoms of lactose intolerance are as follows:

- Bloating (feeling of fullness)
- Abdominal cramps
- Nausea
- Vomiting
- Flatulence
- Diarrhea

Dietary Management

- **Some people with lactose intolerance can tolerate little amounts of lactose but people with lactose intolerance should avoid the following foods:**
  - Milk and milk products
  - Yogurt
  - Whey
  - Ice cream
  - Pudding and custard
  - Toffee, butterscotch and caramels
  - Desserts made up of milk like cakes, cookies, pies, etc.
- **People with lactose intolerance should take lactose-free foods. Lactose-free foods are given as follows:**
  - Fruits and vegetable juices
  - Freshly cooked meat, poultry and fish
  - Nuts, seeds and peanuts
  - Soy cheese
  - Foods made without milk products
  - Soy and tofu products
- **Dietary modifications:**
  - Butter can be substituted with margarine

- Soy milk—people with lactose intolerance can substitute milk with soy milk
- Oat milk
- Rice milk

Protein Intolerance

Many food proteins can act as antigens in humans. Cow milk proteins and soybeans proteins are most common allergen found in children.

Common Signs and Symptoms

- Diarrhea, nausea, vomiting, indigestion, and stomach cramps
- Skin swelling, eczema, and hives
- Wheezing, coughing, congestion and a runny nose
- Anaphylaxis

Dietary Management

Breastfeeding is the first choice in infants without lactose intolerance and foods that contain fewer proteins can be consumed like wheat, rye, oats, buckwheat, barley, yeast, sugars, mushrooms, black tea/coffee yeast, etc.

INBORN ERRORS OF METABOLISM

The term inborn error of metabolism was coined by British physician, Archibald Garrod (1857–1936), in early 20th century (1908). Inborn errors of metabolism are now often referred to as congenital metabolic diseases or inherited metabolic diseases. Inborn errors of metabolism are rare genetic disorders in which the body cannot properly convert food into energy. The disorders are usually caused by defects in specific proteins or enzymes that help to metabolize food.

In other words, inborn errors of metabolism are inherited disorders, which are caused due to defect in protein synthesis. It results in alteration in synthesis, metabolism, transportation and storage of biochemical compounds.

Some of the major classes of inherited metabolic diseases are as follows:

- Disorders of amino acid metabolism, for example, phenylketonuria, maple syrup urine disease, glutaric-acidemia type-I
- Disorders of organic acid metabolism, e.g., alkaptonuria
- Disorders of carbohydrate metabolism, e.g., glycogen storage disease
- Lysosomal storage disorders, e.g., Gaucher's syndrome
- Disorders of purine and pyrimidine metabolism, e.g., Lesch-Nyhan syndrome
- Disorders of steroid metabolism, e.g., congenital adrenal hyperplasia
- Disorders of mitochondrial function, e.g., Kearns-Sayre syndrome
- Disorders of fatty acid oxidation and mitochondrial metabolism, e.g., medium chain acyl dehydrogenase deficiency (glutaric acidemia type-II)

Clinical Manifestations

- Growth failure, failure to thrive and weight loss.
- Deafness and blindness.
- Developmental delay, seizures, dementia, encephalopathy and stroke.
- Low blood pressure, heart failure, enlarged heart, hypertension and myocardial infarction.
- Hypothyroidism, adrenal insufficiency and diabetes mellitus.
- Joint pain, muscle weakness and cramps.
- Hyperventilation and respiratory failure.
- Abnormal behavior and depression, psychosis.
- Liver enlargement, jaundice and liver failure.
- Excessive urination, kidney failure, dehydration and edema.
- Recurrent vomiting, diarrhea and abdominal pain.
- Immunodeficiency, low platelet count, low red blood cell count, enlarged spleen and enlarged lymph nodes.
- Skin rash, abnormal pigmentation, lack of pigmentation and excessive hair growth.
- Developmental delay, seizures, dementia, encephalopathy and stroke.

Management

- Dietary restrictions of proteins are the backbone of treatment for amino acid disorders and phenylketonuria.
- Dietary supplementation of corn starch should be given several times a day to prevent hypoglycemia in people with glycogen storage disease.
- Thiamine supplementation is used to reduce lactic acidosis
- Gene therapy
- Dialysis
- Bone marrow or organ transplantation
- Enzyme replacement therapy
- Symptomatic management and management of complications.

Common Inborn Problems

Phenylketonuria

Phenylketonuria (PKU) is an autosomal recessive genetic disorder, which is characterized by the deficiency of enzyme phenylalanine (PAH). It is necessary for the conversion of amino acid phenylalanine into amino acid tyrosine. It results in the accumulation of phenylalanine in blood and tissues, which is converted into phenylketones (phenylpyruvate), toxic to the brain.

Clinical Manifestations

- Seizures
- Albinism (excessively fair hair and skin)

- Musty odor from baby's urine and sweat
- Microcephaly (abnormally small head)
- Hyperactivity
- Hypopigmentation
- Eczema
- Learning disabilities
- Jerking movements of the arms or legs
- Tremors
- Skin rashes
- Poor bone strength

Dietary Management

- Dietary restrictions of phenylalanine to maintain normal blood phenylalanine level.
- Avoidance of foods high in amino acid, phenylalanine content like meat, fish, nuts, legumes and dairy products.
- Sweetener aspartame containing foods such as jams and jellies and soft drinks must be avoided because it consists of amino acid phenylalanine and aspartic acid.
- Monitoring of starch containing food is must, e.g., potatoes, corn, rice, oatmeal, beans, pasta and bread.
- Breast feeding can be continued with regular monitoring of phenylalanine levels.
- Supplementary infant formulas should be provided to the patients with phenylketonuria because protein-free diet lacks phenylalanine in addition with other amino acids and some nutrients.
- Supplement such as fish oil, which contains long chain fatty acid can be given to improve neurological functions.

Maple Syrup Urine Disease

Maple syrup urine disease (MSUD) is also known as branched-chain ketoaciduria. It is an autosomal recessive metabolic disorder affecting branched-chain amino acids. It is a type of organic acidemia. In this disease the body lacks an enzyme named branched-chain alpha-keto acid dehydrogenase complex (BCKDC). This enzyme is required for processing of 3 important amino acids, i.e., leucine, isoleucine and valine also termed branched chain amino acids. Deficiency of this enzyme results in the accumulation amino acids and keto acids in the body.

Clinical Manifestations

- Sweet smelling urine, which is similar to odor of maple syrup
- Anorexia
- Vomiting
- Dehydration
- Feeding difficulties
- Lethargy
- Seizures
- Hypoglycemia
- Ketoacidosis

- Cerebral edema
- Hypotonia
- Rapid neurological decline
- Coma

Dietary Management

The goal of management is to prevent the accumulation of branched chain amino acid in the blood so as to maintain optimum level of physical and mental health.

- Thiamine supplementation should be given to the individual with thiamine-responsive MSUD.
- A special formula for infants, which contain vitamins, minerals and all amino acids except leucine, isoleucine and valine.
- Some fruits and vegetables such as apples, pineapple, raisins, carrots, cabbage, tomato, pumpkin, turnips and beetroots are permitted to toddlers.

Galactosemia

Galactosemia is rare autosomal recessive genetic disorder, which is characterized by the body's inability to metabolize sugar galactose. As the name suggests it involves the accumulation of galactose in blood. Lactose is broken down into galactose and glucose by the action of intestinal lactase. Enzyme needed for the further metabolism of galactose is absent in individual who is having galactosemia. It leads to the accumulation of galactose in the blood.

Clinical Manifestations

- Lethargy
- Convulsions
- Irritability
- Vomiting
- Poor feeding
- Poor weight gain
- Hypoglycemia
- Brain damage
- Hepatomegaly
- Cataract
- Renal failure
- Failure to thrive
- Jaundice.

Dietary Management

- Avoidance of foods that contain lactose and galactose such as milk, milkshakes, custards, puddings, butter, ice cream, toffees, etc.
- Infants should be given lactose-free milk substitutes, like soy formula and meat-based formula.

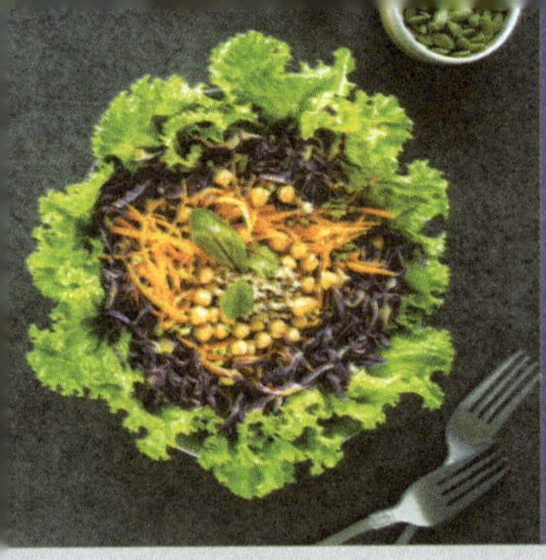

STUDENT ASSIGNMENT

LONG ANSWER QUESTIONS

1. Explain in detail inborn errors of metabolism.
2. What is RDA of pregnant woman? Also write one day menu plan according to dietary requirements.
3. Explain dietary requirements of lactating woman.
4. Discuss protein deficiency diseases.
5. Define BMR and enlist the factors affecting BMR.
6. Define food allergy and discuss the modification in diet required for lactose intolerant person.
7. How nutritive value of the food can be enhanced?
8. Define weaning and enlist the principles for starting weaning.

SHORT ANSWER QUESTIONS

1. Enlist the disorders caused by vitamin deficiency.
2. Define balanced diet and enlist the components of balanced diet.
3. What are the factors to be considered while planning budget for the food?
4. Plan a one day diet plan for school-going child.

MULTIPLE CHOICE QUESTIONS

1. Milk is poor source of:

a. Calcium　　b. Proteins
c. Carbohydrates　　d. Vitamin C

2. The vitamin necessary for coagulation of blood is:

a. Vitamin K　　b. Vitamin D
c. Vitamin B complex　　d. Vitamin C

3. Nutrient with highest calorific value:

a. Carbohydrates　　b. Proteins
c. Fats　　d. Fibers

4. Pernicious anemia is caused by the deficiency of:

a. Vit. B_{12}　　b. Iron
c. Vit. C　　d. Chlorine

5. Deficiency of calcium causes, which of the following symptoms:

a. Rickets in children　　b. Osteomalacia in adults
c. Muscular spasm of hands and feet　　d. All of these

6. **Excessive intake of, which of the following mineral causes pathological changes of bone and teeth?**
   a. Copper b. Chlorine
   c. Iron d. Fluoride

7. **Deficiency of proteins in diet leads to:**
   a. Marasmus and Kwashiorkor b. Anemia
   c. Goiter d. Scurvy

8. **Bitot's spot are caused by the deficiency of:**
   a. Vitamin B complex b. Vitamin A
   c. Calcium d. Phosphorus

9. **Anemia can be caused by deficiency of:**
   a. Iron b. Folic acid
   c. Vitamin B_{12} d. All of these

10. **Blood clotting problem occurs due to deficiency of:**
   a. Vitamin K b. Vitamin C
   c. Vitamin E d. Vitamin A

11. **Deficiency of vitamin C causes:**
   a. Beriberi b. Pellagra
   c. Scurvy d. Osteoporosis

12. **Gradual process of shifting the baby from breast- feeding towards other diet is known as:**
   a. Therapeutic diet b. Weaning
   c. Special diet d. Substitution

13. **Which condition is associated with a deficiency of iodine in the diet?**
   a. Anemia b. Goiter
   c. Night blindness d. Rickets

14. **Which nutrient deficiency is known to cause neural tube defects in newborns?**
   a. Folic acid (folate) b. Vitamin C
   c. Vitamin B_{12} d. Vitamin A

15. **Which disorder is caused by excessive consumption of saturated fats and trans fats?**
   a. Osteoporosis b. Anemia
   c. Type 2 diabetes d. Cardiovascular disease

16. **Which nutrient deficiency is associated with the development of scaly skin and neurological symptoms?**
   a. Vitamin C b. Vitamin D
   c. Vitamin E d. Vitamin B_3 (niacin)

17. **Which condition is caused by inadequate intake of dietary fiber?**
   a. Obesity b. Type 2 diabetes
   c. Constipation d. Osteoporosis

18. **Which mineral deficiency can lead to muscle cramps and irregular heartbeat?**
   a. Potassium b. Magnesium
   c. Iron d. Zinc

19. Which disorder is associated with excessive intake of sugar and refined carbohydrates?

a. Scurvy
b. Diabetes
c. Osteoporosis
d. Beriberi

20. Which nutrient deficiency is linked to the development of pellagra, characterized by dermatitis, diarrhea, and dementia?

a. Vitamin A
b. Vitamin B_{12}
c. Vitamin B_3 (niacin)
d. Vitamin K

21. Which of the following immune responses is characteristic of a food allergy?

a. Delayed onset gastrointestinal symptoms
b. Skin rash and itching
c. Lactose intolerance
d. Difficulty digesting gluten

22. Which of the following condition involves an immune system reaction to specific proteins in food?

a. Celiac disease
b. Lactose intolerance
c. Irritable bowel syndrome (IBS)
d. Heartburn

23. Which of the following symptom is typically associated with lactose intolerance?

a. Hives and swelling
b. Abdominal pain and bloating
c. Wheezing and shortness of breath
d. Dizziness and lightheadedness

24. Which of the following food group should make up the majority of a balanced diet?

a. Fruits and vegetables
b. Dairy products
c. Sugary snacks
d. Red meat

25. What percentage of daily calories should come from carbohydrates in a balanced diet?

a. 10–15%
b. 25–30%
c. 50–60%
d. 70–80%

26. Which nutrient is essential for building and repairing tissues in the body?

a. Vitamin C
b. Protein
c. Iron
d. Calcium

27. Which type of fats should be limited in a balanced diet to promote heart health?

a. Saturated fats
b. Monounsaturated fats
c. Polyunsaturated fats
d. Trans fats

28. What is the recommended maximum daily intake of added sugars for most adults in a balanced diet?

a. <10 g
b. <25 g
c. <50 g
d. <100 g

29. Which eating habit is recommended to promote digestion and prevent overeating in a balanced diet?

a. Skipping meals
b. Eating quickly
c. Eating until 100% full
d. Eating until 75% full

30. Which meal is suggested to be lighter than lunch in a balanced diet?

a. Breakfast
b. Dinner
c. Evening snack
d. Dessert

31. What should be included to ensure a balanced diet with essential vitamins and minerals?

a. Processed foods
b. Supplements only
c. Whole foods from various food groups
d. Beverages with added vitamins

ANSWER KEY

1. d	**2.** a	**3.** c	**4.** a	**5.** d	**6.** d	**7.** a	**8.** b	**9.** d
10. a	**11.** c	**12.** b	**13.** b	**14.** a	**15.** d	**16.** c	**17.** c	**18.** a
19. b	**20.** c	**21.** b	**22.** a	**23.** b	**24.** a	**25.** c	**26.** b	**27.** d
28. c	**29.** d	**30.** b	**31.** c					

4

Food Preparation, Preservation and Storage

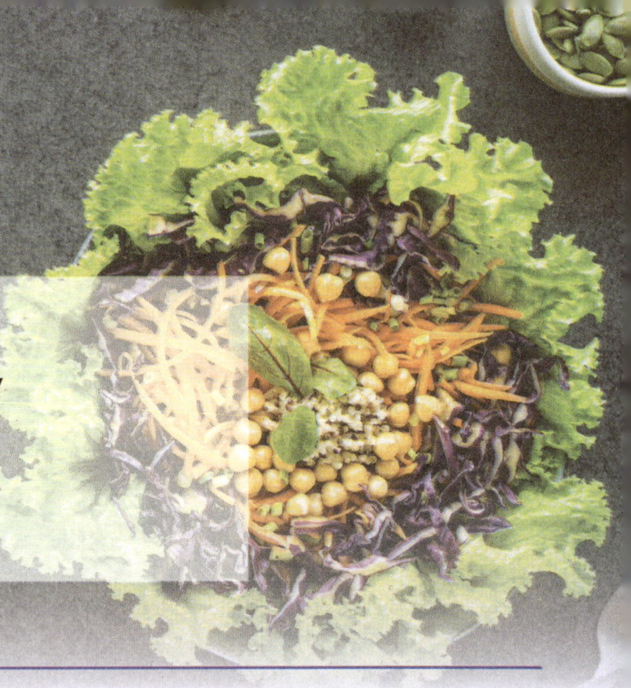

LEARNING OBJECTIVES

After the completion of the chapter, the readers will be able to:
- Discuss principles and methods of cooking.
- Explain methods of food preservation.
- Describe food storage and ill effects of poorly-stored food.
- Explain food adulteration and the related acts.

CHAPTER OUTLINE

- Cooking
- Safe Food Handling
- Preservation of Food
- Storage of Food
- Food Adulteration and Related Acts

KEY TERMS

Cookery: It is the group of methods and techniques, the art and science applied for the process of cooking.
Cooking: It is the process of preparing food particularly by the application of heat.
Cross-contamination: Cross-contamination can occur when microorganisms get spread from one person to another either while preparing the food, distributing or during the time of storage.
Cuisine: It is the type and style for cooking the food particularly for a location or culture.
Foodborne diseases: A foodborne disease refers to the infection or irritation of the gastrointestinal tract caused by the food or beverages that contain harmful bacterias, viruses, parasites or chemicals.
Food preservation: It refers to any one or number of techniques used to prevent food from spoilage
Food safety: The action of monitoring the food to ensure that it will not cause any foodborne illness is known as food safety.
Pasteurization: It is a method to preserve the milk in which milk is heated at temperature of 63–66°C (Holder method) for at least 30 minutes and then quickly cooled to 5°C to destroy the pathogens. It is considered better than boiling as it helps to preserve composition, flavor and nutritive value of milk.

COOKING

Cooking is the art, technology and craft of preparing the food for consumption with the use of heat. Earlier cooking was just considered an art but nowadays it is considered combination of both art and science. Cooking is considered a science because selecting the essential nutrients in right amount can only bring the desired effect on health and on the other hand cooking is also an art because it is symphony of taste, aroma and colors that tickle the senses.

Benefits

Cooking is not preparing the food just to provide energy to the body as it has many other benefits also. These are as follows:

- Cooking increases the variety of food available for consumption as different types of dishes can be prepared by using same ingredients.
- Eating cooked food makes the process of digestion easier and more nutrients can be absorbed by the body as compared to raw food. Certain nutrients are difficult to digest and absorb from raw food and should be properly cooked, for example, it is very hard to consume rice in its uncooked form.
- Cooking adds taste and aroma to the food.
- Cooking makes the mastication easier and saves the amount of energy required for chewing and digesting the food.
- Heating the food during the process of cooking kills the pathogens (*Salmonella, Staphylococcus,* etc.) and makes the food safer for consumption.
- Cooking also makes the preservation of food easier as storage of cooked food is convenient and also prevents spoilage of food.
- Cooking makes the food more presentable by improving its appearance and palatability.

Principles

It is a well-known fact that some nutrients are lost during the process of cooking. Some principles must be followed to minimize the loss of nutrients while cooking. These are as follows:

- While cooking the food, it is always good to cover the container with the lid as it helps to preserve the nutrients dissolved in water. Otherwise in case of open container all the nutrients would get evaporated with water.
- Food should be cooked by steaming method instead of boiling the food as steaming is very effective in retaining the nutrients. If the food needs to be boiled, sufficient water must be taken instead of using excessive water. In any case if the food is cooked in large amount of water, the excess of water may be used for preparing soups, sambar or for other such gravy items. In this way, the nutrients lost in one item can be used in preparing another item.
- Temperature, while cooking is another factor that must be kept in mind as cooking on high temperature results in the loss of nutrients. So try to keep the flame as low as possible to retain the nutrients in the food.
- Avoid deep frying of the food items. Though deep fried items are more crispy and tasty but are deprived of nutrients. Instead of deep frying, choose broiling or baking method that helps in retaining the nutrients.

- Always wash vegetables and fruits before peeling or cutting them as afterwards water soluble vitamins get dissolved into water. Use only sufficient water for washing instead of using excessive water.
- While picking up the food items from refrigerator, allow it to come to room temperature before cooking or consuming such items.
- It is also advised to prepare the food in iron pot as it provides elemental iron.
- Try to consume any vegetable or fruit within two days to avoid getting stale and deficient of nutrients.
- In case of dairy products like milk, sudden changes in temperature must be avoided as it destroys all the nutrients.
- Always pick whole grains over the refined grains. For example, brown rice have their bran intact and thus have more fibers, vitamins and other micronutrients (zinc and calcium).
- Cut fruits and vegetables for salads just before they are to be served and store in a cool place.
- Do not use excessive condiments like salt or red pepper, etc. as it may lead to common problems like hypertension or piles.
- Try to use organic food items to get maximum amount of nutrients.
- Cooking should always be done in hygienic place. The place for handling and storing the food should be hygienic.

Increasing the Nutritive Value of Food

There are various methods for increasing the nutritive value of food:

- Fermentation of the cereals and pulses increases the content of vitamins as done in South India for the preparation of idli and dosa.
- Pulses can be sprouted to increase the content of vitamin B and C. Sprouting not only increases the nutrient contents but also increases the digestibility of pulses. These can be consumed raw or by cooking lightly.
- Mixing the pulses with cereals adds in the nutritive value especially in the protein contents, for example, khichdi. The protein value can also be increased by adding dal, groundnuts to rice, roti or chapati.
- Addition of milk in place of water also increases the content of proteins and calories, for example, milk porridge for the children.
- Using millets such as ragi, jowar or bajra together with staple food as cereals add extra nutrients to the diet.
- The green leafy vegetables can be pounded either fresh or dried. It can be added to the dough for making chapatis. It increases the protein as well as iron content of the food item, for example, palak and dhania.

Methods

The commonly used basic cooking methods are divided into dry heat and moist heat cooking method based upon the type of heat used and way of cooking the food.

Dry Heat Method

In this method, the food being cooked does not use water to cook the food. The food is left dry and heat is applied to cook the food. The juices or water present in the food gets evaporated during heating process, which helps in cooking the food.

The following are the methods of dry heat cooking:

- **Baking (Fig. 4.1):** Food is cooked using convection heating. The food is put into an enclosed area where heat is applied within the confined space that helps the food to cook. Temperature required for baking is 250–255°F. Food prepared by this method is bread, pastry and cake.
- **Steaming (Fig. 4.2):** To steam food, water is added to a pot and then a stand is placed inside the pot. Food is placed on the stand and heat is applied. The hot steam rising from the boiling water acts on the food and helps it get cooked (there is not any contact between the food and water inside the pot). This method is very effective for cooking vegetables as the food does not lose its flavor and much of nutrients are retained during the cooking process.
- **Grilling and broiling (Fig. 4.3):** It is a dry heat cooking method. In the grilling method, food is cooked either directly or in the grill. The flavor and nutrients of the food is not much affected. In this method, heat is applied below the food and the heat seals the outside part of the food and juices inside the food cook it. Food is frequently turned over to prevent it from burning and to ensure that equal heating and cooking time is applied to both sides of the food. Foods like brinjal, tomato, cheese and kebab are cooked by this method. In broiling, heat source for cooking the food is above the food instead of below the food as in case of grilling method and it is also useful for preparing different types of meat.
- **Roasting (Fig. 4.4):** While roasting the food, direct heat is applied to the food. The action of direct heating makes the food tender. Again there is very little nutrient loss and flavor is not spoilt. This is mainly used for the flesh food like fish, meat or chicken.
- **Barbecue (Fig. 4.5):** It is also a dry method of cooking like grilling. The duration of cooking and type of heat used is the main difference between barbecue and grilling method. Grilling is generally done quickly over moderate to high direct heat that produces little smoke while barbecue is done slowly over low, indirect heat and food is flavored by the smoking process. This is mainly used for preparing meat or chicken.

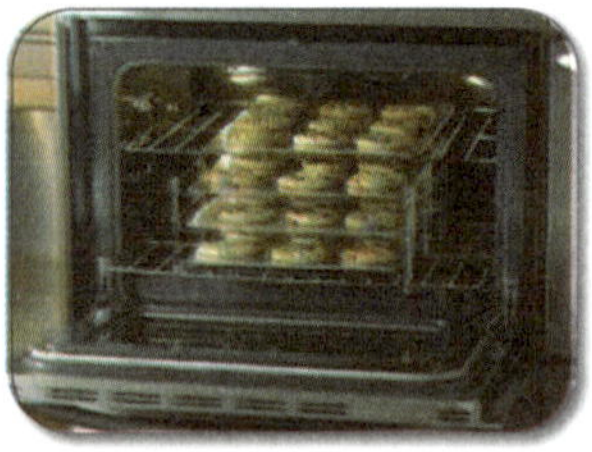

Fig. 4.1: Baking

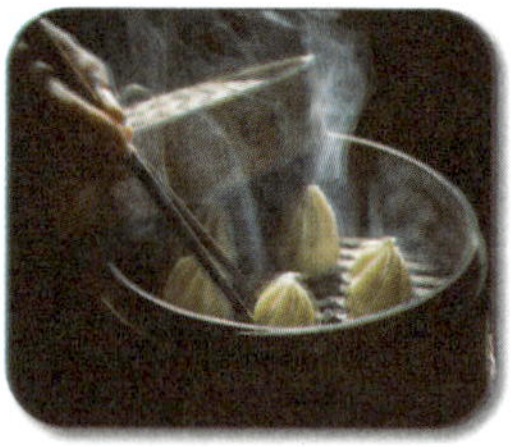

Fig. 4.2: Steaming

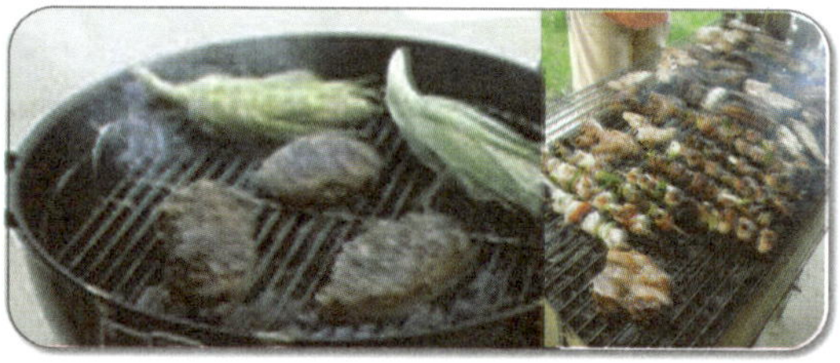

Fig. 4.3: Grilling and broiling

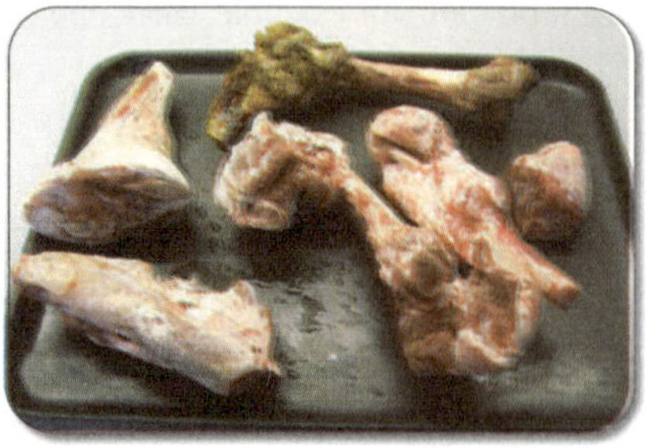

Fig. 4.4: Baking

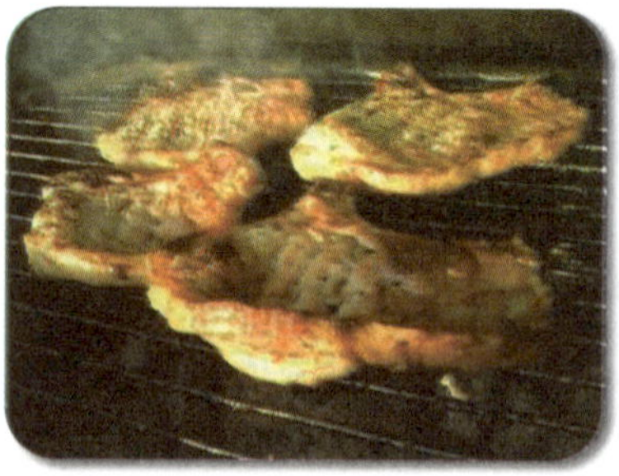

Fig. 4.5: Barbecue

Moist Method

In this method, liquids, such as water, oil or coconut creams are used as a medium to cook the food. These liquids are added before the food is added to the cooking utensils.

- **Boiling (Fig. 4.6):** It is a very common and simple method of cooking. Enough water is added to the food and then cooked over the fire over 100°C. The action of the heated water makes the food cooked, for example, cooking the rice, beans, grams and pulses. Specific time must be kept for boiling these commodities otherwise excessive boiling results in the loss of essential vitamins and minerals.

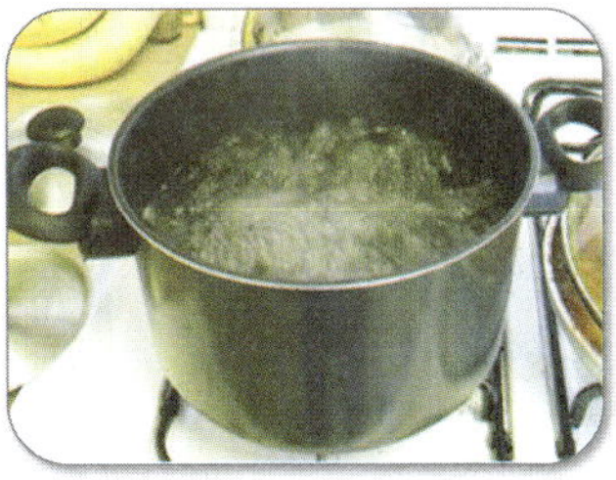

Fig. 4.6: Boiling

- **Simmering (Fig. 4.7):** This method includes cooking below 80°C approximately. It helps in preserving the essential vitamins and minerals. It is used for cooking fish and meat where hardening of fibers occurs at high temperature.
- **Stewing (Fig. 4.8):** In this method, food is cooked by using a lot of liquid. Different kinds of vegetables are chopped or diced and mixed with water then put into the container with well-fitted lid to prevent evaporation. The only disadvantage is that some of the vegetables may be overcooked and nutrient may be lost. It is, therefore, important that the vegetables that took the longest time to cook must be put into the pan first and the ones that need least cooking should be put in the last and in this way nutrients can be preserved.

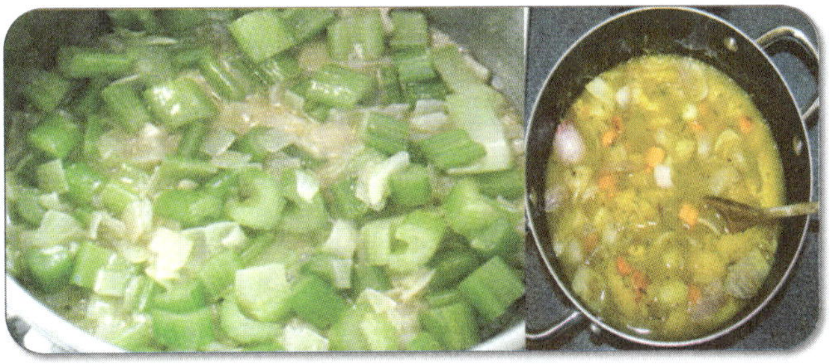

Fig. 4.7: Simmering

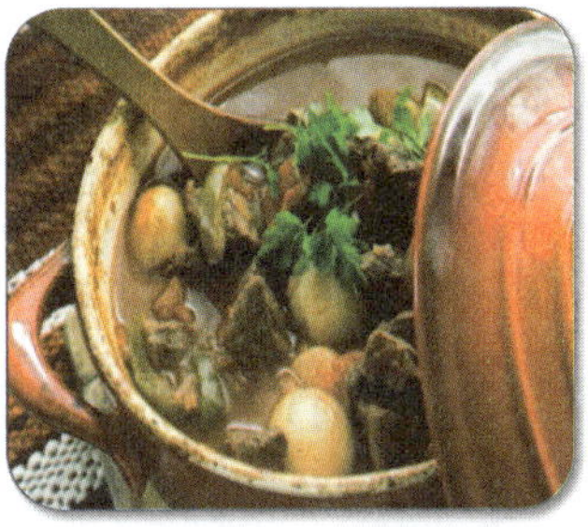

Fig. 4.8: Stewing

- **Frying (Fig. 4.9):** Food is fried using oil and solid fat. It is of further two types:
  i. **Shallow frying:** Food is cooked with a little amount of oil or fat, for example, to make parantha, egg (omelette), dosa or chilla.
  ii. **Deep frying:** Lots of oil or fat is used to cook the food. Food is cooked by putting into hot boiling oil. For example, potato chips and meat balls are cooked by this method.

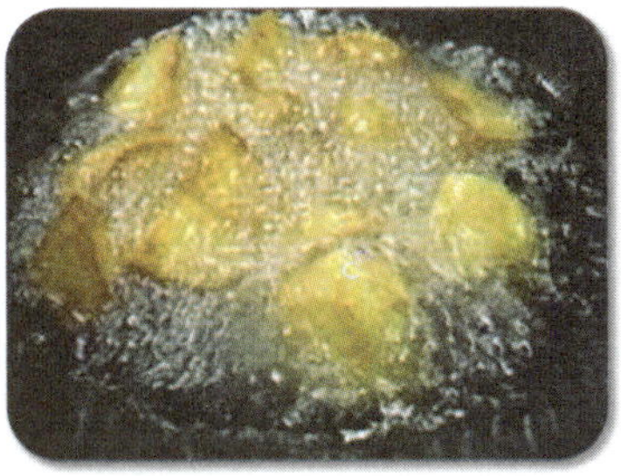

Fig. 4.9: Frying

Effects of Cooking on Food Constituents

- **Carbohydrates:** Starch, sugar, gum and cellulose are important carbohydrates found in food. On cooking, the starch granules in food swell as they absorb water, this process is called gelatinization. Gelatinization also increases the volume of the food as may be seen in case of rice, when it is cooked there is bulk increase in the volume. When the sugar in the carbohydrates gets browned, this process is called caramelization, for example, when bread is heated its color changes to golden brown.

- **Proteins:** On heating, the proteins get hardened and solidified. The liquid inside the protein changes into solid with the effect of heat and this process is known as coagulation. It is very important to cook proteins on right temperature as excessive temperature makes them hard, dry and indigestible.
- **Fats:** Ordinary cooking has no effect on fats but prolonged heating as in case of frying for long periods thickens and darkens the fats. A part of essential fatty acids present in fats are destroyed, toxic polymerized products are formed and a change in flavor also occurs with prolonged heating.
- **Vitamins:** Thiamine and vitamin C are two vitamins which are much affected by the process of cooking. Loss of water soluble vitamins is mainly due to excessive heating or dissolving in excessive water.
- **Minerals:** There is no loss of mineral in normal cooking process but if food is overcooked or water used in cooking is discarded a small fraction of minerals may be lost.

Effects of Cooking on Different Types of Food

- **Cereals:** Cereals are the main staple food consumed for obtaining desired calories in India. Cereals are cooked mostly before consumption for easy digestion. Cereals are mainly rich in starch with a little protein within the cell wall. There are many methods of cooking the cereals. All cereals absorb water during cooking and starch granules swell up and burst, this process is called gelatinization. After gelatinization the protein content on the cell wall of cereals coagulates that improves the process of digestibility. Excessive use of water during cooking leads to loss of water soluble vitamins and minerals, therefore, cooking must be done with sufficient water that gets absorbed in the end of cooking process.
- **Pulses:** Pulses are a rich source of proteins and also contain little amount of carbohydrates, starch fats and fibers. Pulses also contain an antitrypsin substance that hinders the absorption of proteins, vitamins and minerals that get destroyed by proper cooking. Therefore, pulses must be properly cooked before consumption but excessive washing of pulses must be avoided to preserve essential nutrients.
- **Vegetables:** Vegetables are great sources of vitamins and minerals. The application of heat has a definite impact upon vegetables, the cellulose of vegetables gets softened by the heat process and is easier to digest as compared to raw vegetables. Cooking the vegetables in a closed vessel helps to retain flavor as well as essential nutrients. It is also very important to cook the vegetables in sufficient amount of water with sufficient time to avoid destruction of the micronutrients.
- **Meat:** Food of animal origin like meat is rich source of both macro and micro nutrients. Cooking has a major effect on the connective tissue of meat. Cooking results into contraction and gelatinization of collagen fibers, which convert the meat into jelly (very soft)-like structure. The fat of the meat is also melted by heat, which makes it chewable and easy to digest. Cooking also kills the pathogens and makes the meat safer to consume.
- **Milk:** Milk is a rich source of many nutrients like proteins, fats, calcium and phosphate but lacks in Vitamin C and iron. When milk is heated a layer full of fats gets accumulated on the surface, which can be removed easily that reduces the fat and protein content of the milk. Boiled milk is easier to consume as compared to raw milk. Boiling destroys enzymes, thiamine and useful lactic acid bacteria present in the milk. Pasteurization is another alternative method to preserve the milk in which milk is heated at temperature of 63–66°C for at least 30 minutes and then quickly cooled to 5°C to destroy the pathogens. It is considered better than boiling as it helps to preserve composition, flavor and nutritive value of milk.
- **Fish:** It is a rich source of proteins, vitamins and minerals. On heating, the proteins of the fish get coagulated. Cooking makes it chewable and easy to digest.

- **Eggs:** Eggs are the rich source of proteins. The albumin (white portion) of egg begins to coagulate and solidify and gets tough upon heating but much of the nutrients within the egg are not affected by the process of cooking. Raw eggs are very difficult to digest and there are many methods to consume the eggs in various forms that make the digestion of the eggs easier.

SAFE FOOD HANDLING

Safe steps in cooking, distributing and storage are essential to prevent foodborne diseases. Harmful bacteria cannot be seen with naked eyes so it is always better to have precautions.

To handle the food safely, special attention must be given upon **4 Cs.** These are cleanliness, cross- contamination, cold or chill (maintenance of temperature) and cooking at safe temperature. These are as follows (Fig. 4.10):

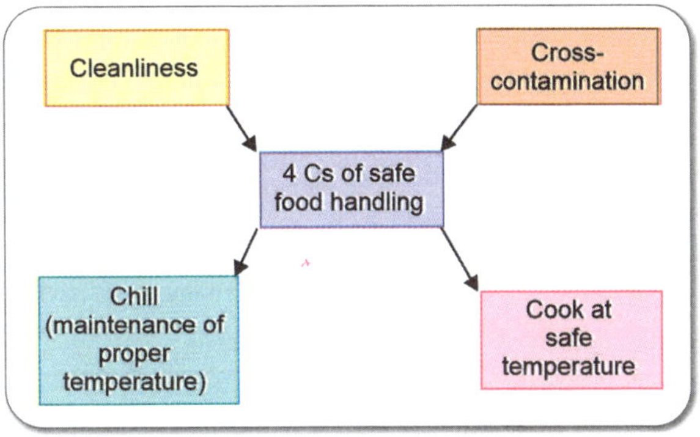

Fig. 4.10: 4 Cs to handle the food safely

- **Cleanliness:** Cleanliness of eating places is very important to prevent foodborne diseases. To maintain proper cleanliness of eating places, following facilities must be there:
  - Eating places should not be near the open drains, manure pits or other sources of infection.
  - Rooms where meals are served must be well ventilated and with adequate lighting facility. Walls of the eating room must be smooth and easily washable. Floors should be higher than the adjoining land and made up of such material that would be easy to clean.
  - Kitchen where the food is prepared must have adequate facilities like ventilation, self-closing doors, proper water facility for drinking and washing the utensils along with adequate facilities for disposal of waste.
  - There must be separate rooms for storage of cooked and uncooked food with adequate facility for maintaining the temperature.
  - The whole area where the food is being prepared, served or stored must be free from rats, flies, cockroaches and other vectors.
- **Cross-contamination:** Cross-contamination can occur when microorganisms get spread from one person to another either while preparing the food, distributing or during the time of storage. Cross-contamination can lead to infection and serious diseases. To prevent cross-contamination, following measures must be adopted.
  - Always wash hands before and after handling the food. Hands must be washed after using the toilets, changing the diapers, handling the pets, after coughing, sneezing and smoking. Use personal towels to rub the hands.
  - Avoid contact with hair, saliva, mucus, sweat, blood, nails, clothes, jewelry or bandages while handling the food items.
  - Food should not be handled by the person suffering from vomiting, diarrhea, sore throat, foodborne diseases, flu, cold, and discharge from ear, eye or any infection on the hands or skin. If in any case such person is handling the food then cover the skin and use mask to prevent cross-contamination.

- Wash cutting boards, dishes, utensils with hot and soapy water before and after preparing the food items.
- Use paper towels for cleaning the kitchen surface. If cloth towels are used then it must be washed properly.
- Always separate raw meat from other food items as their juices may contaminate the other food items. Use separate knives and cutting boards for preparing meat to avoid contamination.
- Always rinse fresh fruits and vegetables under running tap water and lid of the canned food items must be cleaned before opening.

- **Chill (maintenance of proper temperature):** Refrigerate the food items quickly because cold temperature slows the growth of harmful bacteria. There are different temperatures for storing various food items as some are essential to be stored in freezer at a very low temperature.
  - Do not over stuff the refrigerator as cold air must circulate to keep the food items safe.
  - Separate raw meat and other food items even while keeping them in the refrigerator.
  - After removing the food from refrigerator if it looks or smells bad never taste it just discard the food.
  - Do not consume the food items immediately after removing from refrigerator, allow it to come to room temperature.
  - Cooked food that has been frozen and removed from freezer must be reheated and eaten immediately once fully defrosted.
  - Clean the fridge regularly to ensure that it remains hygienic and in good working condition.
- **Cook at safe temperature:** Cooking must be done at adequate temperature as overcooked food may result in loss of nutrients whereas undercooked food may lead to indigestion and many food-borne diseases might occur due to contamination by the microorganisms.

Health of Food Handlers

Food handler is the person who either prepares, cooks, serves, packs, displays, stores, delivers or preserves the food items. The chances of food contamination depend greatly upon the health status of the food handlers, their hygiene behavior and practices. The diseases that are likely to spread by the food handlers are diarrhea, dysentery, common flu, typhoid, paratyphoid, viral hepatitis, intestinal worms, tuberculosis, staphylococcal and streptococcus infections. To prevent such diseases following measures must be taken:

- Food handlers must undergo medical examination at the time of employment. Any person suffering from typhoid, paratyphoid, tuberculosis, chronic diarrhea or dysentery should not be employed.
- Person suffering from wounds, skin or ear, eye infections should not be permitted to handle the food or utensils.
- Day to day health appraisal of the food handlers must be done and if they are found sick they must be excluded from handling the food. Any illness that is occurring in the family of food handler must be notified at once.
- Education of the food handlers is a very important aspect to prevent foodborne diseases. They must be educated regarding personal hygiene, food handling, utensils, dish washing, insects and rodents control. Special emphasis must be given on the following aspects.
  - **Hands:** Always wash hands before and after handling the food. Hands must be washed after using the toilets, coughing, sneezing and smoking. Use personal towels to rub the hands. Finger nails must be trimmed and should be free from dust.

- **Hair:** Head should be covered to prevent loose hair entering to the foodstuffs.
- **Overall:** Clean white overalls must be worn by all food handlers to avoid cross-contamination by the clothes.

PRESERVATION OF FOOD

Preservation of food is done to keep the food safe for a long time. Preservation prevents the food from deterioration and also makes the food safe for consumption. There are many methods to preserve food that can be used single or in combination.

Household Methods (Fig. 4.11)

- **Refrigeration (at low temperature):** It is widely used household method for preserving the perishable items. At low temperature microorganisms are less active and prevent food from spoiling. Foods can be stored either at low temperature between 1°C and 4°C to preserve the food for short time or at freezing point, which is between –18°C and –28°C to preserve the food for long time period.

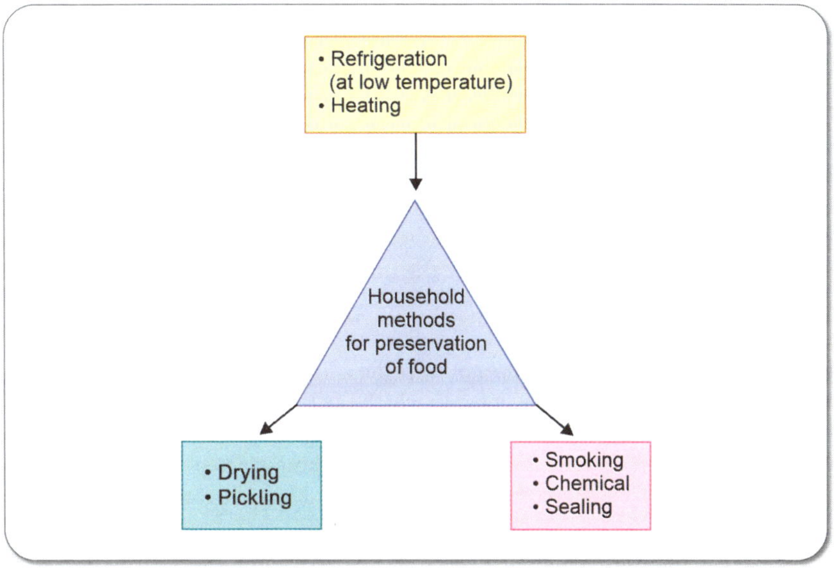

Fig. 4.11: Household methods for preservation of food

- **Heating:** Food is also preserved by the application of heat. The heat is applied at a very high temperature that helps to destroy the pathogenic organisms associated with the food. Another method of applying the heat for preservation of food is known as blanching, which is performed by dipping the food product in boiling water for 2–3 minutes. It also helps to minimize the growth of microorganisms by inactivating their enzymes.
- **Drying and pickling:** This is age-old method of preserving the food by the use of salt and sugar. Salt is considered a valuable preservative, which is used mainly in pickling as it helps to remove moisture and stops the microbial growth. Similarly fruit pulps are preserved in the form of jam by adding sugar.

- **Drying:** It is also an ancient and natural method of preserving the food. In this method, moisture from food content is removed that helps to retard the growth of microorganisms. Moisture can be removed either by sun drying or using by mechanical methods. Fruits, vegetables and fish can be preserved by this method.
- **Smoking:** It is a complementary process that not only preserves the food but also improves flavor and appearance. Temperature control is very important to maintain the texture. Meat is commonly preserved by this method.
- **Chemical:** Various chemicals like vinegar, citric acid, sodium, benzoate, acetic acid, etc. can be used to preserve the food as it retards the growth of microorganisms by decreasing the pH of food and prolongs the shelf life of food.
- **Sealing:** It is the process of covering food to keep the air and moisture out of food items. This process delays the microbial activities but does not kill the microorganisms that spoil the food. Nuts and grains can be preserved by this method.

Commercial Methods

- **Canning and bottling:** It involves the process of storing the foodstuffs in sealed containers. It is based upon the process of sterilization; firstly the microorganisms are killed by the application of heat then sealed in sterilized and air tight container to prevent any further attack of microorganisms. Fruits, jams, pickles, cheese, butter, meat and fish are preserved by this method.
- **Machine drying:** Dehydration in sunlight is an ancient method of preserving the food at home. Various machines are used for different foodstuffs that operate at different temperatures. Commercially special type of steam roller is used for drying milk to reduce it into powdered form. Similarly special ovens are used for drying vegetables at a specific temperature. This method is found better than the traditional method.
- **Preservatives:** Adding preservatives to reduce the microbial growth, such as sugar or salt concentrate, oil and sodium benzoate.
- **Freeze drying:** During drying vegetables or fruits by mechanical methods or by direct sunlight, these foodstuffs get too much squeezed and do not take the original position when used again. In order to modify this defect, freeze drying was invented in which the foodstuffs are kept at –20°C temperature for some time to convert the water content of the food into ice particles and then dried with the machines under low pressure. When foodstuffs are to be used again these are kept under hot water for sometime. This method helps to retain the shape and color of foodstuffs, which got damaged by the simple drying process.
- **Cold storage:** This is the most popular method to preserve the food in rural as well as urban areas based on the principle of refrigeration. Vegetables, fruits, eggs, fish, meat are kept under cold storage and according to the demand of market are carried to the places of requirement.
- **Irradiation:** This is new technique of preserving the food, which still is in an experiment phase. World Health Organization (WHO) has advised the use of this process only for few food items like wheat, onions and potatoes. In this method, gamma rays or high speed electrons, which are termed as ionizing radiations, are used to destroy the microorganisms. The best advantage of this technique is that food can be stored without refrigeration.
- **Use of antibiotics:** These are very often sprayed on the crops as well as used in the animal feeds or in treating infections. When animals are fed with antibiotics their residues may be found in milk. Food and drug administration specifies that milk from such animals should not be used for at least three days

following the treatment with antibiotics. Fishes and poultry items are also treated with antibiotics to increase their shelf life. The effective method of cooking destroys the antibiotics residual from fish or poultry items and makes them harmless for human consumption.

- **Pasteurization:** This method is only applicable for milk. In this method, milk is heated at temperature of 63-66°C (Holder method) for at least 30 minutes and then quickly cooled to 5°C to destroy the pathogens. Milk is pasteurized at a very large scale to safeguard any bacterial infections. The pasteurized milk is then filled in sterilized bottles, which are sealed and can be preserved for 5–6 days. It is considered better than boiling as it helps to preserve composition, flavor and nutritive value of milk.

Precautions to be Taken While Preserving the Food

Food safety is the major concern of the day to day life as poorly preserved food may lead to foodborne diseases, which are sometimes very serious and even results in death.

The following precautions must be taken while preserving the food:

- Keep food surfaces clean. Wash the utensils, plates as soon as used.
- Use safe water and raw material.
- Always separate raw food from the cooked one.
- Keep food at safe temperature. Pathogens grow well between the temperatures 4° and 6°C. Therefore, proper temperature must be maintained.
- Wash the vegetables to remove soil and contamination. Drain completely and place in air tight containers.
- Use proper canning jars for storing the food and never use old lids as it becomes inadequate after use.
- Check from time to time that adequate temperature has been maintained.
- Cool the leftover food as soon as possible and refrigerate it.

STORAGE OF FOOD

Household Storage of Raw Food

Storage of the food items in an effective way prevents the spoilage of the food and makes it safer for consumption. Different food items require different storage conditions depending upon the type, texture, temperature and humidity conditions of the food items. The following points must be kept in mind while storing the raw food at home.

Fruits and Vegetables

- Fruits and vegetables stored at room temperature should be removed from any packing and must be kept loose as the packets/bags traps ethylene gas that causes premature ripening of these food items.
- Green leafy vegetables must be rinsed and dried properly. These items must be wrapped in a paper towel before placing them into fridge.
- Do not store fruits and vegetables together as fruits give off high level of ethylene (ripening agent) that can premature ripen and spoil the surrounding vegetables.
- Before storing the vegetables remove any tie or rubber band. Ensure that the bag in which the vegetables are being stored has some holes to allow for good air flow. Keep the vegetables loosely and separately in the fridge as closer they are greater are chances of spoilage.

- Vegetables can be washed with water before storing them in refrigerator but soft herbs and mushroom should not be washed until these are to be used.
- Fruits like grapes, apples, berries, mangoes ripen very fast at hot temperature so they must be either consumed within two days or must be stored in refrigerator immediately.
- Vegetables must be fresh and unbruised at the time of purchase.
- Potatoes, onions should be kept at cool temperature in a well-ventilated space and frozen vegetables like peas should be placed in the freezer of the refrigerator.
- Fruits when purchased should not be over-ripened, if these are under-ripen they can be kept at room temperature for 2–3 days and when get ripened naturally can be consumed.
- Fruit juices should be consumed immediately as delay may alter the taste as well as nutritive value of the fruit juices.

Cereals

Keeping in mind the importance and high demand of cereals for daily consumption, it is important to store these food items in a proper way as they may be attacked by pests, bacteria or fungi. From ancient times many natural resources are being used for the safe storage of grains as they are considered safer than the chemicals available in the market. These are as follows:

- Neem leaves are widely used to repel pests from stored food grains. Pluck the fresh neem leaves and shade them dry and crush them in the powdered form. Make pouches of the muslin cloth and fill it with neem leaves or powder and keep these pouches inside the container where grains have been stored.
- Turmeric, garlic, cloves, red chillies and camphor have strong smell and insecticide properties, which not only keep the insects away but also are equally safe for the consumption.

Rice and Grains

Rice and grains should be put into clean container that is completely dry as moisture provides a very good medium for the microorganisms to grow.

Pulses

Pulses should be dried in the sunlight and must be stored in the airtight container. Pulses can also be roasted in an open vessel by stirring continuously to avoid burning that helps to remove moisture and make it safer for storage. Roasted dal is also better in taste when cooked.

Peanuts

Peanuts can be stored along with the mint leaves to keep them moisture free. If the storage place is too humid it must be stored in freezer.

Suji

Suji (semolina) and dalia (broken wheat) can be roasted on slow fire in a heavy bottomed vessel or in a microwave and can be stored in air-tight container after cooling to prevent these items from insects attack.

Milk and Milk Products

Milk should not be stored for long time. Dry milk if used should be kept free from moisture in an air-tight container and must be consumed before expiry date. Dairy products should be kept in cool and clean places, whereas cheese, butter and ice creams or deserts must be stored in the freezer.

Meat, Fish and Poultry

Uncooked meat fish or poultry products have higher chances of getting contaminated so these products must be kept away from the cooked items and stored at low temperature in refrigerator after covering them properly. Always store eggs in the available boxes in the fridge.

Household Storage of Cooked Food

Storage of cooked food is mainly done in the refrigerator at household level.

The following points must be kept in mind while storing the food in fridge:

- Cool down the left over food as quickly. It must be ensured that food has been cooled before putting it into the fridge otherwise it can promote bacterial growth.
- Always keep cooked food away from raw food even in the refrigerator.
- Cooked meat must be stored in a sealed container to avoid contamination.
- Never put the open cans in the fridge as the metal may get transferred to the food content, if necessary, place the contents of the can in a storage container or in a covered bowl.
- When food has been prepared try to consume within two hours, if not possible, then it must be kept out of fridge for the minimum possible time.
- Cooked food that has been frozen and removed from the freezer must be reheated and eaten immediately once fully defrosted.
- Defrosted food must be reheated only once because frequent cooling and reheating increase the chances of contamination of food. The bacteria can grow and multiply very fast when food is cooled too slowly or reheated at inappropriate temperature.
- Food stored in freezer such as ice cream and dessert if removed should not be returned in the freezer, so only required amount of items should be removed.
- Food can look or smell fine even after expiry date (packed food) but it is not safe to consume them as there are still chances that the food may be contaminated.
- Keep the temperature of the fridge at 5°C or below.
- Refrigerator must be cleaned regularly and it must be ensured that it remains hygienic and in good working condition to safely store the food items.

Commercial Storage of Food

Food at large level is stored in the cold storage that includes temperature, humidity control, air circulation and maintenance of proper space between the containers for adequate ventilation. A cold store is any building used for storage at controlled temperature. The following facilities must be available in the cold storage:

- The storehouse must be protected from rodents and insects by keeping it clean and free from trash.
- It must be equipped with rat guards, concrete floors, adequate number of doors and windows for proper ventilation and drainage. Building of the store house must be properly insulated.
- Onions, garlic and other food items can be stored safely at low humidity in the stores, if these items are stored in the containers then adequate supply of air must be provided at the bottom of the container and it must be well ventilated, whereas fresh fruits need very low temperature for storage to slow down their metabolic process responsible for ripening the fruits.
- Reusable containers should be disinfected in the chlorinated or boiling water before every use.

Harmful Effects of Poorly Stored Food

Food is a potential source of infection as it can be contaminated at any point during its journey from producer to the consumer. Poorly stored food is one of the common means by which the foodborne infections such as dysentery, cholera, typhoid, etc. may occur. Foodborne diseases or food poisoning is the infection or irritation of the gastrointestinal tract caused by the food or beverages that contain harmful bacteria, viruses, parasites or chemicals. Common signs and symptoms of these diseases include vomiting, diarrhea, abdominal pain, fever or chill. Raw foods such as milk, fish, meat or dairy products if stored poorly may get contaminated very easily and cause foodborne diseases. If the food is not stored at appropriate temperature that may also be a common factor responsible for foodborne infections as under such conditions microorganisms multiply very quickly. Cross-contamination of the food is another major reason for foodborne diseases. Good hygiene practices before, during and after preparation of food can reduce the chances of getting an illness. The action of monitoring the food to ensure that it will not cause any foodborne illness is known as food safety. It includes hygiene in the production, handling, distribution and serving the food.

FOOD ADULTERATION AND RELATED ACTS

Food Adulteration

Food adulteration is a legal term that means the food products get failed to meet the mandatory standards set by the state or any legalized agency. Food adulteration consists of a large number of practices that include mixing, substitution, concealing the quality, putting up decomposed food for sale, misbranding or giving the false labels and addition of toxicants. When the consumer gets adulterated food he is not only paying the extra money for the substandard products but also it can be injurious to his health and even may lead to death, for example, adulteration of mustard oil with argemone oil causes epidemic dropsy.

Food adulteration is a very old problem and its practice varies from time to time and from one place to another place across the world. Food adulterant is any substance that is used unnecessarily to spoil the nature and quality of food items. The common adulterants used to adulterate the food is listed in Table 4.1.

Table 4.1: Common adulterants used in food materials

Food materials	Common adulterants
Cereals such as wheat and rice	Mud, grits, soapstone bits
Dals	Coal tar dyes, kesari dals
Haldi (turmeric powder)	Lead chromate powder
Dhania powder	Starch, cow dung or horse dung powder
Black pepper	Dried seeds of papaya
Chilli powder	Saw dust, brick powder
Tea dust/leaves	Black gram husk, tamarind seeds powder, saw dust, used tea dust
Coffee powder	Date husk, tamarind husk, chicory
Asafetida (Hing)	Sand, grit, resins, gums, soap stones
Mustard seeds	Seeds of prickly poppy, argemone
Edible oils	Mineral oil, argemone oil

Contd...

Food materials	Common adulterants
Butter	Starch, animal fat
Ice creams	Cellulose, starch, non-permitted colors
Fresh green packed peas	Green dye
Milk	Extraction of fat, addition of starch and water
Ghee	Vanaspati, mashed potatoes, sweet potatoes
Sweet wines	Diethylene glycol
Honey	High fructose syrup, cane sugar, jaggery
Alcoholic liquors	Methanol
Wheat flour	Excessive sand, dirt, bran and chalk powder
Cumin seeds	Grass seeds colored with charcoal dust

Types of Food Adulteration

- **Physical adulteration:** Mixing substances like stones, sand, or non-edible colors.
- **Chemical adulteration:** Adding harmful chemicals like artificial colors, pesticides, or preservatives.
- **Biological adulteration:** Contamination with pathogens or microorganisms.

Tests to Detect Common Adulteration

- **Ghee:** Boil 5 mL of the sample in a test tube. Cool and add a drop of iodine solution. Blue color indicates presence of starch. Color disappears on boiling and reappears on cooling.
- **Honey:** Take 5 mL of honey in a dish. Add aniline chloride solution and stir well. Orange red color indicates presence of sugar.
- **Pulses:** Add 50 mL of diluted HCl to a small quantity of dal and keep on simmering water for about 15 minutes. Development of pink color indicates the presence of kesari dal.
- **Black pepper:** Pour the seeds in a beaker containing carbon tetra chloride. Black papaya seeds float on the top while the pure black pepper settles down.
- **Coriander powder:** Soak in water. Dung will float and can be easily detected by its foul smell.
- **Chillies:** Pour the sample in a beaker containing a mixture of chloroform and carbon tetrachloride. Brick powder and grit will settle at the bottom.
- **Wheat flour:** Sprinkle on water surface, bran will float on the surface. Shake sample with dilute hydrochloride effervescence indicates chalk.
- **Turmeric powder:** Dissolve the sample in 1:7 sulfuric acid and filter it. Add 1–2 drops of 0.1% diphenylcarbazide. A pink color indicates presence of lead chromate.
- **Cumin seeds (*Jeera*):** Rub the cumin seeds on palms. If palms turn black, adulteration is indicated.
- **Asafetida (*Heeng*):** Shake a little quantity of powdered sample with water. Soap stone or other earthly matter will settle at the bottom.

Food Adulteration Act (1954)

This Act was passed by the Indian Parliament in 1954 and later on amended in1964, 1976 and lately in 1986 to make it more stringent. Rules are framed, which are revised from time to time by an expert body called **Center Committee for Food Standards** constituted by the Indian government. Although it is a central Act, its implementation is largely carried out by the state governments and local bodies in their respective areas. Center plays a vital role in coordination, monitoring and surveillance of the Act throughout the country with the help of food laboratories and four regional central laboratories (Kolkata, Mysore, Ghaziabad and Pune).

Food Adulteration Act has the following objectives:

- To protect the public from poisonous and harmful foods.
- To prevent the sale of substandard food.
- To protect the interests of the consumers by eliminating fraudulent practices.

Concept of Adulteration

According to PFA (Prevention of Food Adulteration Act), an article of food shall be deemed to adulterated in the following case:

- If the article sold by vendor is not of the nature, substance or quality demanded by the purchaser.
- If the article contains any other substance, which affects the quality of food item.
- If any constituent of the food has been fully or partly extracted to affect the quality of the product.
- If the article has been prepared, packed under unsanitary conditions whereby it has become contaminated or injurious to health.
- If the article is obtained from diseased animal.
- If the article contains any poisonous or other ingredient which is injurious to health.
- If color is used that was not prescribed or color which is present in the article is not within prescribed limits.
- If the article contains any prohibited preservatives in excess of the prescribed limit.
- If the quality or purity of the article falls below the prescribed standards or its constituents are present in the quantities not within the prescribed limits and injurious to health.

Penalties

Guilty will be punished with minimum imprisonment of six months with fine up to ₹1000. Whereas for the cases of adulteration, which may render the food injurious to cause death or such harm may amount to grievous punishment going up to life imprisonment and a fine not less than ₹5000. With the amendment of the Act in year 1986, the consumer and voluntary organization have been empowered to take samples of food.

Food Safety and Standards Regulation Act 2011

Prevention of Food Adulteration Act (PFA) was replaced in 2006 by the Food Safety and Standard Act 2006 and again in 2011 certain amendments were done for laboratories and sample analysis. According to this Act, the sample of any imported article will be sent by the authorized officer for analysis in the central laboratories like Central Food Laboratory at Kolkata, Ghaziabad, Mysore and Pune.

- **Food Safety and Standards Alcoholic Beverages Regulations 2018:** This regulation specifies the requirements for labeling of alcoholic beverages that includes declaration of alcoholic content, not to write any nutritional information, no health claim and restriction of the word nonintoxicating on alcoholic beverages.
- **Food standards:** Food adulteration is a social problem. Certain food standards have been made to combat with this problem. These are as follows:

- **PFA Standards:** Under the Act of Prevention of Food Adulteration (1954), standards have been established, which are revised from time to time by the central committee of food standards.
- **Food Safety and Standards Authority of India (FSSAI):** It has been established under the Food Safety and Standard Act **2006** as a statutory body for lying down science-based standards articles of food regulating, manufacturing, processing, distribution, sale and import so as to ensure safe and wholesome food for human consumption. It was formed in **2011** and its headquarter is in New Delhi. It is an agency of Ministry of Health and Family Welfare of Government of India. It is responsible for protecting and promoting public health through regulations and supervision of food safety.
- **Food Safety and Standards (Foods for Infant Nutrition) Regulations, 2019:** The Food Safety and Standards (Foods for Infant Nutrition) Regulations, 2019 are specific regulations aimed at ensuring the safety and nutritional quality of foods meant for infants and young children. The regulations apply to foods specifically meant for infants and young children, including infant formula, follow-up formula, foods for special medical purposes, and processed cereal-based complementary foods. The regulations set out specific standards and specifications for these categories of foods, including requirements for ingredients, composition, nutritional content, labelling, and packaging. Clear and informative labelling is mandated to provide consumers (parents and caregivers) with essential information about the product, including ingredients, nutritional information, usage instructions, storage conditions, and any warnings or precautions.
- **The AGMARK Standards (Fig. 4.12):** It is a certification mark employed on agricultural products of India and these standards are set by the directorate of marketing and inspection of the government of India. The AGMARK is legally enforced in India by the Agricultural Produce (Grading and Marking) Act in 1937 and amended in 1986. The term AGMARK was coined by joining the words 'AG' that means agriculture and 'MARK' for certification mark. The AGMARK assures the quality of the various food products being delivered to the consumer.

  The commodities certified under AGMARK are whole spices, vegetable oils, pulses, ghee, wheat, honey, etc. Importance of AGMARK is that it not only ensures the quality of the product but also assures that the product has been produced in hygienic condition and is safe for human consumption.

Fig. 4.12: Logo of AGMARK

Benefits of AGMARK:

- Farmers benefit from increased subsidies for products carrying the mark.
- Products receive a marketing boost.
- Product quality is ensured through legal compliance measures.

Differences between FSSAI and AGMARK:

- The FSSAI mark is mandatory, while AGMARK certification is voluntary.
- FSSAI licensing applies to all food processing and packaging, encompassing all types of food items. AGMARK, however, is specifically designed for agricultural products.
- FSSAI licensing operates under the Food Safety and Standards Act, 2006, while AGMARK operates under the Agriculture Produce (Grading and Marketing) Act of India, 1937.

- **Bureau of Indian Standards (BIS):** It is the national standard body of India working under ministry of consumer affairs, food and public distribution and government of India. It was established by the Bureau of Indian Standards Act in 1986. Its headquarter is at Manak Bhawan, Old Delhi. **Indian Standard Institutions (ISI) (Fig. 4.13)** mark on any article of food assures about the quality of the food product prescribed by the Bureau of Indian standards. BIS certification is mandatory for certain products taking into consideration of public health whereas ISI mark is mandatory on all the industrial and electronic appliances of India.

Fig. 4.13: Logo of Indian Standard Institutions

  BIS Act, 2016: The BIS Act, 2016 is a pivotal legislation that reconstituted and empowered the Bureau of Indian Standards (BIS), India's national standards body. The Act was notified on March 22, 2016, and came into effect on October 12, 2017.It replaced the previous legislation governing BIS, namely the Bureau of Indian Standards Act, 1986.The BIS Act establishes BIS as the main authority responsible for creating and enforcing standards across different industries in India. Its goal is to align Indian Standards (IS) with global benchmarks to improve the quality, safety, and effectiveness of products, processes, and services.

  Powers and functions: BIS, according to the Act, has the legal power to:

  - Develop Indian Standards (IS) based on science and industry requirements.
  - Issue certification marks like the ISI mark, Hallmark, etc., to indicate compliance with Indian Standards.
  - Set up systems to check if products meet specified standards.
  - Monitor, test, and inspect certified products to ensure they maintain quality and are safe for consumers.

- **Codex Alimentarius (Fig. 4.14):** It is a collection of internationally recognized standards, guidelines and recommendations related to food production. It was established in 1961 by Food and Agriculture Organization (FAO) of UN and later on was joined by World Health Organization (WHO) in 1962. The main objective of this organization is to protect the health of consumer and ensure fair practices in the food trade at international level. It is a world trade organization that helps in the resolution of disputes related to food safety and consumer protection at international level. As per 2020, there are 189 members in the Codex Alimentarius commission.

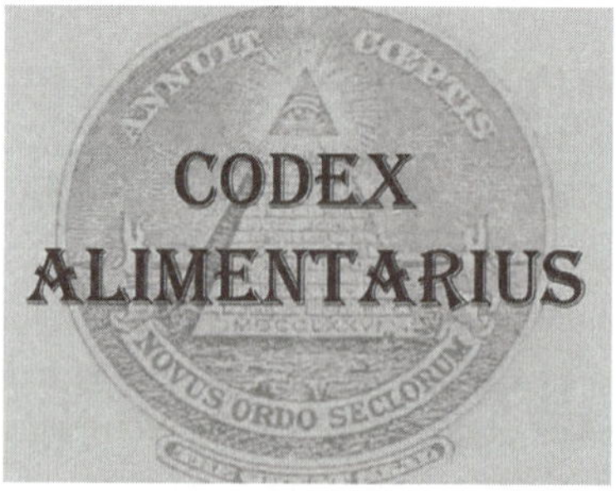

Fig. 4.14: Codex Alimentarius

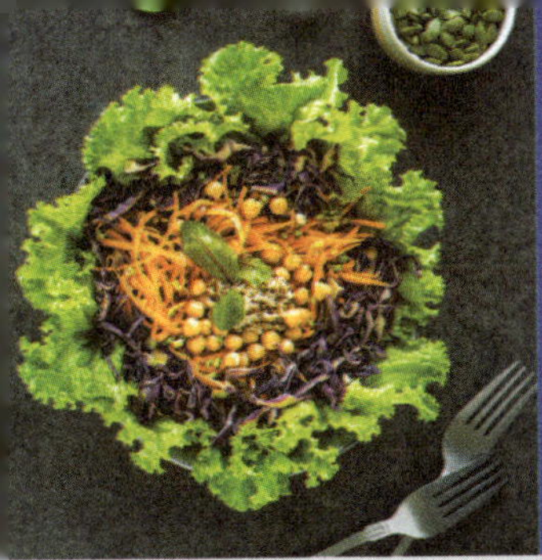

STUDENT ASSIGNMENT

LONG ANSWER QUESTIONS

1. What are the precautions to be taken while preserving the food?
2. How the food can be stored at commercial level?
3. Explain the effects of cooking on different types of food.
4. Explain various food standards to ensure the quality of food.
5. What is food adulteration and what are the main laws to prevent adulteration of food?

SHORT ANSWER QUESTIONS

1. Discuss the principles of cooking.
2. Explain the household method of preservation of food.
3. Enlist the methods of cooking food.
4. What is safe food handling and what are the ill effects of poorly stored food?

MULTIPLE CHOICE QUESTIONS

1. **The full form of PFA is:**
   a. Prevention of Food Act
   b. Protection of Food Act
   c. Prevention of Food Adulteration Act
   d. None of these
2. **Which of the following is an adulterant?**
   a. Pesticides
   b. Urea
   c. Iron fillings in the tea
   d. All of these
3. **Pasteurization is the process of heating milk:**
   a. Above 100°C
   b. Above 500°C
   c. Above boiling point
   d. Below boiling point
4. **Which of the following is a food preservative?**
   a. Sodium benzoate
   b. Alenine
   c. Ergot
   d. All of these
5. **Which of the following is a food adulterant?**
   a. Saffron
   b. Argemone oil
   c. Vanilla
   d. All of these
6. **While planning a balanced diet which of the following is essential?**
   a. Knowledge about the food group
   b. Knowledge about food exchange system
   c. Knowledge of RDA
   d. All of these

7. **Which of the following is used to check the quality of meat?**
   a. Bright pink color
   b. Firm and elastic in touch
   c. Agreeable odor
   d. All of these
8. **Which of the following is not a household method of preservation of food?**
   a. Refrigerator (cold storage)
   b. Smoking
   c. Irradiation
   d. Salting and pickling
9. **Food Adulteration Act was passed by the Indian Parliament in the year:**
   a. 1954
   b. 1965
   c. 1970
   d. 1960
10. **Adulteration of mustard oil with Argemone oil causes:**
   a. Diarrhea
   b. Epidemic dropsy
   c. Anemia
   d. Peptic ulcer
11. **The following are the food standards to ensure quality of food:**
   a. PFA standards
   b. AGMARK standards
   c. Bureau of Indian Standards (BIS)
   d. All of the above
12. **Which cooking method involves cooking food in an oven using dry heat?**
   a. Grilling
   b. Roasting
   c. Boiling
   d. Steaming
13. **In which cooking method is food submerged completely in hot oil or fat?**
   a. Baking
   b. Poaching
   c. Frying
   d. Braising
14. **What cooking method involves cooking food by exposing it directly to a flame or hot coals?**
   a. Boiling
   b. Grilling
   c. Sautéing
   d. Steaming
15. **Which method of cooking uses a combination of dry and moist heat?**
   a. Roasting
   b. Poaching
   c. Sautéing
   d. Broiling
16. **What method of cooking involves cooking food by placing it directly under a heat source?**
   a. Baking
   b. Grilling
   c. Steaming
   d. Stewing
17. **Which cooking method is used to cook food slowly and gently in water or broth that is just below boiling point?**
   a. Boiling
   b. Poaching
   c. Frying
   d. Roasting
18. **In which method of cooking is food cooked quickly in a small amount of oil or fat over high heat?**
   a. Sautéing
   b. Braising
   c. Baking
   d. Broiling

19. **What is the recommended temperature for storing refrigerated foods?**
    a. Below 0°C (32°F)
    b. Between 4°C to 60°C (39°F to 140°F)
    c. Below 4°C (40°F)
    d. Room temperature

20. **When should you wash your hands while handling food?**
    a. Only before touching raw meat
    b. Only after handling raw meat
    c. Before and after handling any food, especially raw meat
    d. Only after cooking is complete

21. **How should you store leftover food in the refrigerator?**
    a. Cover loosely with aluminum foil
    b. Leave it uncovered to cool faster
    c. Store it in shallow containers with lids
    d. Stack containers on top of each other

22. **Which surfaces should be sanitized regularly in a kitchen to prevent cross-contamination?**
    a. Only cutting boards used for raw meat
    b. Only the sink where raw meat is washed
    c. Any surface that comes into contact with food, including countertops and utensils
    d. None of the above

23. **How often should you change dishcloths and kitchen towels to prevent bacterial growth?**
    a. Once a week
    b. Once a month
    c. Daily
    d. Only when visibly dirty

24. **Which of the following is NOT a safe practice for storing leftovers?**
    a. Leaving food uncovered in the refrigerator
    b. Storing leftovers in airtight containers
    c. Labeling containers with the date of preparation
    d. Placing leftovers in the refrigerator within 2 hours after cooking

25. **Which of the following is an example of food adulteration?**
    a. Adding salt to enhance flavor
    b. Mixing pure honey with sugar syrup
    c. Adding vitamins to fortified cereals
    d. Using organic ingredients in cooking

26. **What is the purpose of food adulteration?**
    a. To improve nutritional content
    b. To increase shelf life
    c. To deceive consumers and increase profits
    d. To enhance flavor

27. **Which agency is primarily responsible for monitoring and preventing food adulteration in India?**
    a. World Health Organization (WHO)
    b. Food Safety and Standards Authority of India (FSSAI)
    c. Centers for Disease Control and Prevention (CDC)
    d. United Nations Educational, Scientific and Cultural Organization (UNESCO)

28. **What is the term used to describe the addition of non-permitted substances to food?**

a. Fortification b. Dilution
c. Adulteration d. Preservation

29. **Which of the following is a common form of food adulteration in milk?**

a. Adding sugar b. Adding water
c. Adding vitamins d. Adding preservatives

30. **How can consumers detect the presence of chalk powder in spices such as turmeric?**

a. By visual inspection for an unnatural brightness
b. By tasting for a bitter aftertaste
c. By smelling for a strong odor
d. By checking the expiry date

31. **Which of the following is an example of physical adulteration?**

a. Adding artificial colors to fruit juices
b. Adding water to milk
c. Adding synthetic preservatives to pickles
d. Adding stones to rice

32. **What health risks are associated with consuming adulterated food?**

a. Allergic reactions b. Food poisoning
c. Long-term health problems d. All of these

33. **Which test can be used to detect the presence of starch in milk to check for adulteration?**

a. Iodine test b. pH test
c. Benedict's test d. Biuret test

34. **Who is responsible for penalizing offenders involved in food adulteration?**

a. Local grocery stores
b. Food inspectors and regulatory authorities
c. Manufacturers' associations
d. Consumer advocacy groups

ANSWER KEY

1. c	**2.** d	**3.** d	**4.** a	**5.** b	**6.** d	**7.** d	**8.** c	**9.** a
10. b	**11.** d	**12.** b	**13.** c	**14.** b	**15.** a	**16.** b	**17.** b	**18.** a
19. c	**20.** c	**21.** c	**22.** c	**23.** c	**24.** a	**25.** b	**26.** c	**27.** b
28. c	**29.** b	**30.** a	**31.** d	**32.** d	**33.** a	**34.** b		

5

Therapeutic Diet

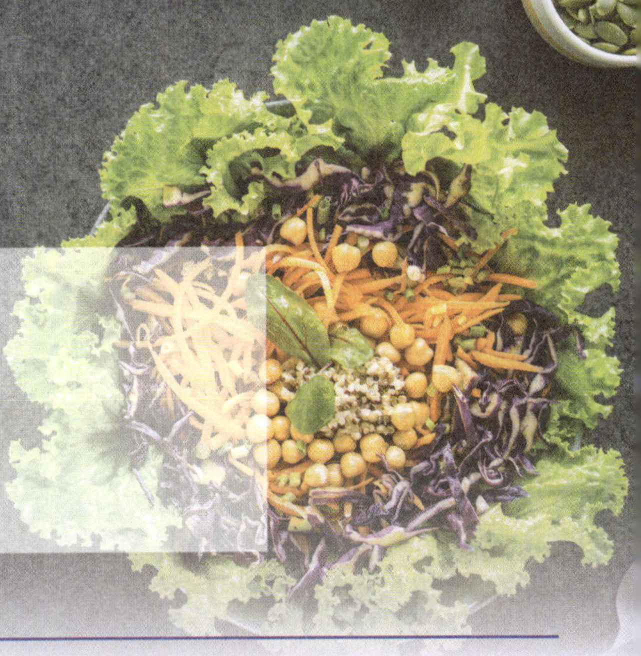

LEARNING OBJECTIVES

After the completion of the chapter, the readers will be able to:

- Discuss diet modifications in relation to medical and surgical conditions.
- Explain about special diet.
- Discuss factors affecting diet acceptance.
- Discuss health education on nutritional needs.

CHAPTER OUTLINE

- Definition
- Purposes
- Dietary Modifications
- Protein Energy Malnutrition
- Diabetes Mellitus
- Cardiovascular Diseases
- Hepatitis
- Renal Diseases
- Gout Disease
- Irritable Bowel Syndrome
- Obesity
- Cholecystectomy
- Gastrectomy
- Bariatric Surgery
- Peptic Ulcer
- Colostomy
- Special Diets
- Geriatric Nutrition
- Clear Liquid Diet
- Full Liquid Diet
- Semisolid Diet
- Soft Diet
- High Fiber Diet
- Factors Affecting the Diet Acceptance in Patients
- Feeding the Helpless Patients
- Nutritional Education

KEY TERMS

Bland diet: This diet is free from spices, condiments, and low in fiber.

Diabetes mellitus: This is a group of metabolic disorder characterized by elevated blood glucose level.

Gastrostomy: It's an opening into the stomach from the abdominal wall, made surgically (stoma) for the introduction of food. A feeding device or a tube is inserted into the stomach when there is problem in taking nutrition by mouth, for example, deformity of mouth or esophagus. A bland diet and medications are given through the tube. A bland diet is designed primarily to help patients recover from gastrointestinal conditions or other medical circumstances in which improved digestion would be essential. It is generally soft, low in dietary fiber, properly cooked rather than raw, and not spicy.

Gastrostomy feeding: It is a method through which a tube is placed in opening of the stomach. This method is rarely used. This method of feeding is used in the clients with esophageal surgery.

Gout: It is a form of inflammatory arthritis characterized by recurrent attacks of pain, red, tender, hot, and swollen joints.

Liquid diets: Liquids are used in that condition where the patients are not able to take solid diet. These diets are free from the chemical and mechanical irritants.

Obesity: It is a medical condition in which excess body fat accumulates to the extent that it may have an adverse effect on health.

Protein energy malnutrition: This term is used to describe clinical disorder, resulting from deficiency of protein and energy.

Therapeutic diet: It is a planned meal that controls or maintains the intake of certain foods or nutrients.

DEFINITION

A therapeutic diet is defined as a planned meal that controls or maintains the intake of certain food or nutrients. It is the part of treatment of disease conditions and are normally prescribed by the doctor and planned by the dietitian.

PURPOSES

- To maintain and restore the nutritional status of an individual.
- To modify the nutritional needs, for example, decrease or increase calories for adequate weight maintenance.
- To provide texture modification for the patients who have chewing and swallowing problem.
- To change the consistency of food, for example, liquid, semiliquid, solid as per health status of the individuals.
- To include or exclude specific nutrient in the diet, for example, in case of certain food allergies, high protein for PEM, salt-restricted diet for hypertensive patient.

DIETARY MODIFICATIONS

In certain conditions, individuals cannot tolerate the regular diet so modification in normal diet is required. These modifications are based on texture or consistency of food items such as liquid diet, soft diet, solid diet, semisolid diet. Modification is also based on the disease condition of the patients, age, income, socio-economic status and various methods of introduction of the food.

- **Dietary modification in medical condition:** Medical conditions such as heart disease, gastrointestinal disease or endocrinal disorder need some modifications in the normal diet. In medical condition, the body metabolic rate changes hence, the diet of a normal person cannot fulfill the basic need for providing enough calories and nutrients. Thus modification in the diet is necessary as per the metabolic rate of the person.
- **Diet modification in surgical condition:** Surgery brings about greatly increased need for nutrients as a result of loss of blood, plasma or pus from the wound surface, hemorrhage from the gastrointestinal or pulmonary tract, etc. Some nutrients may be supplied immediately after surgery by parenteral feeding but the complete need of the body usually cannot be met by that means alone. So the main purpose of dietary management after surgical condition is to maintain correct nutrition and to assure better wound healing and fewer postoperative complications, shorter and mortality.

Types of Modifications (Fig. 5.1)

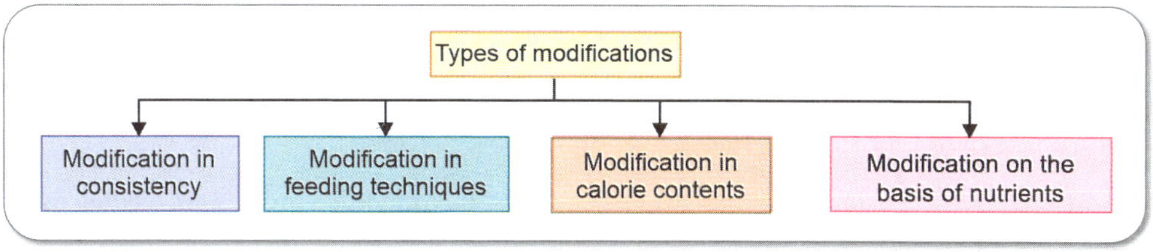

Fig. 5.1: Types of modifications

Modification in Consistency

This modification includes liquid diet, solid diet, and semisolid. The consistency of this diet is soft and they are easy to digest and nonirritating.

Liquid Diets

Liquids are used in that condition where the patients are not able to take solid diet. These diets are free from the chemical and mechanical irritants. Liquid diet is mainly used in fever, vomiting, diarrhea, postoperative patients. Liquid diets include fruit juice, coconut water, barley water, rice kanji, clear vegetable soup, dal soup, tea, coffee. It is of two types:

Clear Liquid Diet

- It includes minimum residue fluids that can be seen through. Examples are juices without pulp, broth, etc.
- It is often used as the first step for restarting oral feeding after surgery or an abdominal procedure.
- It can also be used for fluid and electrolyte replacement in people with severe diarrhea.
- It should not be used for an extended period as it does not provide enough calories and nutrients.

Full Liquid Diet

- It includes fluids that are creamy.
- Some examples of food allowed are ice cream, pudding, thinned hot cereal, custard, strained cream soups, and juices with pulp.
- It is used as the second step for restarting oral feeding once clear liquids are tolerated.
- It is used for people who cannot tolerate a mechanical soft diet.

Soft Diet

Soft diet is soft in texture and consistency, easy to chew and digest with no fiber. Soft diet used in gastrointestinal problem such as peptic ulcer, ulcerative colitis, acute infection.

Semisolid Diet

It is soft than normal diet. Semi solid diet is given to the patients who have no problem in digestion but difficulty in chewing. It includes khichdi, dalia, upma, soft rice, curd, pudding and cornflakes.

Bland Diet

The diet, which is mechanically, thermally, chemically, nonirritating is called bland diet. Food items are free from spices, condiments, and are low in fiber. Foods include milk and milk-based preparations, refined cereals, butter, dehusked pulses.

Modifications in Feeding Techniques

If the person is unable to take food by mouth, there are some other modified methods of feeding used to feed the patients.

- **Tube feeding:** It is a method of feeding through which a tube is inserted from nose to stomach called nasogastric tube. There are different sizes of the tube used according to age. An expert practitioner should insert the tube as there is risk of choking. Clear liquids such as milk, fruit juice, dal soup, etc. are given through this method. This method is used when patients are unable to feed by mouth, for example, in mouth surgery or altered conscious level.
- **Gastrostomy feeding:** It is a method through which a tube is placed in the opening of the stomach. This method is rarely used. This method of feeding is used in the clients with esophageal surgery.
- **Jejunostomy feeding:** In this method, tube is inserted directly into jejunum. A special type of diet is given through this method in small and frequent amounts.
- **Intravenous feeding/Parenteral feeding:** It is defined as the provision of nutrients directly into the blood stream through peripheral or central access.
  - **Peripheral access:** The feed can be infused through a peripheral intravenous catheter placed in a vein. It provides support for mildly malnourished and can be used as a supplement along with the enteral feeding.
  - **Central access:** Catheter is inserted into the subclavian vein and continues until the catheter tip reaches the superior vena cava. After inserting the tube successfully in the right place, total parenteral nutrition (TPN) can be started.

Modification in Calorie Contents

- It includes high calorie and low calorie diet.
- High calorie diet gives 3,000–4,000 kcal. It is mainly used in malnourished patients or in recovery phase after the disease.
- Low calorie diet gives 1,100–1,300 kcal energy and it is used in obesity, hepatic diseases and in patients in coma stage.

Modification on the Basis of Nutrients

It is based on both macronutrients (carbohydrate, protein, fat) and micronutrients (protein and vitamin) Table 5.1.

Table 5.1: Diet modification in particular disease conditions

Nutrients	Disease conditions
High-carbohydrate diet	Liver disease
Low-carbohydrate diet	Obesity, diabetes mellitus
High-protein diet	Burn, Protein Energy Malnutrition (PEM), tuberculosis, liver cirrhosis

Contd...

Nutrients	Disease conditions
Low-protein diet	Acute renal diseases, hepatitis, jaundice
High-fat diet	Marasmus, underweight
Low-fat diet	Obesity, cardiac disease
High-calorie diet	Fever, acute infection, after surgery
Low-calorie diet	Hepatic coma
Low-sodium diet	Hypertension
Fiber-rich diet	Constipation, to prevent colon cancer
Low-fiber diet	Diarrhea, gastrointestinal disease
Low-vitamin diet	Hypervitaminosis

PROTEIN ENERGY MALNUTRITION

Protein energy malnutrition is a term used to describe clinical disorder, resulting from deficiency of protein and energy. It primarily occurs in young children living in poverty. It mainly occurs in preschool children.

Risk Factors

- Poor socioeconomic condition
- Inadequate intake of protein and energy in diet
- Unhygienic living conditions
- Maternal malnutrition
- Infection

Types

It includes:

- Kwashiorkor
- Marasmus

Kwashiorkor

Deficiency of proteins in diet leads to kwashiorkor.

Clinical Features

- Muscle wasting
- Pitting edema of feet, and ankles, which eventually spreads to rest of the body due to reduced plasma proteins
- Moon-shaped face
- Hair are sparse, silky and easily pulled out

- Hyperpigmentation of the skin
- Dermatosis
- Stunt growth
- Weight loss
- Delayed puberty
- Poor appetite
- Impaired immunity

Marasmus

It is a severe form of protein energy malnutrition. It is caused by deficiency of both protein and calories.

Clinical features

- Skin is thin, flaccid, dry and wrinkled
- Face looks like little old man or monkey
- Bitot's spots (spots on the conjunctiva)
- Weight loss
- Dizziness
- Fatigue
- Chronic diarrhea
- Distended abdomen
- Growth retardation
- Lethargy
- Hypotonia (decreased muscle tone)

The differences between kwashiorkor and marasmus is given in Table 5.2.

Table 5.2: Differences between kwashiorkor and marasmus

Kwashiorkor	Marasmus
It is caused due to deficiency of proteins only	It is caused due to deficiency of both proteins and calories
Pitting edema is present	Edema is absent
Face is moon-like	Face is monkey-like
Distended abdomen is present	Distended abdomen is not present
Skin is hyperpigmented	Skin is thin, flaccid, dry and wrinkled
Child with kwashiorkor has poor appetite	Child with marasmus has good appetite
Child is irritable and apathetic	Child is alert

Dietary Management

Energy: 3,000 kcal–3,300 kcal/day (twice the normal requirement)

Protein: 80–100 calories/day (twice the normal requirement)

Food High in Protein

Beef, chicken, lamb leg, kidney beans, soy product, cottage cheese, yogurt, roasted soynuts, tofu, peanut and egg. Protein rich food items and menu planning have been listed in Tables 5.3 and 5.4.

Table 5.3: The National Institute of Nutrition, Hyderabad formulated a mixed diet high in energy and protein (nutritious laddu)

Food items	Quantity (g)
Whole wheat roasted	40
Bengal gram	16
Groundnut	10
Jaggery	20
Total	**86 g (total energy 330 kcal, 11.4 g protein)**

Table 5.4: Menu planning and selection of food items according to time

Meal	Menu
Early morning	Full fat milk one glass
Breakfast	Stuffed parantha + butter + curd
Midmorning	Soup (vegetable)
Lunch	Cheese/tofu vegetable + dal (bengal gram) + roti + brown rice and salad
Evening time	Fruit chat or nutritious laddu with milk
Dinner	Mix vegetable + dal (or soybeans), salad + chapati/rice
Bedtime	Milk shake

DIABETES MELLITUS

Diabetes mellitus is a group of metabolic disorder characterized by elevated blood glucose level resulting from defect in insulin production, insulin action. Insulin is necessary for metabolism of the carbohydrate. Deficiency of insulin leads to hyperglycemia.

Clinical Manifestations

- Mainly characterized by 3Ps:
    - i. **P**olyuria (excessive urine output)
    - ii. **P**olydipsia (excessive thirst)
    - iii. **P**olyphagia (excessive appetite)
- Fatigue, drowsiness
- Tingling sensation and numbness in hands and feet
- Weight loss
- Itching
- Blurred vision

Dietary Management

- **Calories:** Requirement of the calories depends on the weight of the diabetic patients. Depending on the body weight, the requirements of calories are calculated as given in Table 5.5.

Table 5.5: Requirement of calories as per the body weight

Categories	Calories requirement
Overweight	20 kcal/kg body wt/day
Normal weight	30 kcal/kg body wt/day
Underweight	40 kcal/kg body wt/day

- **Carbohydrates:** Simple carbohydrates as glucose, sucrose, fructose and lactose, etc. are not usually advised as they are very quickly absorbed and raise the blood sugar level so complex carbohydrates should be consumed.
- **Fats:** Food rich in saturated fats and cholesterol intake must be limited.
- **Proteins:** The protein amount should be normal, i.e., 1 g/kg of body weight
- **Fibers:** Diet should be rich in fibers as they delay the passage of food through stomach and small intestine thus delaying these in reabsorption of carbohydrate.
- **Vitamins:** Diet should be rich in vitamin B complex as it avoids the development of diabetic neuritis.
- **Minerals:** Food rich in potassium such as tomato, etc. should be taken as it helps in releasing insulin from the pancreas.
- Sweetening agents such as saccharine must be avoided as it is 300–350 times sweeter than sugar. It is used as artificial sweetener in the form of tablet.
- Daily calorie requirement in case of diabetes mellitus is given in Table 5.6.

Table 5.6: Recommended daily allowance (RDA) for diabetes mellitus

RDA	Sedentary worker	Moderate worker	Heavy worker
Energy	1300 kcal	1600 kcal	1900 kcal
Protein	60 g	60 g	70 g
Carbohydrate	170 g	223 g	232 g
Fat	33 g	39 g	39 g

Recommended Dietary Products for Diabetic Patients

- Whole wheat, its product, beans, barley, lentils and other whole grain.
- Vegetables such as carrot, broccoli, peanuts, pumpkin, onion, garlic, cantaloupe, cucumber, mushroom, radish.
- Fruits such as apple, peaches, avocados, cherries, plums, kiwi, orange and other citrus fruits.
- Skimmed milk.
- All soy products such as soy nuts, soybeans, soy beverages, soy cheese.
- Fish with omega 3 fatty acids.

A sample menu plan for diabetes mellitus is given in Table 5.7.

Diabetic patients should avoid following foods:

Simple sugar products, white bread, whole milk, refined flours, red meat, vegetable such as potato, chukander and, fruits such as mango, papaya, melon, bananas and packed fruit juices must be avoided.

Table 5.7: Sample menu plan for diabetic mellitus

Meal	Menu
Early morning	Methi pani/lemon water
Breakfast	Vegetable upma
Midmorning	Salted lassi/citrus fruit juice without sugar
Lunch	Brown rice + missi roti + vegetable (carrot, broccoli, peanuts, pumpkin) + besan kadhi + salad
Evening time	Tea + salted biscuit 2
Dinner	Chapati + salad + dal + curd
Bedtime	Skimmed milk

CARDIOVASCULAR DISEASES

Cardiovascular disease (CVD) is a class of diseases that involve the heart or blood vessels. Cardiovascular disease includes coronary artery diseases such as angina and myocardial infarction (commonly known as a heart attack). Other CVDs are stroke, heart failure, hypertensive heart disease, rheumatic heart disease, cardiomyopathy, heart arrhythmia, congenital heart disease, valvular heart disease, carditis, aortic aneurysms, peripheral artery disease, and venous thrombosis atherosclerosis.

This may be caused by high blood pressure, smoking, diabetes, lack of exercise, obesity, high blood cholesterol, poor diet, and excessive alcohol consumption. It is estimated that 90% of CVD is preventable. It involves improving the risk factors through: healthy eating, exercise, avoidance of tobacco smoke and limiting alcohol intake.

Common Signs and Symptoms

A crushing, squeezing or burning pain, pressure or fullness in the center of the chest. The pain may radiate to the neck, one of the arms and shoulder and the jaw.

- Shortness of breath
- Loss of consciousness
- Sweating
- Fatigue
- Fainting
- Rapid and irregular heart beat
- Nausea
- Dizziness

Dietary Management

Low calorie, low fat diet particularly low in saturated fats, low in cholesterol, high in polyunsaturated fatty acids, low in carbohydrate, with normal protein and vitamin, mineral diet is suggested for the cardiac patients. High fiber diet is also recommended. Desirable range of lipoproteins and daily dietary allowances and food item to be included and avoided and sample menu are given in Tables 5.8 to 5.11.

Recommendations for nutrients are as follows:

- **Carbohydrate:** Simple carbohydrate is replaced by complex carbohydrate. The sources of simple carbohydrates are sweets, biscuit, white refined flour, candies, and chocolate and sweet cookies. They are harmful for heart disease. So, complex carbohydrates such as whole wheat flour, oats, ragi and green leafy vegetables must be consumed.
- **Proteins:** Replacing animal protein with plant protein to decrease low density lipoproteins, cholesterol levels in the body.
- **Fat:** Food generally contains two types of fat—visible and invisible fat. Visible fat sources from plant origin such as vegetable oil (mustard oil, olive oil and sunflower oil) are used in the place of animal sources such as butter and ghee.
- **Vitamins:** Vitamins are rich sources of antioxidants. Antioxidants thus can prevent accumulation of fat and cholesterol in the arteries.
- **Minerals:** Potassium is essential mineral that regulates muscle contraction and electrical impulses between the cells. It also lowers the blood pressure, which in turn helps to lower the risk of heart disease. Magnesium is important for proper heart rhythm.

Table 5.8: Desirable range of lipoproteins (National Cholesterol Education Program, 2001)

Lipoprotein	Range (mg/dL)	Risk
Total cholesterol	<200 200–239 >240	Normal Borderline high High
Triglyceride	<150 150–199 200–499 >500	Normal Borderline high High Very high
Low-density lipoprotein	<100 100–129 130–159 160–189 >190	Normal Optimal Borderline high High Very high
High-density lipoprotein Men Women	 >40 >50	 <40 <50
Lipoprotein	<20 20–30 >30	Normal Borderline high High
Very low-density lipoprotein	<30	Normal

Table 5.9: Recommended dietary allowance for cardiac patients

Calories	1800–1900 kcal
Carbohydrates	280–290 g
Fats	40–50 g

Contd...

Protein	70–80 g
Cholesterol	60–65 mg
Sodium	250–270 mg
Dietary fiber	40–50 g

Table 5.10: Food items included and avoided in cardiac diseases

Food Items	Food to be included	Food to be avoided
Breads and cereals	• Bread–whole grains • Breads and cereals • Oats, corn • Multigrain bread • Rava • Ragi	• High fat crackers • Egg noodles • Pasta with egg yolk • Refined flour
Egg	• Egg white	• Egg yolk
Dairy products	• Butter milk • Low fat cheese • Skimmed milk	• Whole milk • Cream • Cheese
Meat and meat products	• Chicken without skin • Fatty fish such as tuna and sardine	• Beef • Lamb • Pork • Mutton • Chicken with skin
Fats and oil	• Sunflower oil • Safflower oil • Olive oil • Rice bran oil • Soy bean oil • Peanut oil	• Butter • Dalda ghee • Ghee • Whole milk coconut • Margarine

Table 5.11: Sample menu plan for patients with cardiac diseases

Meals	Menu
Early morning	Green tea
Breakfast	Sāmbhar idli or poha
Midmorning	Soup (vegetable)
Lunch	Rice/chapati + green leafy vegetable + dal + salad
Evening time	Fruit chat
Dinner	Khichdi + curd or porridge
Bedtime	Skim milk

HEPATITIS

Hepatitis is a group of diseases characterized by inflammation of the liver. Some people have no symptoms whereas others develop yellow discoloration of the skin and whites of the eyes, poor appetite, vomiting, feeling tired, abdominal pain, or diarrhea.

There are five main types of viral hepatitis: Type A, B, C, D, and E. Hepatitis A and E are mainly spread by contaminated food and water. Hepatitis B is mainly spread by blood, during childbirth, or infected blood that may occur during needle sharing or during intravenous drug use. Hepatitis C and D are most commonly spread by blood.

Hepatitis A, B, and D are preventable with immunization. Medications may be used to treat chronic cases of viral hepatitis. Autoimmune hepatitis may be treated with medications to suppress the immune system. A liver transplant may also be an option in certain cases.

Signs and Symptoms

- Poor appetite
- Vomiting
- Tiredness
- Abdominal pain
- Diarrhea
- Fever
- Rapid weight loss

Causes

Causes of hepatitis can be divided into the following major categories: Infectious, metabolic, ischemic, autoimmune, genetic, and other. Infectious agents include viruses, bacteria, and parasites. Toxins, drugs, alcohol, autoimmune and genetic factor may also be the cause of hepatitis. Ischemic hepatitis results from reduced blood flow to the liver as in shock, heart failure, or vascular insufficiency. Viral hepatitis is the most common cause.

Dietary Management

A balanced diet can lead to better liver functioning and lowered risk of cirrhosis (scarring) of the liver. For a patient with hepatitis, food choices are not limited to a few bland dishes. There are plenty of healthy, tasty food options, which are both beneficial for the liver and for the recovery process.

General Dietary Advice

Eat Regular Cereals

Whole grains are very beneficial to consume as part of a healthy hepatitis diet. These can be in the form of bran, whole wheat bread or cereal, brown rice, whole grain pasta or porridge. Brown rice, gram flour, oatmeal, whole oats, whole rye, whole wheat and whole-grain corn.

Eat Lots of Fruits and Vegetables

Fruits and vegetables are important sources of many nutrients, including potassium, fiber, vitamin C, beta-carotene (a form of vitamin A), and folic acid. Some of these substances are antioxidants that can fight cell damage. As a bonus, most fruits and vegetables are naturally low in fat, sodium, and calories. Eat at least 5 servings of fruits and vegetables a day.

Get Enough Protein

Protein is needed to fight infection and to heal damaged liver cells. Protein helps rebuild and maintain muscle mass and it aids in healing and repair of body tissues. Good protein sources are dairy products that include milk, cheese, yogurt, ice cream, and puddings made with milk and meats, fish, dried beans, soy, nuts, and eggs.

Have Plenty of Fluids

Drink at least 6–8 glasses of fluid a day. Milk, juice, herbal teas, soup, pudding and frozen fruit bars all are counted as fluids.

Healthy Fats

Olive oil, canola oil and flaxseed oil are all healthy fats that are recommended as part of a diet for patients with hepatitis.

Foods to Avoid

It is equally important to avoid certain foods during hepatitis as they can be harmful to the liver. Excessive consumption of these can aggravate the disease and even lead to permanent liver damage. These include pulses, beans, fish, chicken and egg, bakery products, dried nuts, whole milk and pickle. Processed food items are best avoided when recovering from hepatitis. Processed food items include processed ingredients that are harder on the liver and relatively devoid of nutrients.

- Hepatitis patients should also severely limit their salt intake. They should refrain from eating high-sodium foods. This means canned soups or store-bought sauces must be avoided.
- When on a hepatitis diet, avoid eating meat, especially red meats due to their high sodium content.
- Alcohol is a strong toxin to the liver, even in people without hepatitis C. Drinking too much can lead to cirrhosis of the liver, advanced liver disease, or even liver cancer.
- Be careful with dietary supplements.

Recommendation for the Patient with Hepatitis

- **Energy:** A diet that supplies 1,600–2,000 kcal is recommended.
- **Protein:** 1 g/kg/day protein is recommended. In case of severe jaundice 40 g, and in mild case 60 g protein recommended.
- **Fats:** In a severe case 20 g, in mild case 20–30 g fat is given. All fats such as ghee, butter and cream should be avoided.
- **Vitamins:** Vitamins are essential to regenerate the liver. 500 mg of vitamin C, 10 mg of vitamin K and B complex essential.
- A sample of menu plan for patients with hepatitis is given in Table 5.12.

Table 5.12: Sample menu plan for patients with hepatitis

Meals	Menu
Early morning	Orange fruit juice
Breakfast	Cornflakes with skimmed milk
Midmorning	Fruit custard
Lunch	Khichdi + curd
Evening time	Tea with biscuits
Dinner	Rice + mashed potatoes + dal (whole pulses)
Bedtime	Skimmed milk

RENAL DISEASES

The diseases, which affect the functions of kidney or insufficiency of kidney are called renal diseases. Main renal diseases are nephritis, acute and chronic renal failure, acute glomerulonephritis, Nephrotic syndrome and renal calculi. Diet needs to be changed in renal diseases. These changes include limiting fluids, eating a low-protein diet, limiting salt, potassium, phosphorous, and other electrolytes, and getting enough calories.

Dietary Management

Aims

- To maintain normal nitrogen balance so that there is no wasting of body tissue.
- To supply necessary vitamins and other nutrients to maintain general condition of the patients.
- To restrict protein intake since the end products of the protein metabolism cannot be excreted in renal failure.
- To regulate fluid and electrolyte intake.

Food Tips

- Diet has to be low in protein depending upon the urea content in the blood. A moderate-protein diet (1 g of protein per kilogram of body weight per day) is usually recommended.
- Spices and condiments are used in very small quantity.
- To fulfill the need of vitamins and minerals, fruits and vegetables such as lime, mango, plum, sapodilla, tomato and pomegranate are included but it must be ensured that potassium is restricted.
- Amount of dairy products should be limited, because they contain large amounts of phosphorous. This includes milk, yogurt and cheese.
- Carbohydrate can compensate the low protein diet to meet the calorie requirement such as sugar, honey, and jelly.
- Fats can be a good source of calories. But only monounsaturated and polyunsaturated fats (olive oil, canola oil, safflower oil) to protect heart health.
- The minerals calcium and phosphorous must be checked often. Even in the early stages of chronic kidney disease, phosphorus levels in the blood can get too high. This can cause low calcium. This causes the body to pull calcium from bones, which can make bones weaker. Calcium supplements can be used to prevent bone disease.
- In the early stages of kidney failure, there is no need to limit the amount of fluid but, as condition gets worse, or when on dialysis, watch the amount of liquid intake.
- Check all labels to see how much salt or sodium foods contain per serving. Look for products with less than 100 mg of salt per serving.

Healthy Foods for People with Kidney Disease

- Cabbage is high in vitamin K, vitamin C and fiber, and is also a good source of vitamin B_6 and folic acid. Low in potassium and low in cost, it is an affordable addition to the kidney diet.
- Cranberries are known to protect against bladder infections by preventing bacteria from sticking to the bladder wall.

- Cherries have been shown to reduce inflammation when eaten daily. They are also packed with antioxidants and phytochemicals that protect the heart.
- For the kidney diet, egg whites provide protein with less phosphorus than other protein sources such as egg yolk or meats.
- Other foods that can be eaten by the kidney disease patients are red grapes, red bell peppers, strawberry, garlic, cauliflower, cabbage, onion, olive oils, wild salmon, raspberries.

Foods that Need to be Avoided

Avocadoes, bananas, dry fruits, legumes, milk and yogurt, nuts and seeds, citrus fruit juices, potatoes and tomatoes.

Menu Plan

The diet of patient with kidney diseases depends upon the age, type of kidney disease, severity of the disease and general condition of the patient. Generally patient with chronic kidney disease need average amount of calories, limited amount of fluids, proteins, potassium, phosphorus and sodium. A sample menu plan is given in Table 5.13.

Table 5.13: Sample menu plan for kidney diseases

Meal	Food Items
Breakfast	• Vegetable upma with semolina, mixed vegetables, minimal oil • OR Moong dal cheela with grated vegetables, mint chutney Herbal tea (without added sugar) or lemon water
Mid-morning snack	Fresh fruit salad
Lunch	• Brown rice or millet pulao with mixed vegetables (avoid high-potassium) • OR Roti with methi leaves curry, cucumber raita (low-fat curd)
Evening snack	2 rice cakes with 1 tsp jam or 2 renal friendly wheat bran biscuits
Dinner	• Moong dal khichdi with broken wheat, lauki sabzi • OR Palak paneer (low-fat paneer) with roti or bajra roti, cucumber salad

Important notes:

- **Fluid intake:** Follow individualized recommendations from healthcare provider.
- **Protein:** Include high-quality sources like pulses, low-fat dairy, limited lean meat/fish.
- **Salt:** Minimize use; use herbs/spices for flavor.
- **Portion control:** Monitor sizes to manage nutrient intake.

GOUT DISEASE

Gout is a form of inflammatory arthritis characterized by recurrent attacks of a pain, red, tender, hot, and swollen joint. It is a disorder of purine metabolism in which level of uric acid in the blood increases. Normally uric acid level in blood is 2–4 mg/100 mL. But when this level increases, uric acid crystallizes and gets deposited in the joint such as knee joint, at ankle region, at toe, and small joint of the body. This occurs due to a combination of diet and genetic factors. A person who is nonvegetarian, alcoholic and overweight is more prone to develop gout.

Dietary Management

- Both lifestyle changes and medications can decrease uric acid levels.
- Dietary and lifestyle choices that are effective include reducing intake of purine-rich foods of animal origin such as meat and seafood, alcohol, and fructose (especially high fructose corn syrup).

Aims

- To limit the exogenous source of the uric acid.
- As the urate tends to be decreased by fat and enhanced by carbohydrates so the diet should be relatively high in carbohydrate, low in protein and also low in fat.
- Alcohol should be completely restricted.
- Diet should be liberal in the fluid intake.

The following are foods, which have negligible purine contents and they may be used daily.

- Egg, milk and milk products
- All washed pulses, except lentil
- Wheat, rice, suji, maida, maize
- All fruits
- All vegetables, except spinach, mushroom, asparagus
- Tea and coffee
- Pickles and condiments

Foods that should be Avoided

The first focus of a gout diet plan is purine restriction, so cutting out or severely limiting consumption of most animal products particularly fatty fish, red meat, shellfish, and organ meats is essential. Restrict saturated fat also because it reduces the body's ability to get rid of uric acid build-up.

- Red meat
- Organ meat like kidney brain, heart, met extracts
- Yeast (bakery product)
- Whole pulses like rajmah, rongi
- Dried bean
- A sample menu for a gout patient is given in Table 5.14.

Table 5.14: Sample menu plan for gout

Meals	Menu
Early morning	Lemon tea
Breakfast	Bread + fruit jam and tea
Midmorning	Butter milk or fruit juice
Lunch	Washed dal (such as green gram, bengal gram) chapati, mixed vegetable, and salad
Evening time	1 bowl poha or tea with biscuits
Dinner	Rice/chapati, mix vegetable, salad

IRRITABLE BOWEL SYNDROME

It is a group of chronic gastrointestinal disorder in which there is inadequate absorption of the nutrients such as proteins, fats, carbohydrates, vitamins, minerals and water, from the intestinal tract.

Signs and Symptoms

Diarrhea, sometime constipation, distention of abdomen, poor appetite, pallor, weakness, muscle cramps, abdominal blotting, pain in abdomen or mucus in the stool.

Dietary Management

Diet and lifestyle modification play important role in decreasing the frequency and severity of IBS. Such patients should maintain food diary. A high carbohydrate and high protein diet should be provided to the person suffering from malabsorption syndrome.

Avoid gas forming food

- Whole-grain bread
- Nuts
- Legumes
- Seeds
- Brussels sprouts
- Broccoli
- Cauliflower, cabbage
- Coffee, tea

Increase dietary fiber: A regular diet with optimal energy nutrient composition and dietary fiber food source, for example, whole grains, legumes, fruits and vegetables.

Reduce total fat content: Excess fat delays gastric emptying and contributes to malabsorption problems.

Avoid large meals: Large amounts of food in one meal create discomfort from gastric distention and gas. Smaller more frequent meals usually reduce these symptoms.

One may avoid milk and milk products or in case of sensitivity to the protein and in case of gluten allergy, consumption of wheat may be reduced or avoided. A sample menu for irritable bowel syndrome patient is listed in Table 5.15.

Table 5.15: Sample menu plan for irritable bowel syndrome

Meal	Menu
Early morning	Lemon tea/green tea with biscuits
Breakfast	Dalia/porridge
Midmorning	Vegetable soup
Lunch	Brown rice/chapati + pumpkin vegetable + dal (washed pules)
Evening time	Mixed fruit juice
Dinner	Khichdi + curd
Bedtime	Skim milk

OBESITY

Obesity may be defined as abnormal growth of the adipose tissues due to an either enlargement of fat cell size or increase in fat cell number. Obesity is most commonly caused by a combination of excessive food intake, lack of physical activity, and genetic susceptibility. Obesity is a medical condition in which excess body fat has accumulated to the extent that it may have an adverse effect on health.

Factors that Contribute to Obesity

- Economic status: It is found more common among high income groups as they consume excess food and do less physical work.
- Endocrine disruptors such as Cushing's syndrome, deficiency of growth hormone, thyroid insufficiency, etc.
- Physical activity: It is very common in those who have sedentary lives.
- Insufficient sleep is an important factor in weight gain.
- Increased use of medications that can cause weight gain (e.g., atypical antipsychotics).
- Pregnancy at a later age (which may cause susceptibility to obesity in children).
- Epigenetic risk factors passed on generationally.
- Stress is also an important factor in obesity.
- Consumption of sweetened drinks such as soft drinks, fruit drinks, iced tea, and energy and vitamin water drinks is believed to be contributing to the rising rates of obesity.

Assessment of the Obesity

There are various methods of assessment of the obesity.

- **Visual inspection:** It is a simple method that does not require any formula or aid. Deposition of fat on certain body parts such as abdomen and thigh is visible.
- **Standard weight for height measurement:** It is defined by body mass index (BMI) and further evaluated in terms of fat distribution via the waist–hip ratio and total cardiovascular risk factors. BMI is closely related to both percentage body fat and total body fat, given in Table 5.16.

Table 5.16: Classification of body types based on body mass index

Body mass index (kg/m^2)	Classification
Less than 18.5	Underweight
18.5–25.0	Normal weight
25.0–30.0	Overweight
30.0–35.0	Class I obesity
35.0–40.0	Class II obesity
More than 40.0	Class III obesity

- **Waist circumference:** It is used to evaluate abdominal fat. The normal value in men is <40 inches and in women <35 inches.

- **Measurement of body fat:** Various skinfold calipers are available to measure body fat. Caliper measures subcutaneous fats at the triceps, abdomen, and subscapular and subcostal sites.

Dietary Management

Changes to diet and physical therapy are the main treatments. Diet quality can be improved by reducing the consumption of energy-dense foods, such as those high in fat and sugars, and by increasing the intake of dietary fibers as shown in Table 5.17. Medications may be taken, along with a suitable diet, to reduce appetite or decrease fat absorption.

Table 5.17: Daily menu for obese person

Serving	Food items
Early morning	Lemon water or lemon tea without sugar/green tea—1 cup
Breakfast	Dalia/upma—1 bowl
Midmorning	Butter milk/lassi without sugar or citrus fruits juice—1 glass
Lunch	Chapati (without ghee/butter) -2 + green leafy vegetable—1 bowl + black gram —1 bowl and curd ½ bowl + salad—1 plate
Evening tea	Tea/coffee without sugar—1 cup with digestive biscuits—2 (with high fiber contents) or any seasonal fruit
Dinner	Vegetable soup—1 bowl, chapati-2, steamed carrots/cauliflower vegetable/dal —1 bowl
At bedtime	Skim milk—one glass

CHOLECYSTECTOMY

Cholecystectomy is a surgical procedure to remove gallbladder, a pear-shaped organ that is just below the liver on the upper right side of abdomen. Gallbladder collects and stores bile, a digestive fluid produced in liver. It is a common treatment of symptomatic gallstones and other gallbladder conditions. Surgical options include the standard procedure, called laparoscopic cholecystectomy, or an older more invasive procedure, called open cholecystectomy.

Dietary Management

For the first few days after surgery, stick with clear liquids and broths and after that, gradually more solid foods can be added back into diet. Diet must be low in fat content and fried foods. High-fat foods, foods with strong odors and gas-causing foods must be avoided. The following foods should be avoided to prevent discomfort.

- French fries and potato chips
- High-fat meats, such as ground beef
- High-fat dairy, such as cheese, ice cream and whole milk
- Pizza
- Creamy soups and sauces, butter, ghee
- Meat gravies

- Chocolate
- Oils, such as coconut and palm oil
- Chicken or turkey skin
- Spicy foods
- Gas producing foods such as broccoli, cauliflower and cabbage
- **Gradually increase the fiber in diet:** This can help normalize bowel movements. Add soluble fiber, such as oats and barley, fruit and vegetables, wholegrain rice, whole wheat pasta and bread, seeds, nuts and oats, but increase the amount of fiber slowly, such as over several weeks, because too much fiber at initial stage can make gas and cramping worse.
- **Eat smaller, more-frequent meals:** This may ensure a better mix with available bile. A healthy meal should include small amounts of protein, such as poultry, fish or fat-free dairy, along with vegetables, fruits and whole grains. A sample menu plan for cholecystectomy patient is given in Table 5.18.

Table 5.18: Sample menu plan in cholecystectomy

Serving	Food items
Early morning	Fruit juice
Breakfast	Dalia
Midmorning	Seasonal fruit (apple/orange)
Lunch	Khichdi, curd
Evening time	Upma or suji kheer
Dinner	Vegetable soup or thin dal

GASTRECTOMY

Gastrectomy is the removal of part or all of the stomach. In severe duodenal ulcers, it may be necessary to remove the lower portion of the stomach called the pylorus and the upper portion of the small intestine called the duodenum.

Types

- A **partial gastrectomy** is the removal of a part of the stomach. It is usually the lower half that is removed.
- A **full gastrectomy** is the removal of the entire stomach.
- A **sleeve gastrectomy** is the removal of the left side of the stomach. This is usually performed as part of a surgery for weight loss.

Dietary Management

To ensure for healing and recovery after surgery, it will be necessary to follow a complete nutritional menu plan. To prevent over-stretching of the pouch, discomfort, improper healing, or malnutrition, special focus must be given for proper amount of proteins and dense nutrients, hydration and taking essential bariatric vitamins and minerals. The management is divided into four phases.

Phase 1: Clear Liquids (1–5 days)

This period will start when the patient is in the hospital. The diet is started with clear liquids. A clear liquid is anything that is transparent, like broths and vitamin water. The purpose of this phase is to make sure that the patient gets the proper hydration.

Guidelines

- Take small amounts of fluid whole day.
- Sip 4–8 ounces per hour.
- Daily goal is 64 ounces.
- In the beginning, water may irritate the pouch. Warm temperature fluids will soothe and relax the pouch muscles.

Recommended liquids

- Water
- Clear broth/bouillon: chicken, beef, vegetable
- Sugar-free vitamin water
- Unsweetened, caffeine-free herbal tea
- Sugar-free Jell-O
- Sugar-free popsicles
- No carbonated beverages

Phase 2: Full/Thick Liquid Diet (5–14 days)

This phase focuses on staying hydrated and increasing fluids along with incorporating protein, vitamin, and mineral supplementation.

Guidelines

- Begin vitamin and mineral supplementation.
- Give 60–80 g of protein per day (aim for 20 g of protein per meal.)
- Choose a protein supplement with at least 20 g of protein and less than 10 g of total carbohydrates.
- Avoid using a straw; it will increase the chance of air swallowing, which causes distension of the pouch.
- For gastric bypass patients, eat <15 g of total carbohydrates per sitting to prevent dumping syndrome.
- Avoid all carbonated beverages.

Recommended liquids

- All liquids from the previous clear liquid phase
- Protein shakes/powders
- Pureed soups with added unflavored protein
- Clear fluid proteins
- Sugar-free pudding with added protein

Phase 3: Soft Solids (Day 15–30 days)

The purpose of the phase is to introduce slowly soft foods, continues to heal and adjust to the changes.

Guidelines

- Add only one food at a time.
- The recommendation is 4 ounces of food (by weight) per meal (3 ounces of protein and 1 ounce of something else).
- Stop drinking 30 minutes before eating and do not drink until 30 minutes after a meal.
- Chew food thoroughly and slowly to apple sauce consistency before swallowing.
- Eat three meals a day and at least one protein shake per day.
- Protein intake needs to be approximately 60–80 g a day.

Recommended foods

- Scrambled eggs
- Cottage/ricotta cheese
- Pureed beans
- String cheese
- Soft tofu
- Greek yogurt (chobani or fage)
- Chicken, egg, shrimp salads

Phase 4: One Month and Beyond

At this period, solid foods should be started. Start with 2–4 ounces of solid food per meal and then slowly increase the amount of solid food per meal until eating at least 4 ounces per meal but no >6 ounces. In the beginning, protein source is given.

Recommended foods

- **Eat protein first:** Best food tolerated are fish, shrimp, eggs, chicken, tofu, meatless products, beans, cottage cheese.
- **Raw vegetables/salads:** It should be avoided.
- **Citrus fruits:** Such fruits include includes fresh fruit, peeled with no skin, canned fruit in water or natural juice that has been drained.
- **Starches:** There are two types of carbohydrates: whole grains and simple sugars. Focus on eating whole grains, such as whole grain bread, oatmeal and sweet potatoes.
- **Oils and essential fats:** It is important to include essential fats in daily meal plan to prevent deficiencies. Examples of healthy fats are avocado, olives, a variety of nuts, oils, like olive, grape seed or coconut.
- A sample menu plan for gastrectomy patient is shown in Table 5.19.

Table 5.19: Sample meal plan for a gastrectomy patient

Meal	Food Items
Breakfast	• Rava (semolina) upma with finely chopped vegetables, cooked soft • OR Khichdi made with rice and moong dal, well-cooked and mashed • Herbal tea or masala chai (lightly brewed, without milk)
Mid-morning snack	Soft ripe banana or mashed papaya

Contd...

Meal	Food Items
Lunch	• Soft roti with dal (pulses) that is well-cooked and mashed • OR Daliya (broken wheat) khichdi with vegetables, cooked soft
Evening snack	Vegetable soup
Dinner	Soft cooked moong dal with mashed potatoes or lauki (bottle gourd) sabzi

Important considerations:

- **Texture:** choose for softer textures and smaller portions to aid digestion.
- **Spices:** Use mild spices to enhance flavor without causing discomfort.
- **Hydration:** Sip fluids throughout the day, but avoid large amounts during meals.
- **Nutrient density:** Ensure meals are nutrient-dense to support healing and overall health.
- **Frequent meals:** Aim for 5–6 small meals/snacks per day rather than 3 large meals.

BARIATRIC SURGERY

Bariatric surgery (weight loss surgery) includes a variety of procedures performed on people who have obesity. Weight loss is achieved by reducing the size of the stomach with a gastric band or through removal of a portion of the stomach (sleeve gastrectomy or biliopancreatic diversion with duodenal switch) or by resecting and rerouting the small intestine to a small stomach pouch (gastric bypass surgery).The National Institute of Health recommends bariatric surgery for obese people with a body mass index (BMI) of 35–40, and serious coexisting medical conditions such as diabetes.

Dietary Management

- After bariatric surgery, the patient should be kept NPO (nothing per oral) for 24 hours. Afterwards clear liquid diet, which includes foods such as clear broth, diluted fruit juices or sugar-free drinks can be started.
- Within the first month after surgery, in order to prevent fluid volume depletion and dehydration, a minimum of 48–64 fl oz should be consumed by repetitive small sips all day.
- Patient must eat and drink slowly to avoid dumping syndrome. Dumping syndrome is the group of symptoms, for example, nausea, vomiting, dizziness, sweating and diarrhea that can arise when food is consumed too quickly. To avoid it patient must eat and drink slowly and must avoid heavy food. Drinks must be taken at least 30–45 minutes after the meal.
- Patient should eat several small meals a day and sip liquids slowly throughout the day (not with meals). First start with six small meals a day, then move to four meals and finally, when following a regular diet, decrease to three meals a day.
- Food must be taken in small bites and chewed properly before swallowing as larger pieces of food may block the site of surgery and can lead to GI problems like vomiting, nausea and abdominal pain.
- Foods high in proteins must be consumed after surgery as eating high-protein foods not only help in early healing but are also easy to digest as compared to foods that are high in fat or sugars.
- Many patients need to take a daily multivitamin pill for life to compensate for reduced absorption of essential nutrients. Because patients cannot eat a large quantity of food. A diet that is relatively high in protein and low in fats is recommended.

- Some foods must be avoided after bariatric surgery that include nuts and seeds, popcorn, dried fruits, carbonated beverages, stringy or fibrous vegetables, such as celery, broccoli, corn or cabbage, tough meats, fried foods and bread.
- Postsurgery, overeating is curbed because exceeding the capacity of the stomach causes nausea and vomiting. Three to four months after weight-loss surgery, patient may be able to start eating a normal healthy diet, depending on situation of the client.

PEPTIC ULCER

Peptic ulcer is defined as a break in the lining of the stomach, first part of the small intestine, or occasionally the lower esophagus. An ulcer in the stomach is known as a gastric ulcer while that in the first part of the intestines is known as a duodenal ulcer. The most common symptoms are waking at night with upper abdominal pain or upper abdominal pain that improves with eating. The people who are at risk for peptic ulcer are who consume too much alcohol, persons who are on long-term medication (aspirin, ibuprofen, naproxen, or other nonsteroidal anti-inflammatory drugs), smoking cigarettes or chewing tobacco and having radiation treatments.

Symptoms

- Abdominal pain is a common symptom
- Feeling of fullness
- Hunger and an empty feeling in the stomach, often 1–3 hours after a meal
- Mild nausea that may go away with vomiting
- Discomfort in the upper abdomen
- Pain in the upper abdomen that wakes you up at night
- Bloody or dark tarry stools
- Chest pain
- Fatigue
- Vomiting, possibly bloody
- Weight loss

Dietary Management

A diet for ulcers and gastritis does not include foods that irritate stomach and increase stomach acid. Drinks and foods that cause stomach pain, heartburn, or indigestion must be limited or avoided. The following are some foods that must be avoided.

- **Beverages:**
  - Hot cocoa and cola
  - Whole milk and chocolate milk
  - Peppermint and spearmint tea
  - Regular and decaf coffee

- Green and black tea with or without caffeine
- Drinks that contain alcohol
- Orange and grapefruit juices

- **Spices and seasonings:**
  - Black and red pepper
  - Garlic powder
  - Chili powder
- **Other foods:**
  - Dairy foods made from whole milk or cream
  - Spicy or strongly flavored cheeses
  - Highly seasoned, high-fat meats and sausage
  - Tomato products, such as tomato paste, tomato sauce, or tomato juice.

Foods that should be Taken

Eat fruits, vegetables, whole grains, and fat-free or low-fat dairy foods. Whole grains include whole-wheat breads, cereals and brown rice. Choose lean meats, poultry (chicken and turkey), fish, beans, eggs, and nuts. A healthy meal plan is low in unhealthy fats, salt, and added sugar. Healthy fats include olive oil and canola oil.

Cereals like bread, rice, lean meats, poultry (chicken and turkey), fish, beans, eggs, dehusked pulses, boiled, mashed vegetables and stewed fruits. Food of peptic ulcer patients should be cooked by boiling, baking, stewing and poaching. Other methods of cooking like frying, barbecuing and smoking of food should be avoided. A sample menu plan for peptic ulcer patients is given in Table 5.20.

Table 5.20: Sample meal plan for a peptic ulcer patient

Meal	Food Items
Breakfast	• Poha (flattened rice) cooked with mild spices and vegetables, served lukewarm • OR Idli with sambar (sambar without tamarind, mildly spiced) • Herbal tea or ginger tea with minimal sugar
Mid-morning snack	Soft boiled egg or banana
Lunch	• Khichdi made with rice and moong dal, cooked well and slightly mashed • OR Roti with dal (pulses) that is well-cooked and mashed • Steamed or lightly cooked vegetables
Evening snack	Curd (yogurt) with a pinch of roasted cumin powder
Dinner	• Steamed fish or tofu with mashed potatoes or lauki (bottle gourd) sabzi • OR Soft cooked chapati with dal (pulses) and cucumber raita

Important considerations:

- **Avoid spicy foods:** Minimize or avoid spices that may irritate the stomach lining.
- **Small, frequent meals:** Opt for 5–6 small meals/snacks per day rather than 3 large meals.
- **Hydration:** Drink fluids throughout the day, such as water or herbal tea (non-caffeinated).
- **Avoid citrus fruits:** Skip oranges, lemons, and other citrus fruits that can exacerbate acidity.

COLOSTOMY

A **colostomy** is a surgical procedure in which an opening (stoma) is formed in the large intestine or colon through an incision in the anterior abdominal wall and suturing it into place. This opening, in conjunction with the attached stoma appliance, provides an alternative channel for feces to leave the body (Fig. 5.2).

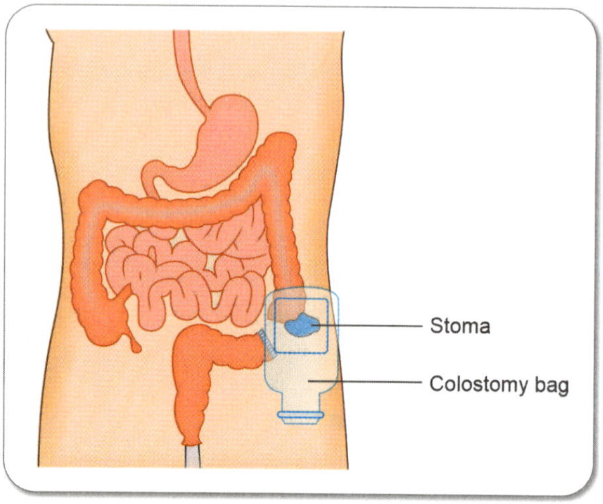

Fig. 5.2: Colostomy

Indications

- Rectal or colon cancer
- Partial or complete intestinal blockage
- Injury to colon or rectum or fistula in the perineum
- Inflammatory bowel disease
- Imperforate anus, severe infection or diverticulitis

Types

- **Loop colostomy:** A loop of colon is pulled out through an incision in the abdomen and then sutured to the abdomen and two openings are created in the stoma.
- **End colostomy:** A stoma is created from one end of the bowel where it is turned like a cuff and edges of the colon are stitched to the skin of the abdominal wall to form an opening called stoma.
- **Double barrel colostomy:** Two separate stomas are created. The proximal stoma, which is functional diverts feces to the abdominal wall.

Dietary Management

- No standard recommendations can be given as each patient and type of surgery is different and most patients return to a fairly normal diet after some time of the surgery.
- Eat foods at a regular time each day. Eating 4–6 smaller meals may help to promote a regular bowel pattern.
- Try to eat the main meal during the day and a smaller meal in the evening. This helps to reduce the stool output at night.
- Food must be chewed properly before swallowing as large pieces of food may block the opening of stoma.
- Colon absorbs water and electrolyte from the stool, when a part of colon is already removed it may lead to dehydration. So plenty of fluids must be taken to keep the stool soft and to prevent dehydration.
- Avoid excessive fats in the diet as extra fat in the abdominal wall create a problem for the stoma to function properly.
- Patient must get educated that color of the stool will change according to the food taken, for example broccoli and spinach can darken the color of the stool.
- One type of food must be given at one time to check the tolerance of food. If it is not tolerated it should be stopped and tried later on.

The following foods that tend to form gas must be avoided or taken in limited amount:

- **Cereals:** Excessive wheat products, including breads and cereals. Check labels for specific grains and breads.
- **Legumes:** Most beans, especially dried beans and peas, baked beans and soybeans.
- **Vegetables:** Cabbage, radishes, onions, broccoli, brussels sprouts, cauliflower, cucumbers and turnips.
- **Fruits:** Excessive amounts of fresh fruits.
- A sample menu plan for colostomy patient is given in Table 5.21.

Table 5.21: Sample meal plan for a colostomy patient

Meal	Food Items
Breakfast	• Soft idli or dosa made from fermented batter, served with coconut chutney • OR Upma made with semolina, cooked soft with vegetables • Herbal tea or buttermilk (diluted with water)
Mid-morning snack	Banana or apple
Lunch	• Khichdi made with rice and moong dal, well-cooked and mashed • OR Roti with mashed vegetables (such as lauki or carrots) and dal • Soft cooked or mashed vegetables (avoiding high-fiber or gas-producing ones)
Evening snack	Yogurt (plain or flavored)
Dinner	• Soft cooked fish or paneer with mashed potatoes or soft roti • OR Rice with dal (pulses) that is well-cooked and mashed

Important considerations:

- **Fiber intake:** Choose low-fiber foods to reduce the risk of blockage or discomfort.
- **Gas-producing foods:** Avoid foods like cabbage, broccoli, and beans that may cause gas.
- **Protein:** Ensure adequate protein intake from sources like eggs, dairy, tofu, or fish.
- **Small, frequent meals:** Choose for 5-6 small meals/snacks per day rather than 3 large meals.

SPECIAL DIETS

Dietary Approaches to Stop Hypertension

Dietary approaches to stop hypertension (DASH) is an eating plan to lower or control high blood pressure. The DASH diet emphasizes foods that are lower in sodium as well as foods that are rich in potassium, magnesium and calcium—nutrients that help lower blood pressure. The DASH diet features menus with plenty of vegetables, fruits and low-fat dairy products, as well as whole grains, fish, poultry and nuts. It offers limited portions of red meats, sweets and sugary beverages.

Fat-Free Diet

A low-fat diet is one that restricts fat often saturated fats and cholesterol. Low-fat diets are intended to reduce diseases such as heart disease and obesity. Reducing fat in the diet can make it easier to cut calories, resulting in weight loss or less weight gain. Foods that are included in low fat diet are beans, lentils, spinach, broccoli, cottage cheese, green tea, fruits such as apples and oranges, skim milk, yogurt, eggs with white portion. A sample menu plan for fat free diet is given in Table 5.22.

Table 5.22: Sample menu plan for fat free diet

Meal	Menu
Early morning	1 glass skim milk
Breakfast	Vegetable upma with green tea
Midmorning	1 bowl mixed fruit chaat
Lunch	Brown rice/chapati, green leafy vegetable, dal, curd(made with skim milk) and salad
Evening time	Sprouted chana (black chickpea)
Dinner	Whole pulses like rongi/rajmah and chapati

Low-sodium Diet

A low-sodium diet is a diet that includes no >1,500–2,400 mg of sodium per day. The human's minimum requirement for sodium in the diet is about 500 mg per day; For certain people with salt-sensitive blood pressure or diseases such as Ménière's disease, this extra intake may cause a negative effect on health.

A low-sodium diet has a useful effect to reduce blood pressure, both in people with hypertension and in people with normal blood pressure. A low-salt diet (approximately 4.5 g/day or 1800 mg/day sodium) in hypertensive people resulted in a decrease in systolic blood pressure by 5 mm Hg and in diastolic blood pressure by 2.70 mm Hg. In people with normal blood pressure, the corresponding decrease in systolic blood pressure was 2.03 mm Hg and diastolic blood pressure 0.99 mm Hg.

Food and Drinks containing Sodium

Sodium occurs naturally in most foods. The most common form of sodium is sodium chloride, which is table salt. Various food groups that are high in sodium content are meats, poultry, fish, legumes, eggs and nuts, smoked or canned meat, fish or poultry, sausage, frozen breaded meats and dinners, such as burritos and pizza, buttermilk, regular and processed cheese. Sodium is also added to various food products. Some of these added forms are monosodium glutamate, sodium nitrite, sodium saccharin, baking soda (sodium bicarbonate), and sodium benzoate.

Guidelines for a Low-Sodium Diet

A main source of sodium is table salt. This is about 20 times as much as the body needs. In fact, our body needs only ¼ tsp of salt every day. Eliminate salty foods from diet and reduce the amount of salt used in cooking. Choose low sodium foods. Low sodium is defined as 140 mg of sodium per serving. Eat more home-cooked meals. Foods cooked at home are comparatively lower in sodium than most instant foods. A sample menu plan for low sodium diet is given in Table 5.23.

Table 5.23: Sample meal plan for a low sodium diet

Meal	Food items
Breakfast	• Vegetable poha (flattened rice) cooked with minimal oil and salt-free spices • OR Oats porridge made with milk and topped with fresh fruits • Herbal tea or green tea
Mid-morning snack	Air-popped popcorn (without butter and salt)
Lunch	• Brown rice with dal (pulses) cooked with turmeric and mild spices • Steamed or lightly sautéed vegetables (such as beans, carrots, or spinach) • Fresh cucumber and tomato salad with lemon juice

Contd...

Meal	Food items
Afternoon snack	Plain yogurt (curd) with a pinch of roasted cumin powder
Dinner	• Baked or grilled fish/chicken marinated with herbs and lemon juice • OR Roti with sabzi (vegetable curry) made with minimal salt • Boiled or steamed green beans or broccoli

Important considerations:

- **Use of spices:** Flavor foods with salt-free herbs and spices like cumin, coriander, ginger, and garlic.
- **Fresh ingredients:** Choose fresh fruits and vegetables over canned or processed options.
- **Avoid processed foods:** Minimize intake of packaged snacks and ready-to-eat meals.
- **Read labels:** Check food labels for sodium content and choose products labeled as low-sodium.
- **Hydration:** Drink plenty of water throughout the day to help flush out excess sodium.

Bland Diet

A bland diet is a diet consisting of foods that are generally soft, low in dietary fiber, cooked rather than raw, and not spicy. Such a diet is called bland because it is soothing to the digestive tract (it minimizes irritation of tissues). A bland diet is designed primarily to help patients recover from gastrointestinal conditions or other medical circumstances in which improved digestion would be essential. It is not especially effective as a long-term weight loss diet, although portion sizes are strictly controlled.

Uses

Bland diets are often recommended for the following:

- Stomach or intestinal surgery
- Peptic ulcers
- Heartburn
- Nausea, vomiting.

What to Avoid

- Fatty dairy foods (butter, whipped cream or high-fat ice cream)
- Strong cheeses, such as blue or Roquefort
- Raw fruits and vegetables, especially berries
- Gassy vegetables (broccoli, cabbage, cauliflower, cucumber, green peppers, and corn)
- Dried fruits
- Whole-grain or bran cereals
- Whole-grain breads, crackers, or pasta
- Vinegar-based foods such as pickles are to be avoided
- Garlic and hot peppers
- Foods with a lot of sugar or honey
- Seeds and nuts
- Highly seasoned, cured or smoked meats and fish
- Fried foods
- Alcohol

Foods to Eat in a Bland Diet

Many milk and dairy products are permissible, even recommended, on a bland diet, but there are a few exceptions.

- **Yogurt:** This includes flavored and plain yogurt, but keep in mind that certain fruits can affect digestion.
- **Cheese:** Some bland diets include all types of cheese.

Most canned fruits and vegetables are fine, with the exception of tomatoes. Bananas are good; however, higher fiber and acidic fruits should be avoided.

In a strict bland food diet, softer protein sources such as smooth butter, eggs and tofu are encouraged over any type of fibrous or seasoned meat.

Certain meats such as poultry or fish are permitted, as long as they are not heavily fried, breaded or processed like sandwich meats.

- **Ice cream:** Due to the fat content in many ice creams, some bland diets will exclude ice cream entirely. Others allow ice cream in moderation or ice creams that do not contain nuts or certain types of fruits.
- **Soy products:** These include tofu, soy yogurts, and soy milk.
- **Baked and grilled meats:** Some bland diets include red meat, but they usually emphasize lean cuts of chicken, pork, and turkey.
- Oatmeal and potatoes
- A sample menu for bland diet is given in Table 5.24.

Table 5.24: A sample menu for bland diet

Meal	Food items
Breakfast	• Plain idli or dosa with coconut chutney • OR Khichdi made with rice and moong dal, cooked soft and lightly seasoned • Herbal tea or buttermilk (diluted with water)
Mid-morning snack	Mashed ripe banana or stewed apple
Lunch	• Soft roti with dal (pulses) that is well-cooked and mildly spiced • OR Steamed rice with mashed potatoes or lauki (bottle gourd) sabzi • Steamed or lightly cooked vegetables (like carrots or beans)
Evening snack	Plain yogurt (curd) or lassi (plain yogurt drink)
Dinner	Non spicy mix vegetable soup or mixed vegetable porridge

Important considerations:

- **Spice levels:** Minimize or avoid spices like chili powder, pepper, and strong herbs.
- **Fats:** Choose cooking methods like steaming, boiling, or baking instead of frying.
- **Avoid acidic foods:** Skip citrus fruits and tomatoes that may irritate the stomach lining.
- **Hydration:** Drink plenty of water throughout the day to aid digestion

High-protein Diet

Protein is a macronutrient to build and repair muscle. It also plays a great role in fat-burning metabolism. Protein also works as secondary source of energy during the deficiency of the carbohydrate. While adequate protein is required for building skeletal muscle and other tissues, there is ongoing debate regarding the use and necessity of high-protein diets in anaerobic exercise, in particular for weight training and bodybuilding.

Some people consume protein supplements after bodybuilding workouts, as they provide a quick and easily consumable protein source (Table 5.25). Alternatively, meat, beans, or other high-protein foods are consumed.

High Protein Recommendation

- Protein 120–150 g
- Calories 3000–3500
- Carbohydrates 250–300 g
- Fat 60–70 g

Indications

- Burn
- Protein energy malnutrition
- Body builders
- Athletes
- Osteoporosis

Sources

- Animal sources, such as meat, fish, poultry, eggs, and dairy products, contain complete proteins—all the amino acids required to form the proteins we need.
- Vegetable sources, such as nuts, seeds, legumes (beans, peas, lentils, and soy products), grains (breads and cereals), and green leafy vegetables, contain incomplete proteins.
- Soybeans and its products.

Table 5.25: Sample menu plan of High-protein diet

Meal	Food Items
Breakfast	• Moong dal cheela (pancake) with mixed vegetables, served with mint chutney or • Vegetable upma made with semolina (rava) Milk or buttermilk
Mid-morning snack	Sprouts salad (moong or chickpea sprouts) with onions, tomatoes, and lemon juice
Lunch	• Grilled chicken breast or paneer (cottage cheese) tikka with mixed salad or • Rajma (kidney beans) curry with brown rice or roti • Steamed or lightly cooked vegetables (like spinach or carrots)
Evening snack	Yogurt or cottage cheese (paneer) with almonds or walnuts
Dinner	• Baked fish or tofu with quinoa or whole wheat roti or • Dal (pulses) tadka with quinoa or millet • Steamed or stir-fried vegetables (like broccoli or beans)
Bed time	Protein shake (made with milk or yogurt, and protein powder)

Important considerations:

- **Protein sources:** Include lean meats (like chicken, fish), dairy products (like yogurt, paneer), legumes (like dal, chickpeas), and nuts/seeds.
- **Balanced meals:** Ensure each meal includes a source of protein, carbohydrates (preferably complex), and vegetables/fruits.
- **Hydration:** Drink plenty of water throughout the day to support protein metabolism.

Low-protein Diet (25–30 g)

A low-protein diet is a diet in which there is reduced intake of proteins (Table 5.26). Though protein is an essential nutrient required for normal functioning of the cells, tissue repair or protection from certain diseases even then it is restricted in the patients of inherited metabolic disorders or the patients of liver and kidney diseases. Proteins are made up of amino acids and it gets delaminated or metabolized in the liver giving urea as the end product of the metabolism. If kidneys are not functioning properly, there is improper excretion of urea. If the person is suffering from such diseases urea or ammonia gets accumulated in the bloodstream, which produces toxic effects in the body, so such patients are advised to restrict their proteins intake.

Fruits and vegetables are the main diet recommended but for the fulfillment of the requirement of the calories, healthy fats can be included in the diet.

Table 5.26: Sample menu for low-protein diet

Meal	Food Items
Breakfast	• Vegetable poha (flattened rice) cooked with minimal oil and spices or • Rava (semolina) upma with mixed vegetables, cooked soft Herbal tea or buttermilk (diluted with water)
Mid-morning snack	A small apple or banana
Lunch	• Roti with Steamed or lightly cooked vegetables (like carrots or beans) or • Rice with sambar (mildly spiced lentil soup) and vegetable stir-fry
Evening snack	Small portion of rice cakes or fiber-rich cookies with herbal tea
Dinner	Chapati with Steamed or stir-fried vegetables (like spinach or cauliflower)

Indications

- Metabolic disorders, such as phenylketonuria,
- Kidney, liver disease
- Glomerulonephritis,
- Chronic uremia
- Jaundice
- Viral hepatitis

Source

- Tomato
- Sweet potato
- Cucumber
- Cauliflower
- Whole meal bread
- Rice vermicelli
- Cornflakes
- Apple
- Banana
- Orange
- Plum
- Strawberry
- Cow milk
- Vegetable oils like olive oil, safflower oil, soybean or sunflower oils are low in proteins
- Nuts like walnuts, almonds and cashews
- Candies, sweeteners and canned fruits

Important considerations:

- **Limit protein sources:** Avoid or minimize high-protein foods like meats, fish, eggs, and dairy products.
- **Carbohydrates and fats:** Focus on complex carbohydrates (like whole grains) and healthy fats (like nuts, seeds, and avocados).
- **Fiber and fluids:** Include fiber-rich foods and drink plenty of water to support digestion and overall health.
- **Supplementation:** Consider vitamin and mineral supplementation as needed to compensate for reduced dietary variety.

Low Calorie Diet

Calories are the most important factor that determines both weight gain and weight loss. The three main sources of calories are fats, carbohydrates, and proteins. Simple carbohydrates like white rice, sugar, white flour, fruit juices and baked goods are high in calories. Complex carbohydrates such as brown rice, wheat flour, beans, lentils, legumes, fruits and vegetables are low in calories. Sources of unhealthy saturated fats are butter, cheese and fatty cuts of meats; whereas sources of healthy unsaturated fats are nuts, vegetable oils, olives and sea food. So, it is important to identify the good and the bad sources of calories and include the right items to make the food healthy and balanced.

It is classified into:

- **Moderately low calorie diet:** It requires 1,200–1,000 kcal/day. It is used mainly for weight loss.
- **Very low calorie diet (VLCD):** It is a diet with extremely low daily food energy consumption. It is defined as a diet of 800 kilocalories (3,300 kJ) per day. VLCDs are formulated, nutritionally complete, liquid meals containing 800 kilocalories or less per day. VLCDs also contain the recommended daily requirements for vitamins, minerals, trace elements, proteins and carbohydrate.

Food Tips for Low Calorie

When calorie intake reduces, stored fat works as a fuel for the body.

- Fruits are given but not more than one serving.
- Sugar and jaggery are not allowed.
- Small amount of fat and oil are used for cooking.
- Cereals are allowed such as wheat in small quantity, ragi, bajra, which contain small amount of starch.
- Food rich in protein is given in measurable amount.

Table 5.27 shows a 1200-calorie diet chart

Table 5.27: Following is a 1200-calorie diet chart

Timing	Foods to eat	Calories
Early morning	Lukewarm water with lemon 1 glass	0
Breakfast	2 scrambled eggs + 1 slice brown bread + skim milk 1 glass (240 g)	315
Midmorning	Any seasonal fruit	80
Lunch	Brown rice 1 cup (195 g) + chicken (100 g) + mixed vegetables ½ cup + salad 1 bowl	360
Evening	Tea without sugar + 2 biscuits	90
Dinner	1 roti + vegetable (50 g) + lentils dal ½ cup + raita 1 small bowl	380
Total		1225

Iron-Rich Foods

Iron is present in all cells in the human body and has several vital functions, such as: Carrying oxygen to the tissues from the lungs. It is an important component of the hemoglobin protein. It facilitates oxygen use and storage in the muscles as a component of myoglobin and as an integral part of enzyme reactions in various tissues. Iron is found in many foods and is present in two forms: Heme and nonheme. Heme iron is better absorbed by the body and is found in animal products such as meat (including poultry) and fish. Nonheme iron is found mainly in plant sources such as beans, pulses and green leafy vegetables. In women, blood loss occurs during menstruation, which is why women need more iron in their diet. Total body iron averages approximately 3.8 g in men and 2.3 g in women.

To improve absorption of iron, it should be consumed along with a good source of vitamin C such as citrus fruits, orange juice, broccoli, or strawberries. Mild iron deficiency can be prevented or corrected by eating iron-rich foods and by cooking in an iron skillet.

Symptoms of Iron Deficiency

- Fatigue
- Lightheadedness
- Hair loss
- Irritability
- PICA
- Impaired immune function
- Dizziness
- Pallor
- Twitches
- Weakness
- Brittle or grooved nails
- Restless legs syndrome.

Sources of Iron in the Diet

- Red meat, beef, lamb, pork, kidneys, liver, heart, black pudding
- **Fish and shellfish:** E.g., sardines, pilchards, crab, anchovies, shrimps, mussels
- Eggs and jaggery
- **Cereal and cereal products:** For example bread, oat, wheat gram, etc.
- **Nuts and seeds:** Such as peanuts, pecans, walnuts, sesame seeds, sunflower seeds, pine nuts.
- **Green leafy vegetables:** Broccoli, spinach, kale, pumpkin, sesame, or squash seeds.
- **Beans and pulses:** Baked beans, peas, lentils, chickpeas, black-eyed beans, kidney beans, lentils, beans.
- **Dried fruit:** Raisins, apricots, prunes, currants, figs.
- Other products like plain (dark) chocolate, cocoa powder, mango chutney, cherries in syrup, ginger nut biscuits, pastry and curry powder.

Table 5.28 shows a sample menu for a patient with anemia.

Table 5.28: Sample menu for a patient with anemia

Meal	Menu
Early morning	2 iron fortified biscuits with herbal tea
Breakfast	• Fortified cereals with milk and nuts (walnuts, almond, cashew) or • Scrambled eggs with brown bread or methi parantha
Midmorning	Seasonal fruit, or orange juice/mixed fruit chaat

Contd...

Meal	Menu
Lunch	• Chapatis made from coarse flour, rajmah/kabuli chana, steamed brown rice, spinach and potato vegetable, salad (lettuce, tomato, cucumber, lemon) • Mixed vegetable cutlets, lauki raita (curd).
Evening	Nutritious laddu or pinnies
Dinner	Pulse/lentil, green beans, peas or cauliflower vegetable, chapatis, salad
Bedtime	Warm milk with added jaggery

GERIATRIC NUTRITION

Geriatrics is a specialty that focuses on health care of elderly people. It aims to promote health by preventing and treating diseases and disabilities in older adults. Elderly people generally want to live independently as long as possible, which requires them to be able to engage in self-care and other activities of daily living.

Geriatric **nutrition** applies nutrition principles to delay effects of aging and disease, to aid in the management of the physical and psychosocial changes commonly associated with growing old.

Changes in Old Age

- **Physiological changes:** Once the body reaches physiologic maturity, the rate of degenerative change exceeds the rate of cell regeneration also decreasing the basal metabolic rate.

  The following are typical physiologic changes that can affect nutritional status:

  - **Musculoskeletal changes:** Progressive drop in bone mass starts when people are in old age making the skeleton more vulnerable to fractures or osteoporosis. Adequate intake of calcium and vitamin D helps to retain bone.
  - **Loss of teeth and sensory changes also occur:** Decrease in all the senses, particularly in the taste buds affects perception of salty and sweet tastes and may affect appetite.
  - **Immunity also decreases with age:** The lower immune function means less ability to fight infections and malignancies. Vitamin E, zinc, and some other supplements may increase immune function.
  - **Gastrointestinal changes:** Gastrointestinal (GI) changes include a reduction in digestion and absorption. Digestive hormones and enzymes decrease, the intestinal mucosa deteriorates, and the gastric emptying time increases. As a result, pernicious anemia and constipation are more likely to occur.
  - **Cardiovascular changes:** Cardiovascular changes may occur. Reduced sodium intake becomes important, as blood pressure increases.
  - **Hormonal changes:** In pancreas, insulin secretion is decreased, which can lead to carbohydrate intolerance, and renal function deteriorates in some people.
- **Psychosocial changes:** A number of changes may occur in the aging person's social and psychological status, potentially affecting appetite and nutritional status. These include:
  - Depression, the most common cause of unexplained weight loss in older adults.
  - Memory impairment caused by various types of dementia, Alzheimer's disease, or other neurological diseases. Weight loss and improper nutrition are potential problems.

Common Problems in Aging

Dysphagia

The incidence of dysphagia, or difficulty in swallowing, increases with age. Dysphagia results from conditions such as stroke, Alzheimer's or Parkinson's disease, multiple sclerosis, or physiological changes such as loss of teeth or poorly fitting dentures.

Fluid Balance

Dehydration is the most common cause of fluid and electrolyte disturbance in older adults. Reduced thirst sensation and fluid intake, medications such as diuretics and **laxatives,** and increased fluid need during illness contribute to dehydration.

Skin Integrity

Skin breakdown is a common problem, particularly in bedridden or immunologically impaired people. The most common skin breakdown is the pressure ulcer.

Malnutrition

While most elderly people require adequate nutritional status, institutionalized and hospitalized older adults are at higher risk for malnutrition than individuals who are living independently.

The following assessment methods are used to assess nutritional needs:

- A thorough medical history, physical examination, and dietary history can provide overview of the individual's nutritional status. Lab values also provide valuable information.
- Weight evaluation may be recommended. Normal weight status guidelines include a BMI of 21–25 (BMI = weight in kg/height in meter^2).
- Dehydration evaluation involves physical assessment (poor skin turgor, dark urine, flushed skin), and assessment of recent fluid and food intake. High laboratory levels of blood urea nitrogen (BUN), albumin, serum sodium, and serum osmolality can indicate dehydration.

Nutrient Needs

Nutrient needs are different in elderly people as compared to younger individuals. This means that seniors need to get a different amount of nutrients while consuming fewer calories. As the age increases, energy requirements progressively decrease. Older individuals are more likely to be deficient in certain nutrients, and they need to make an effort to meet the RDA for these nutrients (Tables 5.29 and 5.30).

Table 5.29: Daily calorie needs of an elderly

Gender	Sedentary lifestyle	Active lifestyle
Elderly women	1,600 calories	2,000 calories
Elderly men	2,000 calories	2,400 calories

Table 5.30: Recommended daily allowances for elderly people

Nutrients	Amount required
Carbohydrate	130 g
Protein	46 g/day in women and 56 g per day in men

Contd...

Nutrients	Amount required
Vitamin A	700–900 IU
Vitamin B_{12}	2.4 µg
Vitamin C	75–90 mg
Vitamin D	800 IU
Fiber	21–30 g
Zinc	8–11 mg
Iron	8 mg
Calcium	1,200 mg, 0.8 g
Folate	400 µg
Sodium	1,500 mg

Points to be kept in mind while meeting nutritional requirements of elderly people:

- They should be given smaller and frequent portions of food to get sufficient amounts of essential nutrients. Because everyone's metabolism is different, the proper portion sizes for seniors will depend on the amount of calories they need to consume to maintain a healthy weight.
- Seniors should prefer more unprocessed foods as they usually contain more nutrients and less fat, added sugar and sodium.
- Calcium and vitamin D play an important role in maintaining bone health. Many older adults do not get enough vitamin B_{12}. Lack of vitamin B_{12} can lead to macrocytic anemia and neurological problems that may affect sensory and motor function. Increasing potassium intake and reducing salt intake can lower your risk of high blood pressure.
- Dehydration is a form of malnutrition and can be a problem in older adults, especially those over the age of 85. Dehydration can lead to constipation, confusion, functional decline and, in some cases, death. Generally, older adults need liquid intake 3.7 liters of fluids a day for men; and it is 2.7 liters a day for women.
- Elderly individuals need fewer calories. They tend to have less muscle mass, which decreases the amount of calories needed to maintain their weight because fat requires fewer calories to maintain the muscle. They also have slower metabolisms, so it takes them longer to burn the calories that they consume through their daily activities.
- The habit of eating fruits and vegetables reduces the risk of chronic diseases and treats them as they provide the body with essential vitamins and minerals. If fruits and vegetables are difficult to eat because of their texture, try purchasing canned items or cooking fruits and vegetables until they are soft.
- A sample diet plan for an elderly man is given in Table 5.31.

Table 5.31: Sample menu plan for an elderly man

Meal	Menu
Early morning	Herbal/green tea, digestive biscuit
Breakfast	Dalia, boiled egg, potato/onion toast with butter
Midmorning	1 bowl of vegetable soup
Lunch	Chapatis/rice, green gram dal, mix steamed vegetables, boondi raita, grated salad

Contd...

Meal	Menu
Evening	Vegetable poha/seasonal fruit
Dinner	• Dal (moong dal), chapatis • Fruit custard • Grated salad
Bedtime	Milk

CLEAR LIQUID DIET

Definition

A clear liquid diet consists of clear liquids—such as water, broth and plain gelatin that are easily digested and leave no undigested residue in intestinal tract. Liquid diet is given to the clients who cannot chew and swallow the food. Clear liquid diet cannot provide adequate calories and nutrients, thus should not be continued for more than a few days. It is free from any solid particles. At beginning, the amount of fluid given to the patients is restricted to about 40–80 mL/hr, then the quantity is increased gradually up to 100–120 mL.

Purposes

- A clear liquid diet is often used before tests, procedures or surgeries that require no food in stomach or intestines, such as before colonoscopy.
- A clear liquid diet helps maintain adequate hydration, provides some important electrolytes, such as sodium and potassium, and gives some energy at a time when a full diet is not possible or recommended.
- It may also be recommended as a short-term diet if the patient has certain digestive problems, such as nausea, vomiting or diarrhea, or after certain types of surgery.
- It is also prescribed pre- and postoperatively to prevent aspiration.

The following foods are allowed in a clear liquid diet:

- Water (plain, carbonated or flavored)
- Fruit juices without pulp, such as apple or white grape
- Fruit-flavored beverages, such as fruit punch or lemonade
- Carbonated drinks, including dark sodas (cola and root beer)
- Gelatin, tea, coffee
- Tea or coffee without milk or cream
- Strained tomato or vegetable juice
- Sports drinks
- Clear, fat-free broth
- Honey or sugar
- Hard candy, such as lemon drops or peppermint rounds
- Ice pops without milk, bits of fruit, seeds or nuts

Sample menu plan for clear liquid diet is given in Table 5.32.

Table 5.32: Sample menu plan for clear liquid diet

Meal	Food Items
Breakfast	• Clear vegetable broth (strained) • Herbal tea or clear coconut water
Mid-Morning Snack	Clear apple juice or lemonade (strained)
Lunch	• Clear vegetable soup (strained) • OR Clear chicken broth (strained)
Evening Snack	Clear herbal tea or clear coconut water
Dinner	• Clear vegetable broth (strained) • OR Clear strained fruit juice

Important considerations:

- **Fluid intake:** Ensure adequate hydration with clear liquids throughout the day.
- **Nutrient supplementation:** Consider vitamin and mineral supplements as this diet lacks essential nutrients.
- **Avoid:** Avoid colored or pulpy liquids, dairy products, and solid foods.

FULL LIQUID DIET

Full liquid diet is composed of solids, which are easily digestible mixed in liquid. This diet is prescribed for severely ill clients who are not able to chew and swallow but need good calories. Full liquid diet is often used after some types of surgery or if patients have certain digestive conditions that do not allow eating solid foods. It is prescribed for the patients who had infection, gastritis, and diarrhea. A full liquid diet is similar to a clear liquid diet, but can also consume milk, vegetable juice, pureed soups and strained cooked cereals if they are thinned with milk or water (Table 5.33).

Table 5.33: Sample menu plan for full liquid diet

Meal	Food Items
Breakfast	• Plain yogurt (curd) blended with water or milk/or • Rice or oats porridge blended with milk or water • Herbal tea or strained fruit juice
Mid-Morning Snack	Vegetable soup (strained and smooth)
Lunch	• Lentil (dal) soup (strained and smooth) • Clear vegetable broth (strained)
Evening Snack	Clear fruit juice or smoothie (strained and without pulp)
Dinner	• Creamy tomato soup (strained and smooth)/or • Mashed potato or sweet potato soup (strained and smooth) • Clear vegetable broth (strained)

Full liquid diets are usually low in calories and nutrients, so liquid dietary supplements such as powdered milk to creamed soups are added to get extra calories, or sweeten foods with sugar or liquid sweeteners such as honey or corn syrup.

Full Liquid Diet Food List

- All kinds of fruit and vegetable juices
- Pureed fruit, or vegetables
- Milk, soy or almond milk
- Yogurt (without fruit chunks)
- Melted cheese
- Eggs can be eaten like a soft custard
- Honey
- Coffee, tea
- Soft drinks, sports drinks
- Strained cooked cereal
- Broth
- Creamed soup (no pieces or chunks of vegetables or meats)
- Pureed meat can be added to soup (again, no chunks)
- Flavored gelatin
- Ice cream (no fruit, chocolate chips, etc.)

SEMISOLID DIET

This diet is softer form of the normal balanced diet. It is given to the patients on way to recovery from acute illness and to patients having chewing problems. This diet is nutritionally adequate and large variety of food can be given.

A semisolid diet includes foods like scrambled egg, low-fat cottage cheese or blenderized lean meats like tuna or chicken (Table 5.34). Blend foods with water, fat-free milk or broth to create a smooth consistency. Additionally, soft fruits and vegetables can be pureed and included into the semisolid diet. Cold semi solid diet is given to patients with tonsillectomy. In this diet, patients continue to gradually add soft, or semisolid, foods into the diet. The semisolid foods stage can last for eight or more weeks. Surgery wounds are nearly healed, but solid, sharp foods can still cause damage. This diet increases the emphasis on low-calorie, high-nutrient choices.

Table 5.34: Sample menu plan for semisolid diet

Meal timings	Foods
Breakfast	Scrambled egg whites with bread topped with low-fat cheese or butter and fat-free milk, ripe banana
Midmorning	Mashed sweet potatoes or fruit custard
Lunch	Well-cooked rice with thin moong dal
Evening time	Oatmeal made with skim milk or 2 tbs dry milk powder
Dinner	Khichdi/upma, curd
Night time	Warm milk/milk shake

List of Foods

- Canned tuna or chicken
- Eggs, egg whites or fat-free, cholesterol-free egg substitute
- Well-cooked rice and pasta
- Fresh, ripe fruit
- Well-cooked vegetables (not broccoli, asparagus, celery)
- Low-fat or fat-free cheese
- Fish be very careful of bones
- Cooked beans and lentils
- Khichdi
- Porridge

SOFT DIET

A soft food diet is basically a diet that contains foods that have been softened by chopping, cooking or mashing and are easy to eat and swallow. Such foods should not be high in fiber content and also not gas inducing. A soft diet menu is not the same as the ones in a bland diet, menu. Examples of such foods are soft breads, muffins, dairy products, scrambled and soft boiled eggs, tomatoes, bananas (Table 5.35).

Table 5.35: Sample menu plan for soft diet

Meal timings	Foods
Early morning	Fruit juice
Breakfast	Scrambled eggs + bread + milk and wheat porridge
Lunch	Khichdi/curd
Evening time	Pudding, mashed banana (or any other fruit)
Dinner	Vegetable soup, mashed potatoes, well cooked rice
Bedtime	Milk

Indications of Soft Diet

- **A soft diet is usually recommended after certain medical procedure such as:**
  - Gastric bypass
  - Mouth surgery
  - Dental procedures
  - Preparation for certain medical tests
  - Patients had surgery of mouth, neck or head
- **Soft diet for old people:** Soft food diets are also recommended for old people because as one grows old it becomes more difficult to eat whole, hard food.
- **Soft diet after surgery:** A soft diet after surgery is recommended as this eliminates certain foods, which are difficult to digest and chew. Patients who have undergone neck or head surgery, intestinal surgery or even those who have undergone chemotherapy or radiation benefit from a soft diet. Foods that should be avoided on this soft diet include gas forming foods such as cauliflower, and broccoli.

Soft Diet Food List

A mechanical soft diet food list comprises the foods given below:

- Pudding
- Canned milk shakes
- Cooked cereal
- Pancakes
- Dairy products such as cottage cheese, yogurt, ice cream and milk
- Soft scrambled eggs
- Fruit sauce
- Pureed vegetables
- Mashed bananas
- Apple sauce
- Mashed potato
- Mashed pumpkin
- Creamed peas
- Broiled or stewed chicken
- Tofu
- Breads: soft breads without crusts.
- Ice cream or custards, soft breads
- Grains: Include cooked cereals
- Foods that should be avoided are hard and thick breads, tough meats, dried fruit, raw fruit and vegetables, fruits with skin or seeds and foods that have nuts or seeds

HIGH FIBER DIET

Diets high in fiber may reduce the risk of obesity, heart disease, and diabetes. Along with fiber and adequate fluid intakes, fiber is responsible for quickly moving foods through the digestive tract, helping it function optimally. Fiber works by drawing fluids from the body to add bulk to the stool. When increasing dietary fiber in diet, it is essential to start slowly, and increase gradually. A sample menu plan for high fiber diet is given in Table 5.36.

Table 5.36: Sample menu plan for high-fiber diet

Meal timings	Foods
Breakfast	Corn flakes, whole grain bread with boiled egg and milk.
Midmorning	1 seasonal fruit apple/guava
Lunch	Brown rice, dal, vegetable spinach with potato, chapati, salad
Midafternoon	Vegetable upma/sweet potato chaat
Dinner	Steamed mix vegetables and chapati and fruit custard

Recommended Daily Fiber

Women: 25 g/day

Men: 35–40 g/day

Types of fiber: Both soluble fiber and insoluble fiber has recently been shown important in helping to control and manage many diseases.

- **Insoluble fiber:** Bulking fibers absorb water as they move through the digestive system, easing defecation. It provides bulk in the intestines, while helping to balance the pH levels in the intestines. It promotes regular bowel movements, and helps to prevent constipation. Insoluble fiber does not dissolve in water, and does not ferment with bacteria in the colon. It helps to prevent diverticulosis and hemorrhoids.
- **Soluble fiber:** Soluble fiber, which dissolves in water, is readily fermented in the colon into gases and physiologically active byproducts, and can be prebiotic and viscous. Soluble fiber helps to lower cholesterol and helps to regulate blood sugar levels for individuals with diabetes. It is present in beans, legumes, oats, barley, berries, and some vegetables. It does ferment in the stomach, which can lead to bloating and gas. Increase these foods gradually, and drink plenty of water.

Benefits of High-fiber Foods

- **High-fiber diets lower the risk:** Risk of some cancers, diverticulitis, heart disease, kidney stones, and obesity are lowered through high-fiber foods. For individuals with digestive tract conditions, dietary fiber may help to relieve symptoms. High fiber helps to shift the balance of bacteria, increasing healthy bacteria, while decreasing the unhealthy bacteria that can be the root of some digestive problems. Prebiotic soluble fiber products, like those containing inulin or oligosaccharides, may contribute to relief from inflammatory bowel disease, Crohn's disease.
- **Dietary fibers help in reducing blood cholesterol level:** Binding of bile acids to fiber or bacteria in the cecum with increased fecal loss from the enterohepatic circulation. The enteric loss of bile acids results in increased synthesis of bile acids from cholesterol, which in turn reduces body cholesterol.
- **Dietary fiber and obesity:** Dietary fiber has many functions in diet, one of which may be to aid in energy intake control and reduced risk for development of obesity.

Sources

Soluble Fibers

- Legumes (peas, soybeans, lupins and other beans).
- Oats, rye and barley.
- Some fruits (including figs, avocados, plums, prunes, berries, ripe bananas, and the skin of apples, quinces and pears).
- Certain vegetables such as broccoli, carrots, and Jerusalem artichokes.
- Root tubers and root vegetables such as sweet potatoes and onions (skins of these are sources of insoluble fiber also).
- Psyllium seed husks (a mucilage soluble fiber) and flax seeds.
- Nuts, with almonds being the highest in dietary fiber.

Insoluble Fibers

- Whole grain foods
- Wheat and corn bran
- Legumes such as beans and peas
- Nuts and seeds
- Potato skins
- Lingams
- Vegetables such as green beans, cauliflower, zucchini (courgette), and celery
- Some fruits including avocado, and unripe bananas
- The skins of some fruits, including kiwifruit, grapes and tomatoes

FACTORS AFFECTING THE DIET ACCEPTANCE IN PATIENTS

A person's dietary pattern is usually slow during his illness because of multiple factors. In hospital, choice of the food by the patient is influenced by various factors that includes environment, psychological, culture, socioeconomic status, satiety value, secondary effect of drug therapy and disease condition of the client.

- **Environmental factor:** Hospital environment is totally different from the home environment. In hospital, there are numerous factors that can affect the intake of diet such as noise, dirt, unpleasant odors, excessive heat or cold, unpleasant objects like sputum cups, bedpans, equipment used for carrying out medical or nursing procedure, etc. Hence attractive surrounding and cheerful environment (must be free from unpleasant odor or sight) must be provided during the meal timings in the hospitals.
- **Psychological factors:** Emotion strongly influences the eating habits of the individuals. Emotional status such as boredom, anger, depression, stress can influence the quality and quantity of the food eaten. For example, in case of depression some people suffer from anorexia and some urge to do overeating.
- **Religious factors:** There are many different customs regarding foods in various religions, for example, Hindus do not eat beef whereas Muslims and Jews do not eat pork. On the other hand, some people are pure vegetarians or some can consume eggs. Therefore, adequate diets must be planned to meet the nutritional requirement of the client by keeping the religion and sentiments of the client in mind.
- **Economical factors:** The adequacy of a person's food budget affects dietary choices and patterns. The increasing cost of food coupled with limited purchasing power may result in a decrease in the nutritional quality of the diet. So while planning diet, economic status of the client must be kept in mind, for example, groundnut can be a substitute for the almonds.
- **Lifestyle factors:** Also has a great impact on eating habits as people who spend enough time at home can prepare healthy meals and take it on proper time. On the other side, people who are always busy and in hurry prefer to buy convenience grocery (fast food) or eat outside that affects their health. Due to busy schedule fast food has become the first choice of many youngsters.
- **Basal metabolic rate:** BMR is the factor that influences the nutritional requirement of the client. During disease condition, Basal Metabolic Rate increases thus high calorie diet is necessary and in other disease condition low calorie diet is needed.
- **Age:** Age also influences nutritional status of the patient. Young children need more energy and protein than adult. In a diseased condition, client needs the food item that are easily digestible and high in nutritive value.
- **Sex:** Sex also makes variation in energy requirements. Women need low calorie as compared to men. Women are more taste sensitive.

- **Cultural factors:** Cultural factor in health and nutrition has also gained the attention of the dietician. Every culture has its own customs and beliefs regarding nutritional practices, for example, papaya is avoided in some societies because it is believed to cause abortion.
- **Satiety value:** Food must also be satisfying. Physical and mental fatigue should be avoided. Physical exhaustion can be relieved by resting before a meal. Mental fatigue can be overcome by arousing a pleasant thought or idea.
- **Availability of food:** Preferred therapeutic diet availability at some seasons may affect the acceptance of the diet.
- **Texture of diet:** Some foods contexts also affect the patient's nutritional status. If a person had lost his denture he would not be able to take solid food.

FEEDING THE HELPLESS PATIENTS

When a client comes in hospital, the nurse must take care of all the basic needs of the client. The most common need is nutritional need that must be planned according to his/her physical condition, metabolic changes, food habits/preferences and socioeconomic status. The following are the points to remember while feeding a helpless client:

- Check doctor's order for any specific precaution regarding the diet, moment or positioning of the client.
- Plan the diet according to the need, likes or dislikes and socioeconomic status of the client.
- Check the general condition of the client and ability to accept feeding.
- Unpleasurable odor or articles like sputum mug, bed pan must be removed from the client unit before serving the meal.
- A helpless client should be fed carefully by placing client into semi-Fowler position to prevent aspiration.
- After feeding, all the dishes should be removed immediately and the client should be helped to wash his hand and rinse mouth or brush the teeth to provide comfort if the client is in his conscious state.
- Diet should not be served immediately after painful procedure.
- Client must be comfortable before feeding. Different comfort devices like cardiac table; side table must be used as an aid to comfort the client.
- Client should be given sufficient time to chew and taste the food. Never feed the client hurriedly.
- Psychological condition of the patient must be kept in mind before feeding as the client is in different environment and he/she may feel insecure, fear, worry, anger, depression, homesickness, pain, etc. that can interfere the process of feeding.
- Sometime a sick person denies to accept the food. Nurse must encourage the client by providing proper knowledge and benefits of taking nutritious food but the client should never be forced to eat.
- In some disease conditions (cardiovascular accident), suction apparatus must be kept aside the client bed to prevent any complication of feeding.
- Fluid requirement should be met to prevent dehydration. Fluids are given at the end of meal or can be given in between the meal in small amounts.
- Meal should be served in clean and covered containers. Care must be taken to prevent transmission of diseases through the food and drinks.
- Create a pleasant environment for the clients.

NUTRITIONAL EDUCATION

Nutritional education is important in improving the health status of the family and community. In community, there are the people that belong to different socioeconomic status. People with low economic status hesitate to purchase qualitative things and high status people eat the things which are not useful for them. Education level, religion, custom, culture also influence the nutritional status of the person. Thus it is the responsibility of the nurse to provide teaching and awareness regarding the balanced diet.

Purposes

- To impart good dietary habits amongst the population.
- To select good and nutritious foods.
- To teach hygienic practices in handling and preservation of the food.
- To budget their menu by using exchange list system.
- To use various methods in cooking.

Principles

- **Understanding the client:**
  - **Cultural sensitivity:** Respect and understand the client's cultural background, including traditions, beliefs, and practices related to health and food.
  - **Food preferences:** Consider the client's likes and dislikes when suggesting dietary changes or improvements.
  - **Religious considerations:** Be mindful of religious dietary restrictions or preferences that may affect food choices.
  - **Socioeconomic status:** Take into account the client's economic situation when recommending foods or health practice.
  - **Educational status:** Determine the client's level of education to provide health information appropriately according to education level of the client.
- **Gradual introduction of new ideas:** Introduce new health concepts gradually, focusing on one topic at a time to ensure understanding and retention.
- **Enhancing communication:** Use local words and terms for food items to improve communication and understanding.
- **Practical tools:** Use real foods, nutritional posters, flip charts, puppets, and role-playing to discuss health issues effectively.
- **Affordable recommendations:** Avoid recommending foods or practices that clients cannot afford or implement due to financial constraints.
- **Supporting families in food preparation:** Offer guidance to families on selecting, storing, and preparing food items to enhance nutrition and food safety.
- **Based on facts:** Provide information that is backed by science and reliable sources.
- **Personalization:** Give advice that fits each person's needs and goals.
- **Practical advice:** Offer realistic tips that can be easily applied in daily life.
- **Active learning:** Encourage participation and interaction to help people learn.

- **Long-term thinking:** Focus on habits that support health over the long term.
- **Empowerment:** Help people feel confident in making healthy choices for themselves.

Methods

- This education must be based on actual needs of the community people and a nurse or health personnel should prepare a proper audio-visual aids for effective health education.
- Practical methods may include short menu plans, budgeting of food and calculating the calorie of the food items, etc.
- Give cooking demonstration of various food dishes, which are useful but not known by the people such as preparing weaning diet for the infant.
- Personal talks means give the information to the person through one to one communication on specific topics regarding the food and nutrition such as menu planning, various food exchange list, balanced diet, high calorie diet, low calorie diet. Personal talks do not need any specific preparation of the person.
    - **Exhibition:** In exhibition, various shows are performed such as practical menus of using fresh vegetables and fruits, how to grow variety of seasonal vegetables. For example, in exhibition of spices various condiments are displayed and their usage, benefits for the health are taught.
    - **Posters:** Through posters calorie value of any food items, any specific diet such as diabetic diet, menu for renal diseases, infant diets can be taught to the community.
    - **Group discussion:** It is a method through which 6–12 members can participate and discuss various nutritional issues and nutritional problems. Here, the participants can clear their doubts regarding any particular topic.

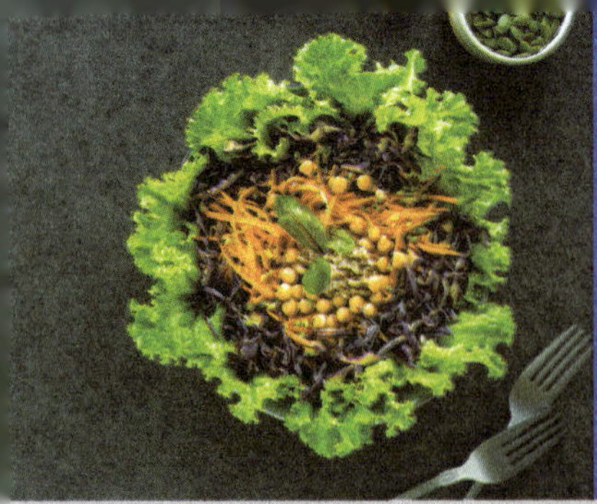

STUDENT ASSIGNMENT

LONG ANSWER QUESTIONS

1. Discuss common problems in old age people and the points to be kept in mind while meeting the nutritional requirements of the elderly people.
2. What is bland diet and why it is recommended?
3. What are the factors affecting the acceptance of diet?
4. Define PEM and write the difference between marasmus and kwashiorkor.
5. Explain the points to be kept in mind while feeding a helpless patient.
6. Define nutrition education and enlist the principles of nutrition education.

SHORT ANSWER QUESTIONS

1. Define Therapeutic diet and enlist the types of modification in the diet.
2. What type of modification in diet is required for the diabetic patient?
3. Plan a one-day diet plan for an anemic patient.
4. Discuss modification of diet for the following conditions:
   a. Obesity
   b. Hepatitis
   c. Irritable bowel syndrome

MULTIPLE CHOICE QUESTIONS

1. Which of the following does not contain fat?

a. Meat
b. Butter
c. Cheese
d. Sugar

2. Excessive energy is stored in the body in the form of:

a. Fat
b. Fiber
c. Water
d. Salt

3. Following food content must be added in the diet:

a. Salt
b. Sugar
c. Fiber
d. Fat

4. Goiter of neck is caused by the deficiency of the following:

a. Iodine
c. Calcium
c. Proteins
d. Chlorine

5. **Therapeutic diet is used:**
   a. To provide change in consistency of food
   b. To include greater or lesser amount of one or more nutrients
   c. To modify the method of feeding
   d. All of the above

6. **Which of the following does not come under liquid diet?**
   a. Fruit juices
   b. Clear vegetable/dal soup
   c. Beverages
   d. Khichdi

7. **In the disease diabetes mellitus, following diet is recommended:**
   a. Low carbohydrate diet
   b. High carbohydrate diet
   c. High fat diet
   d. Low protein diet

8. **Low calorie diet is recommended for the following disease condition:**
   a. Osteoarthritis
   b. Obesity
   c. Malnourished
   d. Gout

9. **Following nutrient requirement is more in females than males:**
   a. Phosphorus
   b. Sulfur
   c. Floride
   d. Iron

10. **Person suffering from cardiovascular diseases must avoid the following:**
    a. Whole grains, cereals and pulses
    b. Green leafy vegetables, high-fiber fruits
    c. Whole milk, cheese, butter, cream
    d. Egg white, lean meat

11. **Normal value of glucose in blood is:**
    a. 80–120 mg/dL
    b. 60–80 mg/dL
    c. 120–140 mg/dL
    d. 150–170 mg/dL

12. **Harmful effects of excessive fat is/are:**
    a. Obesity
    b. Atheriosclerosis and coronary artery disease
    c. Increase risk of cancer
    d. All of the above

13. **Which of the following therapeutic diets is typically prescribed for individuals with hypertension?**
    a. Low-fat diet
    b. Low-sodium diet
    c. High-protein diet
    d. Low-carbohydrate diet

14. **Which type of diet is recommended for individuals with celiac disease?**
    a. Low-residue diet
    b. Gluten-free diet
    c. Ketogenic diet
    d. High-fiber diet

15. **Which types of diet is commonly used for patients with diabetes mellitus?**
    a. Low-sodium diet
    b. Low-protein diet
    c. Low-fat diet
    d. Carbohydrate-controlled diet

16. **Which therapeutic diet is suitable for patients with chronic kidney disease (CKD) who are on dialysis?**

a. High-protein diet
b. Low-potassium diet
c. Low-calorie diet
d. High-sodium diet

17. **Which therapeutic diet is beneficial for individuals with lactose intolerance?**

a. Dairy-free diet
b. High-calcium diet
c. High-protein diet
d. Low-fat diet

18. **Which type of diet is appropriate for patients with cardiovascular disease?**

a. Low-sodium diet
b. Low-cholesterol diet
c. High-potassium diet
d. High-fiber diet

19. **Which therapeutic diet would be recommended for individuals with gastroesophageal reflux disease (GERD)?**

a. High-fat diet
b. Low-fiber diet
c. Low-protein diet
d. Low-acid diet

20. **Which type of diet is commonly prescribed for patients recovering from gastrointestinal surgery?**

a. Clear liquid diet
b. Full liquid diet
c. Soft diet
d. Low-residue diet

21. **Which therapeutic diet is suitable for patients with liver disease encephalopathy?**

a. High-protein diet
b. Low-sodium diet
c. Low-protein diet
d. Low-ammonia diet

22. **What is the primary goal of nutritional education?**

a. Promoting specific diet products
b. Educating individuals on proper nutrition practices
c. Selling nutritional supplements
d. Discouraging healthy eating habits

23. **Which principle of nutrition education emphasizes tailoring information to the specific needs and preferences of individuals or groups?**

a. Accuracy
b. Clarity
c. Relevance
d. Engagement

24. **What is the primary goal of introducing new nutrition-related ideas gradually during education sessions?**

a. To overwhelm participants with information
b. To ensure all topics are covered in one session
c. To reinforce key concepts over time
d. To save time during the session

25. **Why is it important to assess the educational status of participants in nutrition education programs?**

a. To exclude those with lower education levels
b. To customize the delivery of information appropriately
c. To prepare certificates for completion
d. To prioritize advanced topics

26. Which approach improves communication during nutrition education by using local terminology for food items?

a. Respect
b. Engagement
c. Clarity
d. Cultural sensitivity

27. Why is nutrition education particularly effective in schools?

a. Because it is mandatory for teachers to teach it
b. Because children are more likely to change behaviors learned at a young age
c. Because it is easier to monitor children's diets
d. Because schools have better resources

28. During pregnancy, why is nutrition education crucial for both the mother and the baby?

a. To help the mother lose weight
b. To prevent the mother from eating certain foods
c. To improve the mother's health and ensure the baby's healthy development
d. To keep the mother away from eating too much

29. Which teaching method is effective in nutrition education for illustrating healthy food choices?

a. Using theoretical concepts only
b. Using actual foods, especially locally produced ones
c. Using abstract diagrams
d. Using historical data

30. What is an important consideration when recommending dietary changes during nutrition education?

a. Recommending expensive foods
b. Recommending trendy diets
c. Recommending foods not culturally appropriate
d. Recommending foods based on personal preference

31. How can nutrition education support families in improving food preparation techniques?

a. By providing pre-made meals
b. By teaching better selection, storage, and preparation of foods
c. By only giving recipes
d. By providing free cooking lessons

ANSWER KEY

1. d	**2.** a	**3.** c	**4.** a	**5.** d	**6.** d	**7.** a	**8.** b	**9.** d
10. c	**11.** a	**12.** d	**13.** b	**14.** b	**15.** d	**16.** b	**17.** a	**18.** b
19. d	**20.** d	**21.** d	**22.** b	**23.** c	**24.** c	**25.** b	**26.** d	**27.** b
28. c	**29.** b	**30.** c	**31.** b					

Notes

6

Community Nutrition

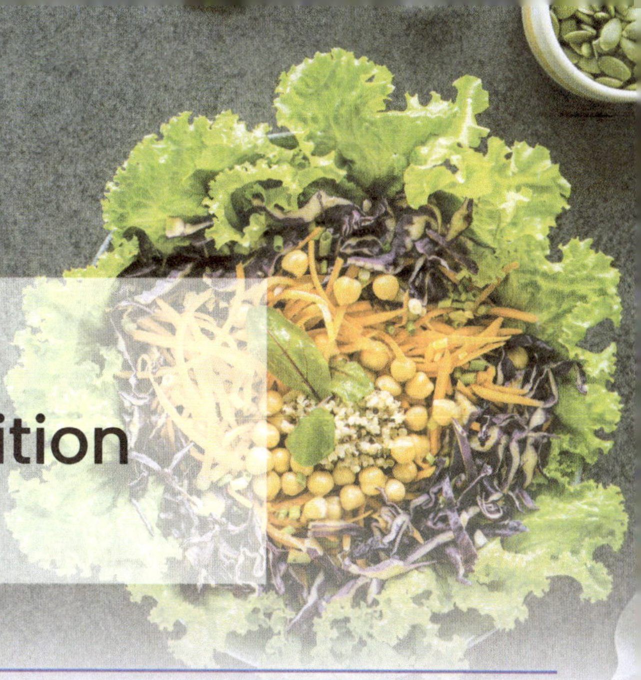

LEARNING OBJECTIVES

After the completion of the chapter, the readers will be able to:

- Explain nutritional problems and programs in India.
- Discuss community food supply and food hygiene.
- Discuss National and International food agencies.

CHAPTER OUTLINE

- Common Definitions
- Nutritional Problems in India
- Community Nutrition Programs
- National Nutrition Policy
- Community Food Supply
- Public Distribution System
- Food Hygiene
- Food-borne Diseases
- Commercially Prepared Food
- Locally-grown Food
- National and International Food Agencies

KEY TERMS

Commercially prepared food: Tertiary processed food that is prepared (often through processing) to optimize ease of consumption.

Food additives: These are chemicals that keep food fresh or enhance their color, flavor or texture.

Food hygiene: It refers to hygiene practices in all the areas that include production, packaging, handling and distribution.

Food toxicants: These are harmful substances found in food.

Meat hygiene: It is the prevention of transmission of disease from animal to man and to provide safe product for human consumption.

Pasteurization of milk: It is the process of heating and cooling of liquids or foods at specific temperature to kill microorganisms.

Slaughter houses: These are the places where animals are killed and the flesh is intended for human consumption.

COMMON DEFINITIONS

- **Food additives:** These are chemicals that keep food fresh or enhance their color, flavor or texture. For example, flavor enhancer monosodium glutamate (MSG) is commonly used in packed foods like maggi.
- **Food toxicants:** These are harmful substances found in food. When such food is ingested, it causes toxic effects that present the risk of death, disease, injury and birth defects. It may be natural or synthetic (man made). For example, neurolathyrism is the disease caused by beta oxalyl amino alanine, which is found in the seeds of pulses (kesari dal).

NUTRITIONAL PROBLEMS IN INDIA

Adequate nutrition is essential for human development. According to population, India is the second largest country in the world and many people in the country belong to low socioeconomic status and are suffering from many nutritional problems. Some common nutritional problems among Indians are as follows:

Nutritional Anemia

It is a worldwide problem with the highest prevalence in developing countries. It can be divided into iron deficiency anemia and vitamin deficiency anemia.

Iron Deficiency Anemia

In India, it is the widespread deficiency that is very common among children and women of reproductive age group (15–49 years). It is seen more frequently in adolescent girls and in pregnant women. World Health Organization (WHO) defines it as a condition in which hemoglobin level of the blood is lower than the normal as a result of deficiency of one or more essential nutrients.

- **Causes of iron deficiency anemia:** Iron deficiency can arise due to inadequate intake of iron and vitamin C as vitamin C helps in the absorption of iron. Anemia is caused due to excess loss of iron from the body as in case of women during menstruation or any other medical condition that leads to heavy blood loss. Some other causes are malaria, hookworm infestation and mothers who have children at very close interval. Any disease or medical condition that prevents the body from absorbing enough nutrients also contributes to anemia.
- **Symptoms of iron deficiency anemia include:**
  - Pale skin and eyes (Fig. 6.1)
  - Spoon-shaped finger nails (Fig. 6.2)
  - Sores or ulcers in the mouth and tongue
  - Hair loss
  - Dyspnea (difficulty in breathing)
  - Changes in the sense of taste
  - Itchiness
  - Menstruation irregularities in females
  - Fatigue and lack of energy
  - Complication of anemia includes the higher risk of maternal and fetal mortality and morbidity

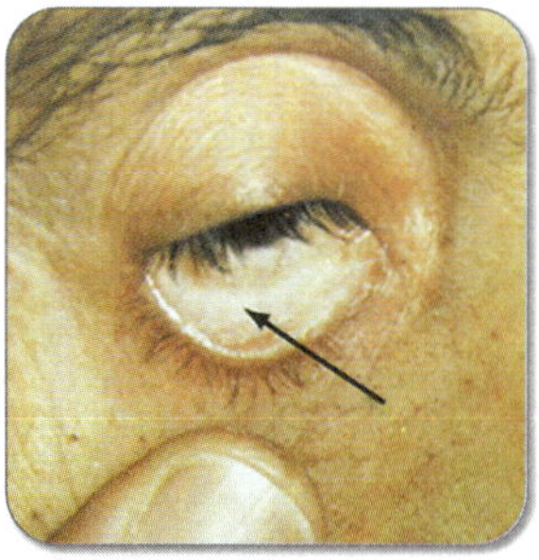

Fig. 6.1: Pale eyes (conjunctiva) in iron deficiency anemia

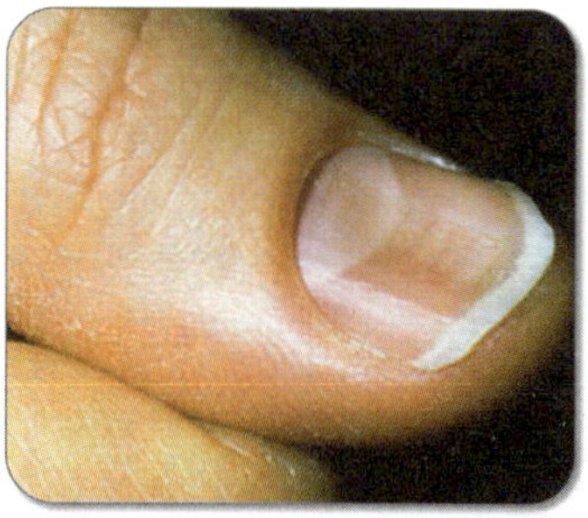

Fig. 6.2: Spoon shaped nails

Vitamin Deficiency Anemia

Vitamin deficiency anemia can develop when a person does not consume or is unable to absorb sufficient amount of vitamin B_{12} or folate (vitamin B_9). Deficiency of vitamin B_{12} is also known as megaloblastic anemia that is not very common in general population but can occur in pregnant women or people with low socioeconomic status.

Symptoms of vitamin deficiency anemia:

- Feeling of tingling sensation (pins or needle)
- Muscle weakness
- Lack of energy
- Difficulty with concentration, thinking and memory, confusion
- Long-term complications include infertility, complication during pregnancy, nervous system disorders and cardiac problems.

Vitamin Deficiency Diseases

Vitamin A Deficiency

Vitamin A is very essential for the formation of rhodopsin (A photoreceptor pigment in the retina). Vitamin A deficiency not only leads to disorder in the eye but also many other problems in the body.

- **Xerophthalmia (dry eyes) and blindness:** Xerophthalmia is a vitamin A deficiency disease in which the eye fails to produce tears. It is seen more common in children age 1–3 years. It is often associated with protein energy malnutrition (PEM). It affects about 8–10 million people worldwide. Poor dietary factors, lack of vitamins and severe malnutrition are the main causes of this disease. If it is left untreated, it may lead to blindness and corneal ulceration (Fig. 6.3).
- **Keratomalacia:** It is an eye condition in which cornea gets cloudy and softens and if this condition is not treated, it can lead to infection, rupture and tissue changes causing blindness (Fig. 6.4).

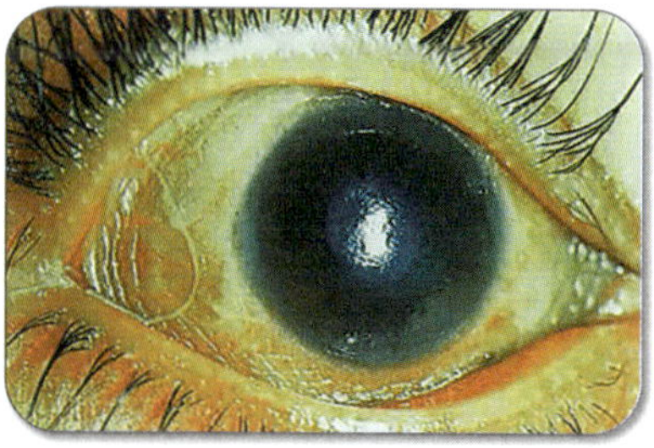

Fig. 6.3: Xerophthalmia

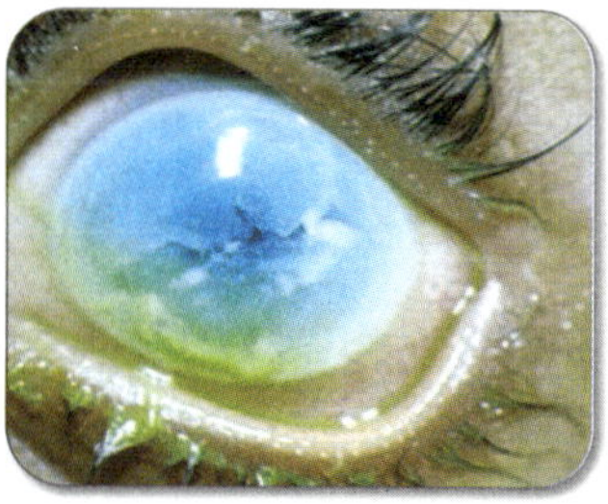

Fig. 6.4: Keratomalacia

- **Night blindness:** Severe vitamin A deficiency can cause night blindness. In this condition a person is unable to adjust the vision during dim or dark light.
- **Other vitamin A deficiency diseases:** Delayed growth in children, infertility, inflammatory skin conditions as vitamin A plays important role in skin repair and helps to fight inflammation. Deficiency of vitamin A can also lead to poor wound healing as vitamin A promotes the formation of collagen.

Vitamin C Deficiency Disease (Scurvy)

A severe form of deficiency of vitamin C is known as scurvy. Its symptoms include dry and splitting hair, bleeding from gum, delay in wound healing, rough, dry and scaly skin (Fig. 6.5). Vitamin C is needed for the health and repair of various tissues including skin, bone, teeth and cartilage.

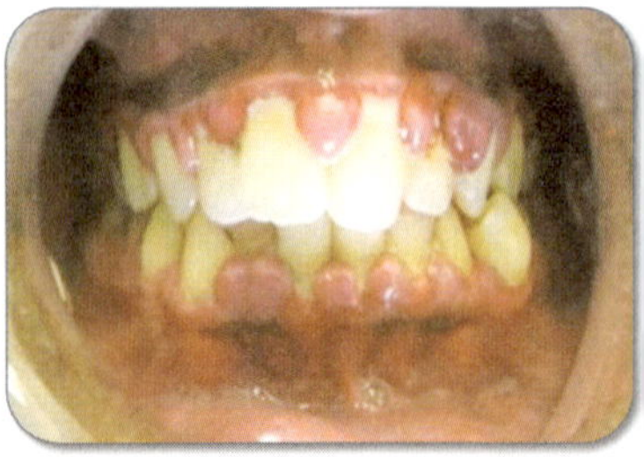

Fig. 6.5: Scurvy

Gingivitis: Gingivitis is a common and mild form of gum disease, characterized by inflammation, redness, swelling, and sometimes bleeding of the gums (Fig. 6.6). It occurs when plaque, a sticky film of bacteria, builds up on teeth and gums. If left untreated, gingivitis can progress to more severe forms of gum disease that can lead to tooth loss and other complications.

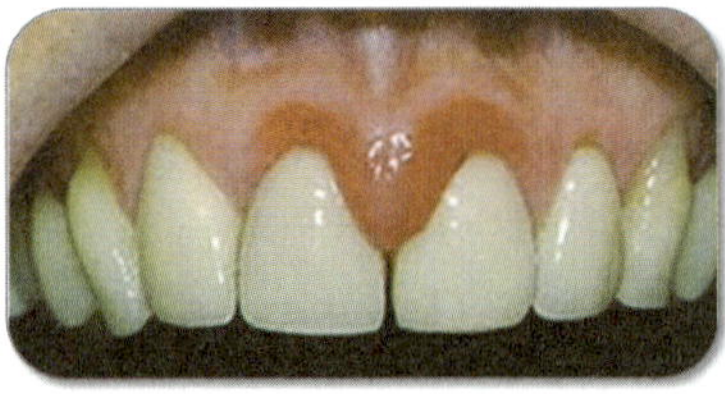

Fig. 6.6: Gingivitis

Vitamin D Deficiency Disease

Vitamin D is essential for strong bones because it helps the body to use calcium. Its deficiency may lead to problems like rickets (children) (Fig. 6.7) and osteomalacia (adults) (Fig. 6.8), diseases in which the softening of the bones and skeletal deformities occur. Symptoms of rickets include delayed growth, bow legs, weakness and pain in the spine, legs and pelvis. Symptoms of osteomalacia include muscular pain, difficulty in walking, spasm in arms and legs and very brittle bones that are prone for fracture. Vitamin D deficiency also causes low calcium and phosphate, which can lead to hyperparathyroidism.

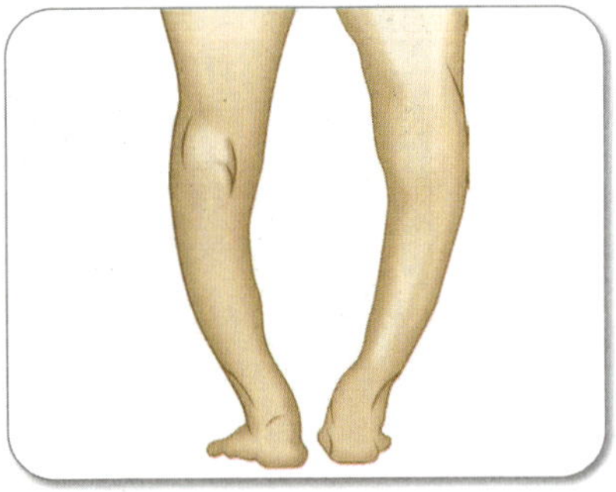

Fig. 6.7: Rickets

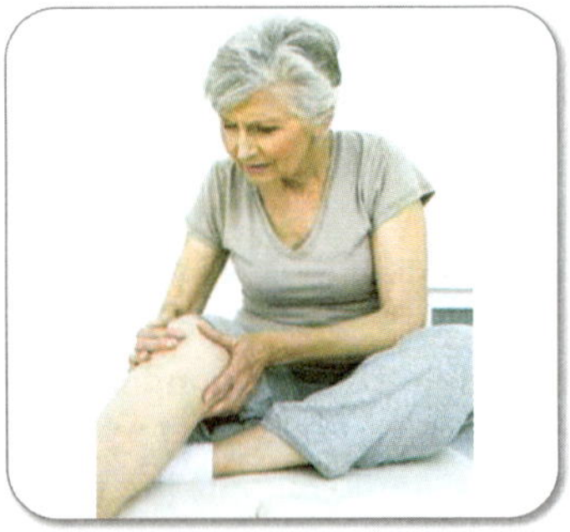

Fig. 6.8: Osteomalacia

Protein Energy Malnutrition

Protein energy malnutrition (PEM) is a major health and nutritional problem in India. It results from deficiency of proteins and calories in the food for longer time. It is very common among young children. It is not only an important cause of childhood morbidity and mortality but also leads to permanent impairment in physical and mental growth. Due to deficiency of proteins, children suffer mainly from two diseases named as marasmus and kwashiorkor (Table 6.1) (Figs 6.9 and 6.10).

Table 6.1: Differences between marasmus and kwashiorkor

Clinical features	Marasmus	Kwashiorkor
Muscle wasting	Seen obviously	Sometime hidden by edema and fat
Fat wasting	Severe loss of subcutaneous fat	Fat often retained but not firm
Edema	Not present	Present in lower legs, in face and forearm
Weight for height	Very low	Low but may be masked by edema
Mental changes	Sometimes quiet and apathetic	Irritable moaning and apathetic
Appetite	Usually good	Poor
Skin changes	Usually none	Diffuse pigmentation and dermatitis
Hair changes	Seldom	Sparse and easily pulled out
Hepatic enlargement	None	Sometimes due to accumulation of fat

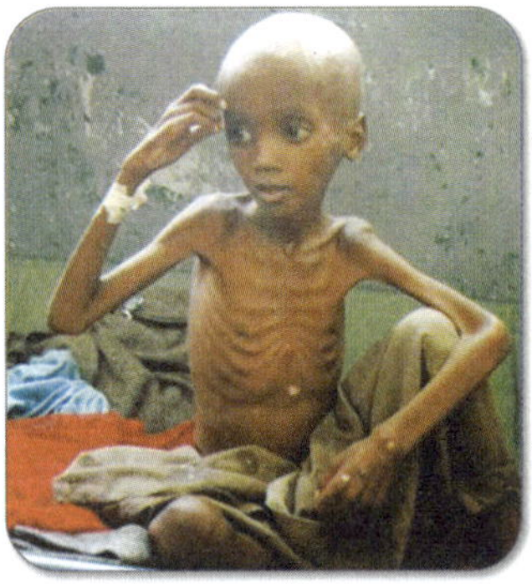

Fig. 6.9: Marasmus

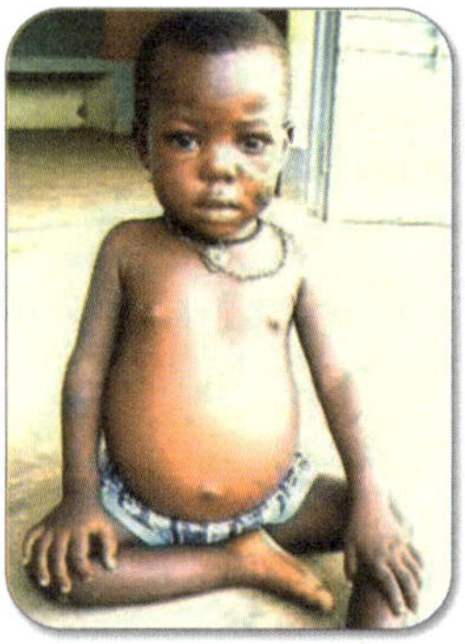

Fig. 6.10: Kwashiorkor

Another method to detect PEM is by the anthropometric measurement that can be seen by various methods and helps to detect the degree of malnutrition.

Low Birth Weight (<2500 g)

It is one of the major health problems in developing countries. Although this is a multifactorial problem, maternal malnutrition and anemia is considered the major cause of low birth weight. Hard physical labor during pregnancy, illness or any infection to the mother, motherhood in very young age, high parity, habits of smoking or alcoholism and close intervals between the births are some other factors responsible for low birth weight in newborn. In India, 28% newborns have low birth weight as compared to western countries where it is only 4% (Fig. 6.11).

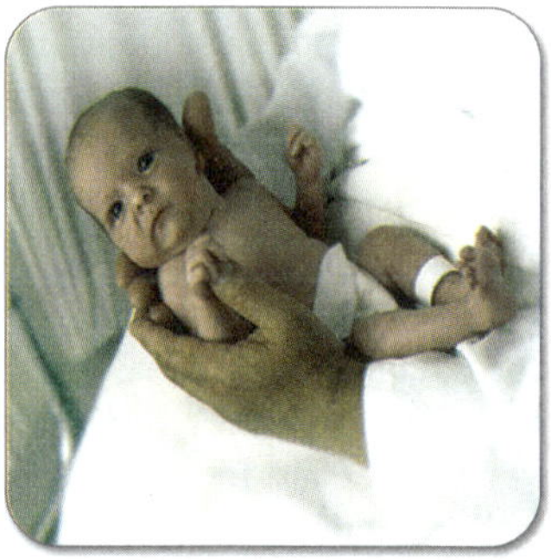

Fig. 6.11: Low birth weight baby

Iodine Deficiency Disorder

This is another major health problem that is endemic in Himalaya belt extending from Kashmir to Naga Hills in the east, about 24,000 km affecting northern states like Jammu and Kashmir, Himachal Pradesh, Punjab, Haryana, Delhi, Uttar Pradesh, Bihar, West Bengal, Sikkim, Assam, Arunachal Pradesh, Nagaland, Mizoram, Meghalaya, Tripura and Manipur. Deficiency of iodine not only causes **goiter** but also the disorders commencing with the intrauterine life and extending through childhood to adult life with serious health and social implications (Fig. 6.12).

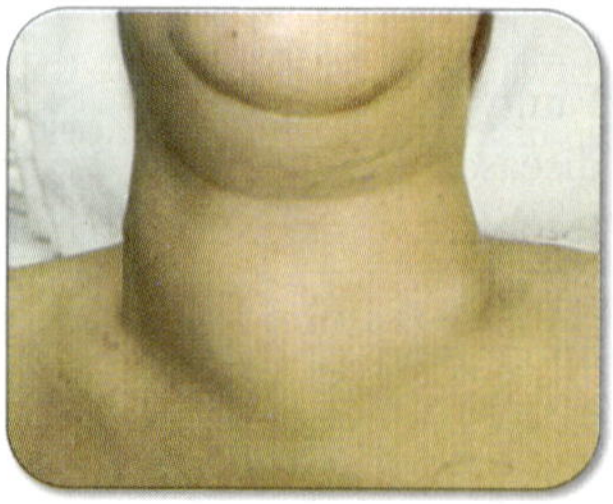

Fig. 6.12: Goiter

Fluorosis

In many parts of the country, where drinking water contains excessive amount of fluorine, an endemic fluorosis has been observed. It is of two types that are dental fluorosis and skeletal fluorosis:

1. **Dental fluorosis:** It is characterized by erosion of enamel of teeth. It results in loss of shiny appearance of the teeth and chalk white patches also develop upon the teeth (Fig. 6.13).
2. **Skeletal fluorosis:** It is a bone disease caused by excessive accumulation of fluorides in the bones. In advance cases, skeletal fluorosis causes pain and damage to bones and joints.

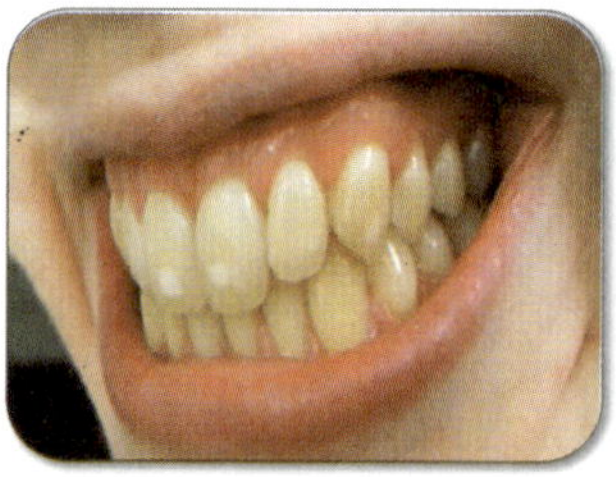

Fig. 6.13: Dental fluorosis

Lathyrism or Neurolathyrism

It is a neurological disease of humans and domestic animals, caused by eating certain legumes of the genus lathyrus (also known as grass pea or kesari dal). The consumption of large quantities of lathyrus grains containing high concentration of glutamate analogue (neurotoxin) causes paralysis characterized by lack of strength or inability to move the lower limbs.

Obesity

Today obesity is a global nutritional concern. Obesity is a public health problem and it has emerged as a global non-communicable epidemic. It is the fifth leading cause of death all over the world. WHO predicts that overweight and obesity may soon replace the traditional public health concerns such as under nutrition and infectious diseases as the most significant cause of poor health. WHO (2000) defines obesity as a medical condition in which excess body fat has accumulated to the extent that it may have an adverse effect on health, leading to reduced life expectancy and/or increased health problems. Genetic and environmental factors have been documented as potential cause of obesity. The rising prevalence of obesity is attributed to the growing urbanization; transition toward high calorie western diet, fast foods and sedentary lifestyles and entertainments such TV, mobile phones or video games (Fig. 6.14).

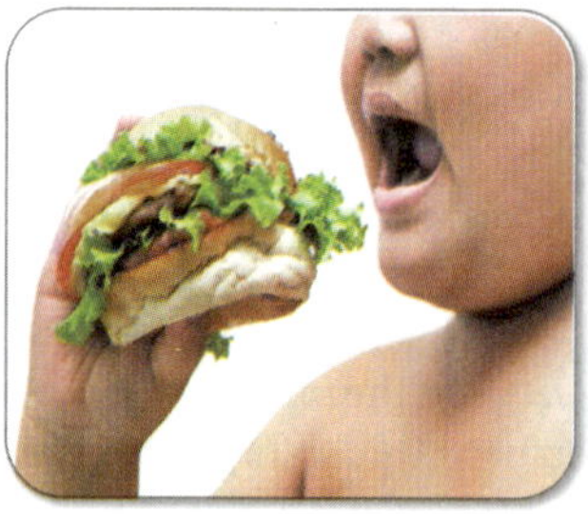

Fig. 6.14: Obesity

Cardiovascular Diseases

Faulty intake of diet is responsible for the onset of many cardiovascular diseases. Various studies support the role of elevated blood cholesterol level and low density lipoproteins in the development of atherosclerosis. Excessive intake of certain nutrients in the diet like cholesterol, lipoproteins, fatty acids, triglycerides, carbohydrates and salt have direct linkage with the onset of certain cardiovascular diseases (Fig. 6.15).

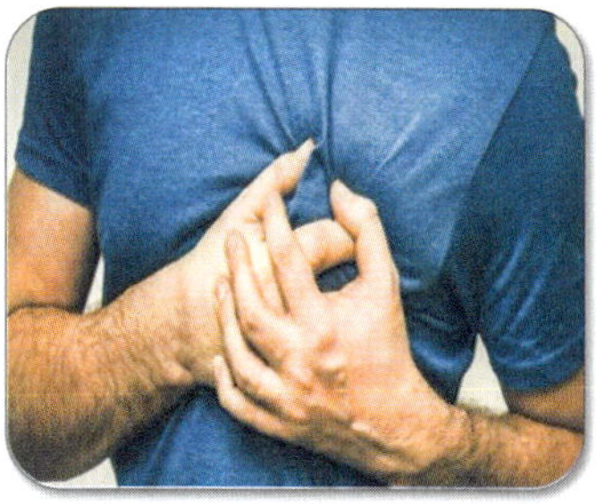

Fig. 6.15: Cardiovascular diseases

COMMUNITY NUTRITION PROGRAMS

The Government of India has initiated several supplementary nutrition programs to deal with specific deficiency diseases. These are as follows:

- **Special Nutrition Program (SNP):** This program was launched in 1970–71 by the Ministry of Social Welfare, Government of India. The main objective of the program was to improve the nutritional level of preschool children, pregnant and lactating mothers of poor socioeconomic group in urban slums, tribal areas and drought-prone rural areas. The beneficiaries are selected according to socioeconomic status. The supplement is provided to them for about 330 days in a year. The food supplement provides **300 kcal** and **10–12 g of proteins per child** and beneficiary **mother receives 500 kcal and 25 g of proteins** per day. The program is being gradually merged into ICDS program.
- **Balwadi Nutrition Program:** This program was started to benefit the children between age groups of 3–6 years in rural areas. The food supplement provides **300 kcal and 10 g of proteins per child** per day. National level organization like Indian council of child welfare and voluntary organizations, which receives the fund are responsible for day to day management of the program. Program is being implemented through balwadis as these also provide preschool education to these children.
- **Wheat-based Supplementary Nutrition Program:** This was a centrally sponsored program introduced in 1986 but now transferred to the states. Under the program, there is supply of free wheat and supportive cost for other ingredients, cooking and transport, etc.
- **Integrated Child Development Program (ICDS):** This program was started in **1975** under the national policy for children. An Anganwadi worker at village level delivers the services. Each Anganwadi unit covers about 1000 population in providing health and nutrition services. Anganwadi workers are supervised by mukhya sevikas and field supervision is done by child development project officer (CDPO).

  Beneficiaries of ICDS: The beneficiaries are preschool children below 6 years, adolescent girls, pregnant and lactating mothers and the women of reproductive age group (15–45 years).

  Objectives of ICDS:

  - To improve the nutritional health status of preschool children in the age group of 0–6 years
  - To lay the foundation of proper psychological development of the child
  - To reduce the incidence of mortality, morbidity, malnutrition and school drop outs
  - To promote the child development by effectively coordinating between different departments
  - To enhance the capacity of the mother to look after the health and nutritional needs of the child

  Services provided under ICDS:

  - Supplementary nutrition
  - Prophylaxis against anemia, goiter and vitamin A

- Immunization
- Treatment for minor ailments
- General health check ups
- Deworming
- Watch over the menarche (adolescent girls)
- Referral services in case of emergency
- Counseling and guidance on family welfare
- Nutrition and health education
- Monitoring of growth and development
- Other supportive services include safe drinking water, environmental sanitation and women empowerment programs

- **Midday Meal Program (MDMP):** Also known as school lunch program, it was launched in 1923 by the corporation schools in Madras city. Later on in 1982, chief minister of Tamil Nadu decided to universalize the scheme for all children in government schools for primary classes. Realizing the need of national nutritional support to primary education, midday meal scheme was formally launched on 15th August, 1995 all over the country.

  Objectives of MDMP:
  - To improve the nutritional status of the school children
  - To improve school attendance and to attract the children for admission to schools
  - To reduce the dropouts and retain them in the schools to improve the literacy rate

  The National Institute of Nutrition, Hyderabad recommends that school lunch must be provided minimum 250 days in a year to get the desired impact on the children.

  The following guidelines must be kept in mind while providing meal in the schools:
  - The meal should provide at least one-third of the total energy requirement and half of the protein need.
  - The meal should be supplement and not the substitute of the home diet.
  - The meal provided in the schools must be of low cost, easily prepared by using locally available food items and should not be monotonous. (Table 6.2)

Table 6.2: Model menu for the school meal

Food stuff	G/day/child
Cereals and millets	75
Pulses	30
Oils and fats	8
Leafy vegetables	30
Non-leafy vegetables	30

- **Vitamin A Prophylaxis Program:** The program was launched by the Ministry of Health and Family Welfare in 1970. It is also an important component of National program for control of blindness. According to this program, a total 9 dosage of vitamin A (200,000 IU) after the six month interval is administered to the preschool child. First dose is administered at the age of 9 months (100,000 IU) with the routine immunization against Measles. These doses are administered by anganwari workers.

- **Prophylaxis against Nutritional Anemia:** This program was launched by the Government of India during the fourth Five-Year plan for the prevention of anemia among children and pregnant women. The program emphasizes distribution of iron and folic acid tablets through maternal and child centers (MCH) in urban areas, primary health centers (PHC) and anganwadis (ICDS) in rural areas. The technique of fortification of salt with iron is also developed by the National Institute of Nutrition, Hyderabad to combat with the problem of anemia.
- **12 by 12 Initiative for Anemia Control:** It was launched at AIIMS, Delhi on April 2007 with the objective that every child should have hemoglobin of 12 g by the age of 12 years. This initiative is jointly taken by Ministry of Health and Family Welfare, Government of India.
- **Control of Iodine Deficiency Disorder:** Also known as **National Goiter Control Program,** it was initially launched by Government of India in 1962 in the Himalayan belt known as endemic area. Later on in 1986, by seeing the extent of the problem the program was renamed as National Iodine Deficiency disease control program.

  Objectives of the program:
  - Surveys to assess the magnitude of iodine deficiency disorders
  - Supply of iodized salt in place of common salt
  - Laboratory monitoring of iodized salt in place of common salt
  - Health education and publicity
- **Anemia Mukt Bharat (AMB):** In 2018, the Government of India launched the AMB strategy with the target to reduce anaemia in the vulnerable age groups such as women, children and adolescents.
- **National Nutrition Mission (Poshan Abhiyan):** The PM-POSHAN scheme, known as PM Poshan Shakti Nirman, provides free, nutritious cooked meals to children in government schools and other centers across India. It aims to enhance enrollment, attendance, retention, and overall health of children, particularly benefiting girls' completion rates in primary education. The scheme has also improved children's attendance, nutritional status, micronutrient intake, cognitive development, academic performance, and social behavior.
- **National Food Security Act (NFSA):** The National Food Security Act (NFSA) of 2013 is legislation aimed at ensuring food and nutrition security for the people of India. It covers approximately two-thirds of the population, providing subsidized food grains through the Targeted Public Distribution System (TPDS). NFSA also offers nutritional assistance to pregnant women, lactating mothers, and children up to 14-year-old. The Act includes provisions for grievance redressal, transparency, and accountability.

NATIONAL NUTRITION POLICY

National Nutrition Policy (NNP) was launched by the Government of India in the year 1993. Nutrition is a multi -sectoral issue, it needs to be tackled at various levels by direct and indirect involvement of various sectors.

Goals of National Nutrition Policy

- Reduction in the incidence of moderate to severe malnutrition and stunted growth among children
- Reduction in the incidence of low birth weight to <10%
- Elimination of vitamin A deficiency blindness

- Reduction in the iron deficiency anemia among pregnant women to 25%
- Universal iodization of salt for reduction of iodine deficiency disorders
- Special emphasis on geriatric nutrition
- Annual production of 250 million tons of food grains
- Promotion of appropriate diet and lifestyle

It comprises the following interventions:

Direct Interventions

- Nutritional interventions for special vulnerable groups
- The universal immunization program, oral rehydration therapy and ICDS services has great impact on improving child mortality rate and malnutrition so it should be implemented strictly
- Improving growth monitoring between age group of 0 and 3 years with the involvement of mothers
- Ensuring the better coverage of adolescent girls and expectant women to make them ready for safe motherhood
- Fortification of food and control of micronutrient deficiency especially among the vulnerable groups

Indirect Interventions

- Basic health and nutrition knowledge
- Prevention of food adulteration
- Land reforms
- Health and family welfare
- Nutrition surveillance
- Monitoring of nutrition programs
- Research into various aspects of nutrition
- Community participation
- Education and literacy particularly of women
- Improvement of the status of the women
- Equal remuneration for women
- Improvement of dietary pattern through production and demonstration
- Intersectoral coordination
- Food security

Source: J Kishore's National Health Programs of India

COMMUNITY FOOD SUPPLY

During the World War II, India faced acute food shortage and to meet the requirement a separate food department was established on 1st December, 1942. The food department was redesignated as Ministry of Food on 29th August, 1947. After undergoing many changes finally on 17th July, 2000, this department was renamed as the Ministry of Consumer Affairs Food and Public Distribution with two departments; namely department of Food and Public Distribution and Department of Consumer Affairs.

Functions

- Implementation of public distribution system with special focus on the poor.
- Provision of storage facility for the central reserve of food grains and promotion of scientific storage.
- Formulation of national policies related to import and export.
- Quality control and specification of food grains.
- Administration of food subsidies relating to rice, wheat grains, etc.
- Price control of interstate trade, supply and distribution of vanaspati, oilseeds and vegetable oil.
- Policy matter related to sugar and sugarcane sectors, fixation of fair and remuneration price of sugarcane and sugar supply for public.

PUBLIC DISTRIBUTION SYSTEM

Public Distribution System (PDS) is an Indian food security system established by Government of India under the Ministry of Consumer Affairs; Food and Public Distribution and jointly managed with the help of state governments. It distributes subsidized food and nonfood items to the poor. This scheme was launched in India in June 1997. Major commodities distributed include staple food grains such as wheat, rice, pulses, sugar and kerosene through a network of fair price shop also known as ration shops. It is maintained by Food Corporation of India (a Government owned corporation). To buy these items one must have ration card (pink card issued by the Government to the poor families). India has 478,000 such shops, making India as the largest distribution network in the world.

FOOD HYGIENE

Food is liable to contaminate with microorganism at any point during its journey from producer to consumer and may become a rich source of infection. Food hygiene implies hygiene practices in all the areas that include production, packaging, handling and distribution. Food hygiene is a broader term that can be further subdivided into the following terms:

Milk Hygiene

Milk can be contaminated at any point in milk production process. The sources of infection may be animal's health or cleanliness, human handler and environment that includes contaminated vessel, water or vectors such as flies, etc.

Safe Milk

Milk is considered sterile when secreted into uninfected udder. Contamination may occur during and after milking. Essential requirement of milk safety is to maintain udder free from infection. Milk equipment used for milking must be with minimal joints and smooth surfaces. If possible milking machines must be used. The milk vessel must be sterile and kept covered. The water supply must be safe from harmful bacteria. Milk handlers must be free from communicable diseases.

Milk-borne Infections

Infectious microbes commonly found in milk:

- ***Bacillus cereus:*** These bacteria produce a toxin that can cause diarrhea and vomiting.
- ***Brucella:*** It causes brucellosis also called undulant fever because of regular reoccurrence of fever.
- ***Escherichia coli:*** It is found in milk responsible for bloody diarrhea.
- ***Mycobacterium tuberculosis:*** *M. bovis* causes tuberculosis in cows and can be passed to human by unpasteurized milk.
- ***Salmonella:*** Contamination of raw milk has been a source of outbreaks that causes diarrhea and high fever.
- ***Staphylococcus aureus:*** It produces toxins that cause explosive vomiting.

Pasteurization of Milk

It is the process of heating and cooling liquids or foods at specific temperature to kill microorganisms. It was developed by Louis Pasteur in 1864 and the practice became commercialized around late 19th and 20th century. It not only improves the consumer safety but also enhances the quality and shell life of food.

Methods

- **High temperature long-term treatment:** Milk is heated at 161°F for 15 seconds
- **Low temperature long-term treatment:** Milk is heated at 145°F for 30 seconds
- **Flash pasteurization:** It involves high temperature for 3–15 seconds followed by cooling. It is used for packaging milk and other liquids that can be stored for longer period without refrigeration.
- **Ultra high temperature pasteurization:** Heating milk to 280–302°F for 1–2 seconds followed by packaging in air tight containers allows storage without refrigeration for some days.

Meat Hygiene

Primary purpose of meat hygiene is to prevent transmission of disease from animal to man and to provide safe product for human consumption. The term meat includes various tissues of animal origin. It must be inspected properly before consumption. A good meat should not be pale pink or deep tint. It should be firm, and elastic to touch and have only agreeable odor.

Aspects of Meat Hygiene

- **Animal care:** Taking care of animals raised for meat involves keeping their living spaces clean, providing enough food and water, and handling them carefully to minimize stress and injuries.
- **Inspection:** Trained inspectors check meat for signs of disease, contamination, or anything that could affect its quality.
- **Processing and packaging:** After slaughter, meat is processed—cutting, removing bones, and packing it. Clean equipment and facilities are important to prevent germs from spreading and to keep meat safe.
- **Cold storage:** Keeping meat at the right temperatures during processing and transportation stops germs from growing and keeps meat fresh until it's sold.
- **Hygiene:** Store owners and butchers need to keep their work areas clean, store meat correctly, and separate raw meat from cooked to avoid spreading germs.

- **Government rules:** Laws set by governments make sure meat is handled safely. They cover how to keep things clean, what temperatures to use, labeling meat correctly, and keeping track of where meat comes from.
- **Testing:** Meat is regularly checked for germs, chemicals, and other things that could be harmful. This makes sure meat is safe to eat and meets safety rules.
- **Consumer information:** Teaching people how to safely handle, store, and cook meat helps prevent sickness and makes sure meat is safe to eat.

Guidelines for Slaughter House

Slaughter houses are the places where animals are killed and the flesh is kept safe for human consumption.

- Slaughter house must be situated away from the residential areas with abundant supply of portable water as well as adequate facility of treatment and disposal of the waste.
- Sufficient space is required to dig the pits for condemned animals and disposal of waste.
- The floor must be made up with hard material with impervious sloping sufficiently toward the drain for easily cleaning.
- Walls of the slaughter house must be made up of the material that is easy to wash such as stone or concrete.
- Slaughter house must be covered by proper fencing and with adequate facilities to control the pests.
- Every slaughter house must be equipped with adequate storage and transport facilities. There should be sufficient space for storage with covered vans to transport the animal products (meat).

Fish Hygiene

Fishery products must be handled and stored properly and must undergo chilling as soon as possible after loading for safe consumption of the human being. Fish deteriorates and loses its freshness because of autolysis by the bacterias. Stale fish should not be consumed as it contains many harmful bacterias. There may be many sources of contamination of the fishery products that includes environment, product handler or the product itself. To preserve the fishery products for long time it must be freezed either by surrounding the fish with a stream of cold air, by placing the fish in contact with cold surface or by spraying it with certain liquid refrigerants. In large amount, fishery products can be stored at –30°C in cold storage.

Egg Hygiene

Careful and hygienic handling of eggs through the supply chain or in kitchen is vital to prevent infections or food-borne diseases. Eggs contain a number of nutrients that include 13 essential vitamins, minerals, high quality proteins, antioxidants and approximately 70 calories. If cooked properly, eggs are a safe, wholesome and convenient food. The following points must be kept in mind while handling the eggs in the kitchen:

- Eggs should be cooked until the white and yolk part of the egg becomes firm so that harmful bacterias get destroyed.
- Utensils or surfaces that come into contact with raw eggs must be cleaned properly.
- Separate eggs from other foods in grocery cart/bag as well as in the refrigerator.
- Eggs accidentally left at room temperature must be discarded as it is not safe for human consumption.

FOOD-BORNE DISEASES

Bacterial Pathogens

- *Clostridium botulinum*
- *Escherichia coli*
- *Listeria*
- *Shigella*
- *Salmonella*
- *Staphylococcus aureus*
- *Vibrio cholerae*
- *Streptococcus*

Commonly caused diseases by these bacteria are typhoid fever, paratyphoid fever, salmonellosis, diarrhea, shigellosis and brucellosis.

Viral Pathogens

- Enterovirus
- Hepatitis A
- Norovirus
- Rotavirus

Commonly caused diseases are viral hepatitis and gastroenteritis.

Parasitic Pathogens

- *Cryptosporidium*
- *Entameba histolytica*
- *Giardia*
- *Trichinella*

Commonly caused diseases are taeniasis, hydatidosis, ascariasis and amebiasis.

Common Food-borne Diseases in India

In India, several food-borne diseases are prevalent due to various factors such as environmental conditions, food handling practices, and dietary habits.

Here are some common food-borne diseases seen in India:

- **Diarrheal diseases:** These are often caused by bacterial infections such as:
    - **Salmonellosis:** Caused by Salmonella bacteria, typically transmitted through contaminated water, poultry, eggs, and dairy products.
    - **Campylobacteriosis:** Caused by Campylobacter bacteria, commonly found in undercooked poultry, unpasteurized milk, and contaminated water.

- **Typhoid fever:** Caused by the Salmonella Typhi bacteria, transmitted through contaminated food and water. Symptoms include prolonged fever, headache, abdominal pain, and diarrhea.
- **Cholera:** Caused by the Vibrio cholerae bacteria, transmitted through contaminated water and food. It leads to severe watery diarrhea and dehydration.
- **Hepatitis A:** A viral infection causing inflammation of the liver, transmitted through contaminated food and water. Symptoms include fever, fatigue, nausea, abdominal pain, and jaundice.
- **Viral gastroenteritis:** Caused by various viruses such as norovirus and rotavirus, leading to symptoms like vomiting, diarrhea, abdominal cramps, and fever.
- **Amoebiasis:** Caused by the parasite Entamoeba histolytica, transmitted through contaminated food and water. It leads to dysentery with bloody stools, abdominal pain, and fever.
- ***E. coli* Infections:** Certain strains of Escherichia coli bacteria can cause severe diarrheal illness and abdominal cramps, often linked to contaminated water or undercooked meats.
- **Food poisoning:** General term for illnesses caused by consuming contaminated food, often due to bacteria (like Staphylococcus aureus or Bacillus cereus) or toxins produced by bacteria in food.

COMMERCIALLY PREPARED FOOD

It is also known as tertiary processed food that is prepared (often through processing) to optimize ease of consumption. Such food is usually ready to eat without any further preparation. It is easily portable and has long shelf life. Type of such food varies from country to country and also by geographic region. Examples of such food are candies, beverages such as soft drink, juices and milk, fast food, nuts, chips and cookies, etc.

- **Production process:** Commercially prepared foods are made using specific recipes and methods in big factories that can make a lot of food at once.
- **Ingredients:** The ingredients used in commercially prepared foods are bought in large amounts, like meat, grains, and vegetables. All items undergo quality control checks to ensure safety and compliance with regulatory standards.
- **Processing methods:** Various processing methods such as cooking, baking, frying, freezing, and canning are employed depending on the type of food product. Each step is carefully monitored to maintain food safety and quality.
- **Packaging:** After processing, foods are packaged in suitable containers or packaging materials that preserve freshness, prevent contamination, and provide information about ingredients, nutritional content, and storage instructions.
- **Regulations and standards:** Commercially prepared foods undergo strict regulations and standards formulated by government agencies to ensure safety, labelling accuracy, and compliance with health and hygiene requirements.
- **Distribution and retail:** Once packaged, commercially prepared foods are distributed through various channels such as supermarkets, convenience stores, restaurants, and institutional food service providers.
- **Consumer convenience:** These foods are designed to offer convenience to consumers by providing ready-to-eat or easy-to-prepare options that save time and effort in meal preparation.
- **Quality control:** Quality control measures, including regular testing and inspections, are implemented throughout the production process to detect and address any issues related to food safety, taste, texture, and shelf-life.

LOCALLY-GROWN FOOD

Locally-grown food initiatives often promote sustainable and organic farming practices. Locally describes the market arrangements directly from regional farmers to the consumers. The term local is widely understood by the general public as a description of regional distribution of food. Locally-grown food may be defined as the food that is grown locally or in the region in which the final product is marketed, so that the total distance of the transportation to market the product is <400 miles (640 km) from the origin of the product or the state in which the product is produced (Bill Text 110th Congress 2007–2008; Thomas Library of Congress). Locally-grown food varies from one place to another as it depends upon climate, culture, ethnic group and society, etc. Examples are rice, wheat, jowar, pulses, jute, coffee, sugarcane, vegetables, fruits and tea that require a particular environment that varies from region to region.

Locally-grown food refers to food that is produced and sold within a specific geographic region, typically not far from where it is consumed.

Aspects of Locally-grown Food

- **Production:** Locally-grown food is grown and harvested by farmers who are nearby, often within the same town, city, or region.
- **Transport:** It travels shorter distances from farm to market compared to food that is transported across long distances or internationally.
- **Freshness:** Because it doesn't travel far, locally-grown food is often fresher when it reaches consumers.
- **Seasonality:** Locally-grown food is seasonal available offering fruits and vegetables that are in particular in that season.
- **Supporting local economy:** Buying locally-grown food supports local farmers and the local economy.
- **Community connection:** Consumers often have a stronger connection to where their food comes from when they buy locally-grown products.

Benefits of Consuming Locally-grown Food

- It is full of flavor and nutrients as it is available in the fresh form.
- It promotes safer food supply as there is less chance of contamination that may occur while transferring the food from one place to another.
- It is also beneficial to the environment as there is no need for longer storage or transportation of food.
- It supports local economy by supporting the local farmers.
- It prevents from many diseases that may occur due to over consumption of commercially prepared food, for example, obesity.

NATIONAL AND INTERNATIONAL FOOD AGENCIES

Central Food Training Research Institute (CFTRI)

The CFTRI is a premier institute under the Council of Scientific and Industrial Research, Ministry of Science and Technology and Government of India, New Delhi. It was established in 1950 in Mysore, Karnataka, a constituent laboratory of council of Scientific and Industrial Research, India. It also has its resource centers in Hyderabad, Lucknow and Mumbai. Over the years, the institute is continuously enhancing its capabilities to achieve high quality research through training, innovation and recruitment of personnel for its research and development activities (Fig. 6.16).

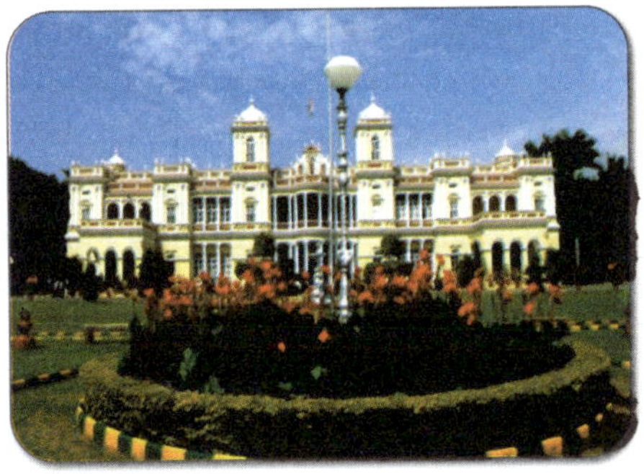

Fig. 6.16: Central Food Training Research Institute

Presently the institute accommodates over 200 scientists, technologists, engineers, skilled workers and supportive staff. There are 16 research and development departments including laboratories focusing on food biotechnology, microbiology and food safety. India is the world's second largest food grains, fruits and vegetables producer and the institute is engaged in research in production and handling of grains, pulses, oilseeds, spices, fruits, vegetables, meat, fish and poultry. The institute develops technologies to increase efficiency, reduce harvest losses, increase export, find new sources of food products, integrate human resources in food industries and reduce cost. The institute has designed over 300 products, processes and equipment. It also holds several patents and releases many publications.

Functions of CFTRI

- Suggest networking with other national laboratories on programs of mutual interest.
- Review research and development activities and research programs and advise for future directions.
- Advise on fostering linkages between laboratory, industry and clients.

Food and Agriculture Organization (FAO)

The FAO was formed in **1945** with the headquarter in Rome. The idea of an international organization for food and agriculture emerged in late 19th and 20th century and is brainchild of US agriculturist and activist **David Labin.** An international conference was held in Rome, Italy, which led to creation of International Institute of Agriculture. Its Latin motto is **fiat panis,** means, **"let there be bread" (Fig. 6.17).**

Fig. 6.17: Logo of FAO

Functions of FAO

- FAO is an agency of the United Nations that leads international effort to defeat hunger serving both developed and developing countries.
- FAO acts as a neutral forum where all the nations meet to negotiate agreements and debate policy.
- FAO is also a source of knowledge and information, and helps developing countries to improve agriculture, forests, fisheries, ensuring good nutrition and food security for all.
- FAO is directed by the conference of member nations, who meet every two years to review the work carried out by the organization and to plan work and budget for the next two-year-period. It is composed of seven different departments.
- FAO also collaborates with other international agencies in the applied nutrition programs and has conducted nutritional surveys, training courses, seminars and coordination of research programs for zoonotic diseases.

Food and Agriculture Organization works in the following areas:

- Helps to eliminate hunger, food insecurity and malnutrition
- Makes agriculture, forestry and fisheries more productive and sustainable
- Reduces rural poverty and helps the rural poor to gain access to the resources and service they need
- Enables inclusive and efficient food systems that support small agriculturists and reduces poverty and hunger in rural areas
- Helps the countries to prepare for national and human aroused disasters by reducing their risk and enhancing the resilience of their food and agriculture system

National Institute of Nutrition

It is an Indian public health, biotechnology and research center located in Hyderabad (India). It is one of the oldest and largest research centers under the Indian Council of Medical Research. The institute was established in 1918 by Sir Robert McCarrison. It was originally a single room lab at Pasteur Institute Coonoor (Tamil Nadu) for the study of Beriberi disease and also known as Beriberi enquiry unit. Later on, the scope of lab was extended to include all the deficiency diseases. In 1928–1929, it became the nutrition research lab with McCarrison as its first director. The lab moved to **Hyderabad** in **1958** and in (Fig. 6.18) **1969** it was renamed as National Institute of Nutrition (NIN).

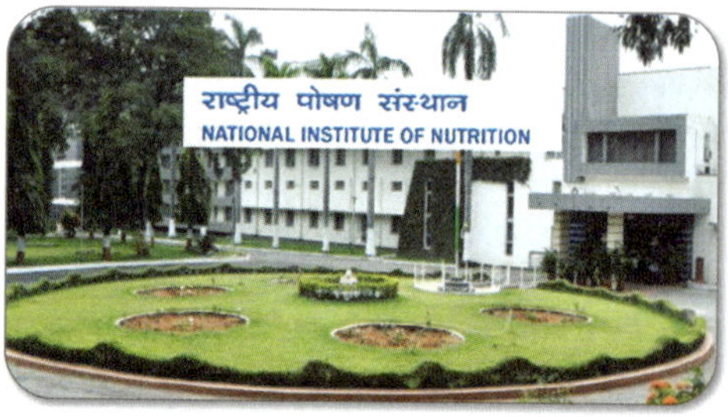

Fig. 6.18: National Institute of Nutrition

Functions of NIN

- To perform periodic assessment of nutrient intake, health and nutrition status of the population and assist the Government and regulatory bodies in policy making.
- To establish recommended daily allowances, dietary guidelines for Indian population and assessment of nutrient composition of food.
- To identify various nutritional deficiency disorders prevalent among different segments of population.
- To develop human resources in nutrition and also provide evidence-based nutrition knowledge to the community.
- To carry out research in clinical nutrition, pathology, food chemistry, endocrinology, regenerative medicines and community nutrition.
- To offer courses for MS, MD and PhD programs for nutrition, biochemistry and dietetics.

Main Achievements of NIN

- Established growth norms for Indian children.
- Emphasized the importance of growth monitoring for early diagnosis and appropriate management of protein energy malnutrition (PEM).
- Developed food-based guidelines and formulated recommended dietary allowances (RDA) for Indians.
- Initiated national prophylaxis programs against blindness due to vitamin A deficiency covering 30 million preschool children in India.
- Recommended appropriate immunization schedule based upon studies of nutrition and infections.

- Identified the causative factor of food-borne illnesses like Epidemic dropsy.
- Helped to improve nutritional status of pregnant and lactating women and birth weight of infants.
- Developed food safety norms for street food and public catering.

Food Safety and Standards Authority of India (FSSAI)

The FSSAI has been established under the Food Safety and Standard Act **2006** as a statutory body for lying down science-based standards articles of food regulating manufacturing, processing, distribution, sale and import so as to ensure safe and wholesome food for human consumption (Fig. 6.19).

Fig. 6.19: Logo of FSSAI

Administrative control

It was formed in **2011** and its headquarter is in New Delhi. It is an agency of Ministry of Health and Family Welfare of Government of India. It is led by a nonexecutive chairperson appointed by the central Government from amongst the persons of eminence in the field of food science or administration who has been associated with the subjects or holding or has hold the position of not below the rank of secretary to the Government of India. The agency has 8 regional offices (located in Delhi, Chandigarh, Lucknow, Guwahati, Mumbai, Kolkata, Cochin and Chennai), 4 referral labs, 72 local labs located throughout India.

Aims of FSSAI

- To lay down science-based standards for articles on food
- To regulate the manufacture, storage, distribution, import and sale of food
- To facilitate the safety of food.

Functions of FSSAI

- Food Safety and Standards Authority of India is responsible for protecting and promoting public health through regulations and supervision of food safety.
- Framing of regulations to lay down the standards and guidelines in relation to articles of food.
- Laying down mechanism and guidelines for accreditation of certification bodies related to food.
- Generate new knowledge that would help continuously updating and upgrading food safety standards that are compatible with international organization.
- Carry out evidence-based studies for improving or building rules and regulations.

The agency is divided into the following main departments (panels) for better functioning and supervision

- Panels for functional food nutraceuticals, dietetics and other similar products
- Panel for method of sampling and analysis
- Panel for food additives, flavoring, processing aids and material in contact with food
- Panel to check contaminants in the food products
- Panel to check biological hazards
- Panel for pesticides and antibiotic residues
- Panel for labeling and claim advertisements
- Panel for genetically modified organisms and food
- Panels for fish and fishery products.

Source: Fssai.gov.in

Cooperative for Assistance and Relief Everywhere

Cooperative for Assistance and Relief Everywhere (CARE) is an international humanitarian agency was founded in **1945**. It is a non-sectarian, impartial nongovernment and one of the oldest and largest humanitarian aid organizations. At present it is working in 90 countries and operating 880 poverty fighting projects and reaching up to 72 million people (Fig. 6.20).

Fig. 6.20: Logo of CARE

Functions of CARE

- It mainly delivers emergency relief and long-term international projects.
- CARE also advocates at local, national and international levels for policy making and rights of poor people.
- It also focuses particularly on empowering and meeting the needs of women and girls for promoting gender equality.
- It provides assistance to disaster affected communities and helps in the distribution of relief assistance, training the people, organization leaders and their members to help in the crisis.

Funding of CARE

It is not a funding agency. It does not provide financial support directly to individual or organizations. It works in partnership with governments, organizations and communities in developing countries to find out solutions to combat with poverty.

Structure of CARE

Cooperative for Assistance and Relief Everywhere (CARE) is an international confederation of fourteen CARE national members coordinated by international secretariat. The secretariat is based in Geneva (Switzerland) with offices in New York and Brussels in order to liaise with UN and European nations respectively. Each CARE national member is an autonomous NGO registered in the country and each member runs programs, fund raising and communication activities both in its own and developing countries where it operates.

Main Projects of CARE:

- **Gender and women empowerment:** CARE list sit as a priority and focuses its programming in the areas toward this goal.
- **Food security:** It provides emergency, food aid and supports the prevention of malnutrition by promoting proper breastfeeding techniques, providing education focusing on the cultivation and preparation of nutritious food and improving infrastructure.
- **Health:** Health programs not only focuses mainly upon maternal health and HIV/AIDS but also addresses other areas such as nutrition, safe drinking water, health education and training of local health workers.
- **Climate changes:** It is engaged in climate changes advocacy and also supports local mitigation strategies such as promoting early warning system, helping communities to draft evacuation plans, providing technical equipment and information supporting reforestation and working with local Government to reduce pollution.
- **Education:** CARE provides economic incentives to assist parents to keep their children in schools, advocates for importance of educating girls and supports programs that ensure that girls receive quality education and engage girls in extracurricular and leadership activities.

- **Water sanitation and hygiene (WASH):** CARE builds and maintains clean water system and latrines. It also provides education about hygiene and waterborne illnesses. These programs aim to reduce the risk of water-related diseases and increase the earning potential of households by saving otherwise spent upon fetching water.
- **Economic development:** It supports increased market linkage, promotes diversified livelihoods, savings at village levels and loan associations.
- **Emergency response:** It supports emergency reliefs as well as prevention, preparedness and recovery programs. CARE sectors for emergency response are food security, shelter, water, sanitation, sexual and reproductive health.

National Institute of Public Cooperation and Child Development

The NIPCCD is a premier organization devoted to promotion of voluntary action research, training and documentation in the overall domain of women and child development. It was established in New Delhi in the year **1966** under Society's Registration Act 1860. It functions under the aegis of ministry of women and child development. In order to cater the region specific requirements of the country, four regional centers at Guwahati (1978), Bengaluru (1980), Lucknow (1982) and Indore (2001) have been established (Fig. 6.21).

Fig. 6.21: Logo of NIPCCD

Functions of NIPCCD

- The institute functions as an apex institute for training of integrated child development services (ICDS).
- It works as a nodal agency entrusted with responsibility of training and capacity building of functionaries at the national and regional level under the new scheme of integrated child protection scheme (ICPS).
- It also imparts training upon two important issues of child rights and prevention of trafficking of women and children by the ministry of women and child welfare.
- Conduct, promote, sponsor and collaborate in research, evaluation studies in child development
- Review programs for children in light of national policy for children
- Review voluntary action in social development

The expertise and performance of the institute were recognized by UNICEF in 1985 when it was awarded Maurice Pate award for its outstanding contributions in the field of child development.

It works mainly under the following areas:

- **Child guidance center (CGC):** It offers family comprehensive diagnostic assessment by qualified team of child development professionals, child counselors, psychiatrists, psychologists and child therapists. It offers specialized screening and diagnosis of children suspected at risk of showing learning, behavior, emotional and development difficulties.
- **Child care center:** It aims at holistic development of child. It follows playway and activity approach to provide stimulating environment for holistic, intellectual, social, emotional, physical development of the child. Annually this center holds 30 children in the age group of 3–4 years from low income group belonging to neighboring localities.
- **Adolescent guidance center:** It was established in 2001 with the vision to build society that ensures a healthy psychological development of young people so that they can experience a sense of well being and grow up as adult with constructive attitude toward self and society.

- **Advance diploma in child guidance and counseling:** It was launched in 2005 to address the need of trained manpower to work in the area of child and adolescents mental health. The course is affiliated with Guru Gobind Singh Indraprastha University and also recognized by rehabilitation Council of India (RIC). This institute has organized ten batches and trained 166 students till date.
- **Nutrition resource platform:** It is an institute of child development and nutrition bureau of ministry of women and child development with aim to collect and make available resources and materials on nutrition and child development. It also functions as a food and nutrition board in Ministry of Women and Child Development

Source: nipccd.gov.in

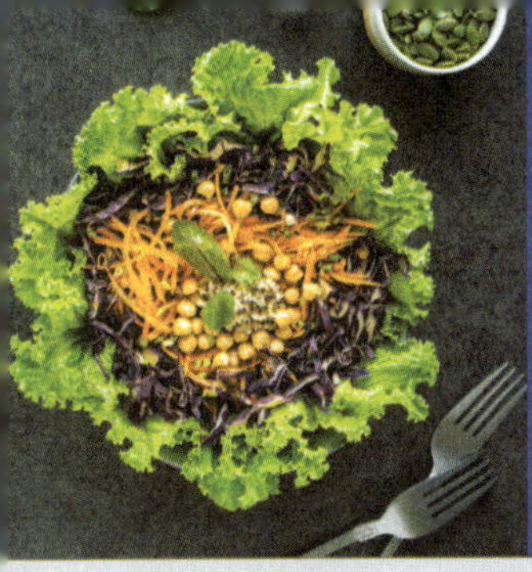

STUDENT ASSIGNMENT

LONG ANSWER QUESTIONS

1. Explain the common nutritional problems in India.
2. How food is supplied in the community?
3. Explain main community nutrition programs in India.
4. What is milk hygiene and explain about pasteurization of milk?

SHORT ANSWER QUESTION

1. Write short notes on the following:
    a. FAO
    b. NIN
    c. CARE
    d. FSSAI

MULTIPLE CHOICE QUESTIONS

1. Which of the following is not a part of midday meal school program?
a. To combat nutritional problem
b. To substitute home diet
c. To attract more children for school
d. To improve literacy rate

2. Midday meal program was initiated in the year:
a. 1973–78
b. 1950–55
c. 1962–63
d. 1958–60

3. Endemic area known for iodine deficiency is:
a. Himalayan region
b. All hilly areas
c. Tribal areas
d. All over India

4. The first indicator for growth retardation in children is:
a. Less intake of food
b. Obesity/over weight
c. Lethargic child
d. Under weight as per age

5. National program for prevention of anemia covers:
a. Pregnant women
b. Lactating mother
c. Adolescents and young children
d. All of these

6. Food and Agriculture Organization (FAO) was established in the year:
a. 1945
b. 1970
c. 1965
d. 1950

7. **Headquarter of FSSAI is in:**
   a. Kolkata
   b. Mumbai
   c. New Delhi
   d. Chandigarh

8. **Which agency in India is responsible for implementing and regulating food safety standards across the country?**
   a. FSSAI (Food Safety and Standards Authority of India)
   b. Ministry of Agriculture and Farmers Welfare
   c. Ministry of Food Processing Industries
   d. Bureau of Indian Standards

9. **Which ministry oversees the implementation of the National Food Security Act, 2013 in India?**
   a. Ministry of Health and Family Welfare
   b. Ministry of Consumer Affairs, Food and Public Distribution
   c. Ministry of Women and Child Development
   d. Ministry of Social Justice and Empowerment

10. **Which agency in India is responsible for the distribution of food grains through the Public Distribution System (PDS)?**
    a. Food Corporation of India (FCI)
    b. National Agricultural Cooperative Marketing Federation of India Ltd. (NAFED)
    c. Ministry of Food Processing Industries
    d. Central Warehousing Corporation (CWC)

11. **Which organization is responsible for promoting agricultural marketing and exports in India?**
    a. Ministry of Commerce and Industry
    b. Ministry of Agriculture and Farmers Welfare
    c. Agricultural and Processed Food Products Export Development Authority (APEDA)
    d. National Horticulture Board (NHB)

12. **Which agency in India is responsible for implementing the Mid-Day Meal Scheme in schools to improve nutrition among children?**
    a. Ministry of Education
    b. Ministry of Women and Child Development
    c. Ministry of Human Resource Development
    d. Ministry of Social Justice and Empowerment

13. **Which international organization sets standards for food safety, quality, and trade?**
    a. World Health Organization (WHO)
    b. Food and Agriculture Organization (FAO)
    c. Codex Alimentarius Commission
    d. World Trade Organization (WTO)

14. **Which organization works to eliminate hunger, achieve food security, and improve nutrition worldwide?**
    a. World Health Organization (WHO)
    b. Food and Agriculture Organization (FAO)
    c. United Nations Children's Fund (UNICEF)
    d. International Labour Organization (ILO)

15. Which institution in India conducts research and provides training in food science and technology?

a. Central Food Technological Research Institute (CFTRI)
b. Food and Agriculture Organization (FAO)
c. National Institute of Nutrition (NIN)
d. Food Safety and Standards Authority of India (FSSAI)

16. Which institute in India provides guidelines on dietary requirements, and promotes nutritional health?

a. Central Food Technological Research Institute (CFTRI)
b. Food and Agriculture Organization (FAO)
c. National Institute of Nutrition (NIN)
d. Food Safety and Standards Authority of India (FSSAI)

17. Which agency in India is responsible for regulating and ensuring food safety standards across the country?

a. Central Food Technological Research Institute (CFTRI)
b. Food and Agriculture Organization (FAO)
c. National Institute of Nutrition (NIN)
d. Food Safety and Standards Authority of India (FSSAI)

18. Which institute provides training and research on food processing, quality control, and safety in India?

a. Central Food Technological Research Institute (CFTRI)
b. Food and Agriculture Organization (FAO)
c. National Institute of Nutrition (NIN)
d. Food Safety and Standards Authority of India (FSSAI)

19. Which of the following is an important aspect of milk hygiene to prevent contamination?

a. Pasteurization
b. Freezing
c. Canning
d. Drying

20. Which organism is commonly targeted during pasteurization to ensure milk safety?

a. Salmonella
b. Listeria
c. Escherichia coli
d. Mycobacterium tuberculosis

21. What is the purpose of meat inspection conducted in slaughterhouses?

a. To improve taste and flavor
b. To increase shelf life
c. To ensure safety and quality
d. To reduce cost of production

22. Which of the following is a common bacterial food-borne disease in India caused by contaminated water or food.

a. Malaria
b. Typhoid fever
c. Cholera
d. Dengue fever

23. Which parasite commonly causes food-borne infections through consumption of contaminated water or undercooked meat?

a. Giardia
b. Plasmodium
c. Taenia
d. Trypanosoma

24. **Which viral infection is transmitted through contaminated food or water causing symptoms such as nausea, vomiting, abdominal pain, and jaundice?**
   a. Hepatitis A
   b. Dengue fever
   c. Chikungunya
   d. Japanese ence

25. **Which method is commonly used to ensure fish hygiene and safety?**
   a. Freezing
   b. Salting
   c. Canning
   d. Drying

26. **Which practice is essential for ensuring egg hygiene and safety?**
   a. Washing eggs with soap and water
   b. Storing eggs at room temperature
   c. Refrigerating eggs promptly after purchase
   d. Boiling eggs for at least 10 minutes

27. **Which bacterium commonly causes contamination of eggs and can lead to food-borne illness if consumed undercooked or raw?**
   a. Escherichia coli
   b. Salmonella
   c. Listeria monocytogenes
   d. Staphylococcus aureus

28. **What is a recommended practice to check if an egg is fresh?**
   a. Shake it vigorously
   b. Check the color of the shell
   c. Place it in a bowl of water (fresh egg sinks, old egg floats)
   d. Smell it

ANSWER KEY

1. b	**2.** c	**3.** a	**4.** d	**5.** d	**6.** a	**7.** c	**8.** a	**9.** b
10. a	**11.** c	**12.** c	**13.** c	**14.** b	**15.** a	**16.** c	**17.** d	**18.** a
19. a	**20.** c	**21.** c	**22.** b	**23.** c	**24.** a	**25.** a	**26.** c	**27.** b
28. c								

7

Cookery Practical

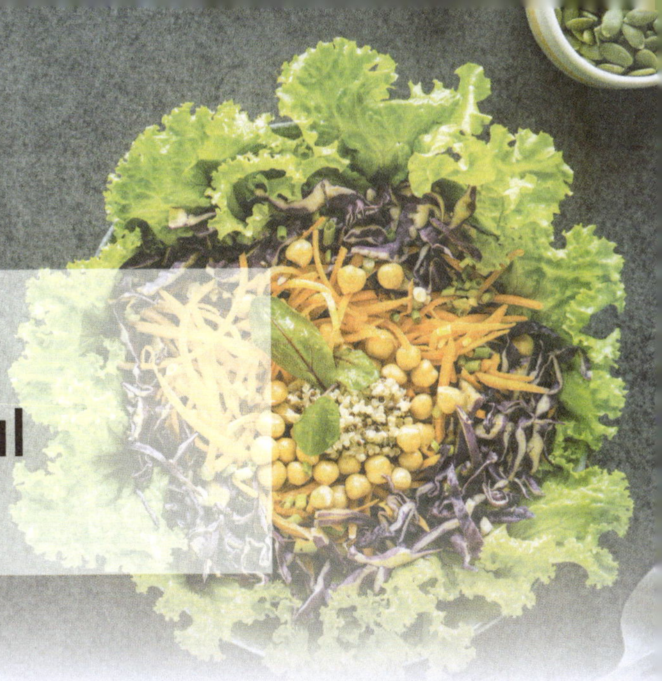

HOUSEHOLD MEASUREMENT

- 1 liter = 1000 milliliter (mL)
- 1 liter = 1 kilograms (kg) = 1000 grams = 1,0000,000 milligrams
- 1 gallon = 4 quarts
- 1 quart = 1 liter
- 1 pint = 500 milliliters (mL)
- 1 cup = 240 milliliters (mL)
- 1 fluid ounce (oz) = 30–32 milliliters (mL)
- 1 ounce = 28 grams
- 1 tbs (tbs) =15 milliliters (mL)
- 1 tsp (tsp) = 5 milliliters (mL)
- 3 tsp (tsp) = 1 tbs (tbs)
- 2.2 pound (lbs) = 1 kilograms (kg)
- 1 quart = 2 pints = 4 cups = 64 tbs (tbs) = 192 tsp
- 1 quart = 16 ounces = 1 pound
- 1 cubic centimeter (cc) = 1 milliliter (mL)

Note: A cubic centimeter (cc) is equal to the volume of a cube with side length of 1 cm.

Commonly used Culinary Terms

- **Bake:** To cook food in an oven using dry heat
- **Beat:** To stir rapidly in circular motion to make smooth mixture, using a whisk, spoon or mixer
- **Broil:** To expose food to direct heat on a rack or spit often used for melting food like cheese
- **Brown:** To cook over high heat to make the food look like brown color
- **Caramelize:** To heat sugar until it liquefies and becomes syrup
- **Chop:** To cut vegetables into large pieces

- **Cube:** Like chopping to cut food into small cubes approximately ½ inch
- **Dice:** To cut into small pieces usually ¼–⅛ chunks
- **Dress:** To coat food with a sauce such as salads
- **Drizzle:** To pour liquid over a dish in a fine stream, usually melted butter or melted chocolates
- **Dust:** To coat lightly with powdery ingredients such as sugar or cocoa
- **Fillet:** To cut the bones from a piece of meat, poultry or fish
- **Grease:** To coat the anterior of a pan or dish with oil or butter to prevent food from sticking during cooking
- **Knead:** The process of mixing dough with the hands or a mixer
- **Marinate:** To soak in a sauce or flavored liquid for a long period of time usually meat or fish
- **Mince:** To cut as small as possible like garlic
- **Parboil:** To partially cook by boiling
- **Poach:** To cook gently over very low heat in simmering water just to cover.
- **Pinch:** 1/16th tsp
- **Puree:** To mash or grind food until completely smooth
- **Roast:** Like baking but concerning meat or poultry, it is to cook food in an oven using dry heat
- **Sauté:** To cook small pieces of food over a medium high heat with oil in a pan, usually to brown
- **Shred:** Done on grater with large holes resulting in long, smooth stripes to cook or melt
- **Simmer:** Bring a pot to boil, then reduce the heat until there are no bubbles
- **Skim:** To remove the fat or foam from the surface of a liquid
- **Steam:** To cook food on a rack or in a steamer set over boiling or simmering water
- **Stew:** To cook covered over low heat in a liquid for a substantial period of time
- **Whip:** To beat food with a whisk or mixer to incorporate air and increase volume
- **Zest:** The outer, colored peel of a citrus fruit

Commonly used Terms in Nutrition

- **Calorie:** A unit of energy provided by food and beverages.
- **Macronutrients:** Nutrients required in large amounts by the body, including carbohydrates, proteins, and fats.
- **Micronutrients:** Essential nutrients required in smaller amounts, including vitamins and minerals.
- **Antioxidants:** Compounds that help protect cells from damage caused by free radicals.
- **Dietary fiber:** Non-digestible carbohydrates that promote digestive health and help regulate bowel movements.
- **Probiotics:** Live microorganisms that provide health benefits when consumed in adequate amounts, often found in fermented foods.
- **Omega-3 fatty acids:** Essential fatty acids important for brain function and heart health, found in fish, flaxseeds, and walnuts.
- **Glycemic index:** A measure of how quickly a carbohydrate-containing food raises blood glucose levels.
- **Recommended dietary allowance (RDA):** The average daily level of intake sufficient to meet the nutrient requirements of nearly all healthy individuals.

- **Daily value (DV):** A reference value indicating how much of a specific nutrient is in a serving of food in relation to a total daily diet.
- **Nutrient density:** A measure of the nutrients a food provides relative to its calorie content.
- **Fortified:** Foods to which nutrients have been added that were not originally present, usually to address deficiencies.
- **Hydration:** The process of absorbing water into the body, essential for overall health and proper bodily functions.
- **Metabolism:** The process by which the body converts food and drink into energy and other essential nutrients for growth, repair, and maintenance.
- **Whole grains:** Grains that include the entire grain seed (bran, germ, and endosperm), providing more nutrients and fiber compared to refined grains.
- **Calorie intake:** The amount of energy derived from food and beverages consumed daily.
- **Macronutrient intake:** The consumption of carbohydrates, proteins, and fats, often measured in grams or as a percentage of total energy intake.
- **Micronutrient Intake:** The consumption of essential vitamins and minerals, measured in micrograms (μg) or milligrams (mg).
- **Body mass index (BMI):** A measure of body fat based on height and weight, used to classify individuals as underweight, normal weight, overweight, or obese.
- **Waist circumference:** A measurement of abdominal fat, which is associated with increased health risks such as cardiovascular disease and type 2 diabetes.
- **Energy expenditure:** The amount of energy expended by the body in daily activities and exercise, measured in calories or kilojoules.

HOT BEVERAGES

Hot Coffee (Fig. 7.1)

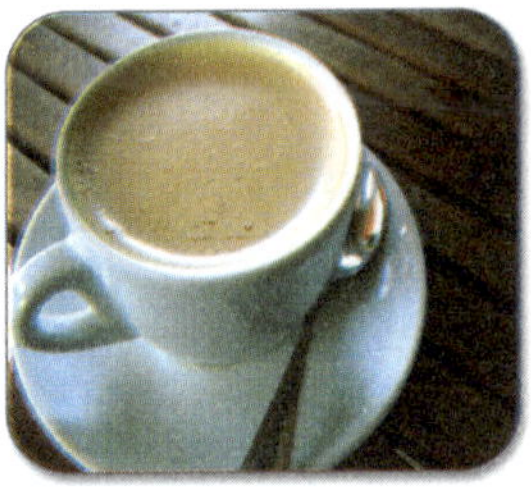

Fig. 7.1: Hot coffee

Ingredients

- Coffee: 2 tsp
- Sugar: 1 tsp
- Milk: 1 cup

Method

- Take the instant coffee powder and sugar in a cup.
- Add a tsp of water or milk and mix the coffee powder and sugar.
- Whisk the mixture with the help of spoon until it becomes light brown in color and creamy.
- Heat the milk and let it come to boil.
- Pour the hot milk into coffee cream prepared earlier. Mix with the help of spoon.
- Mix the milk and coffee cream by transferring between two cups.
- Once done, serve the hot coffee.

Honey Lemon Ginger Tea (Fig. 7.2)

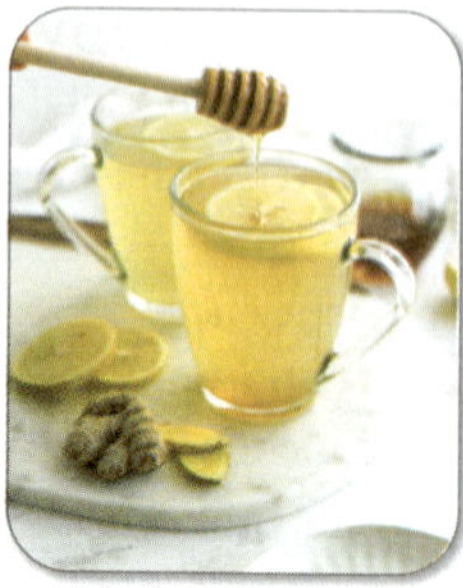

Fig. 7.2: Honey lemon ginger tea

Ingredients

- 1 tsp ginger finely chopped
- 1 tsp tea leaves
- 1 tsp lemon juice
- 1 tsp honey

Method

- Heat 3 cups of water in a pan.
- Before it brings to boil add ginger.
- As it starts to boil add the tea leaves, lemon juice and honey.
- Strain into a cup and enjoy.

Indian Kadha Recipe (Herbal Tea) (Fig. 7.3)

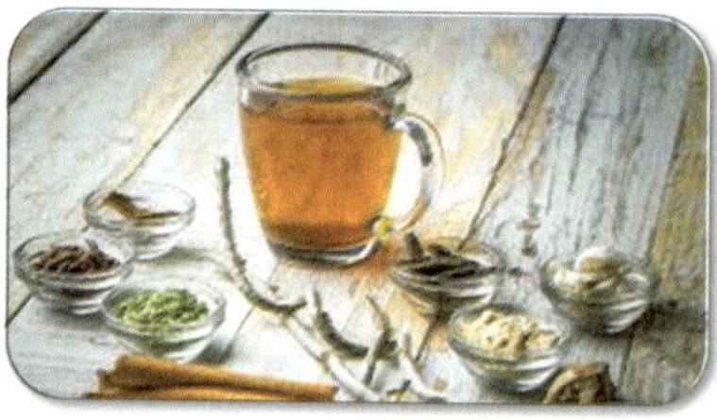

Fig. 7.3: Indian kadha recipe (herbal tea)

Kadha or herbal tea is used commonly to fight with common cold, flu and throat infections. It is very effective in boosting immunity as well as improving metabolism and fighting with stress. This is also considered very effective to fight against COVID-19 infection. Common Indian spices and herbs are used to make this kadha.

Ingredients

- 5 leaves fresh mint (pudina)
- 3–4 basil (tulsi)
- 2 cloves
- 2 cinnamon sticks
- 2–3 pieces of black pepper
- 1 green and 1 black cardamom
- 5 g ginger
- 3–4 big raisins (munnaka) optional

Method

- Crush tulsi, mint and place them in a bowl.
- Crush rest of all the ingredients like cloves, cinnamon sticks, black pepper, green and black cardamom and ginger.
- Take 4–5 cups of water and add all the crushed ingredients in it.
- Simmer it for few minutes until approximately one cup of water is left.
- Strain the water and drink it hot.
- Small amount of salt or honey can also be added.

Note: Some people add other nutrients like giloy, haldi or neem leaves also in the kadha.

Turmeric Milk (Haldi Doodh) (Fig. 7.4)

Turmeric or haldi is an integral part of Indian cooking, without this core spices Indian food cannot be cooked. It not only adds flavor to the food but also increases nutritive value of the food. Turmeric is very well known for its anti-inflammatory properties. It is used to treat common cough, cold, minor injuries and pain. Even in Western countries nowadays, it is consumed in the form of turmeric tablets.

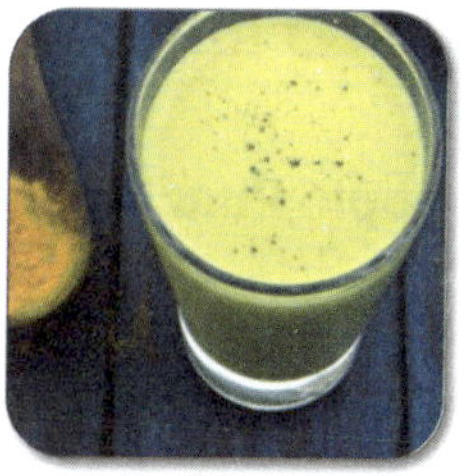

Fig. 7.4: Turmeric milk (Haldi Doodh)

Ingredients

- Milk—250 mL
- Turmeric powder—1 tsp or crushed turmeric if using fresh
- Cardamom—1
- Cinnamon sticks—2
- Black peppercorns—2–3 grains

Method

- Add milk to a pan on medium heat.
- Add turmeric powder or crushed turmeric when the milk is lukewarm.
- Then add crushed green cardamom, cinnamon sticks and black peppercorns.
- Whisk it all together and bring to low simmer for 5 minutes.
- Strain the golden milk and serve it hot.
- Cardamom or cinnamon powder can be sprinkled before serving.
- Honey or sweetener can also be added.

Kahwa (Fig. 7.5)

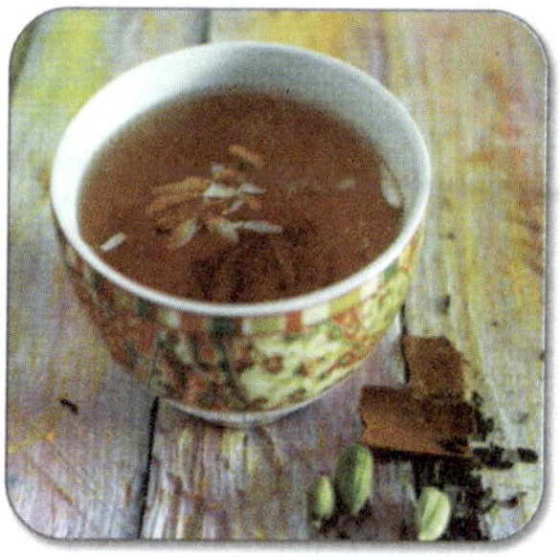

Fig. 7.5: Kahwa

Ingredients

- 1 L water
- 75 g sugar
- 20 g cinnamon sticks
- 10 g cardamom powder
- 40 g kahwa tea
- 50 g almonds

Method

- Boil the water with sugar, cinnamon and cardamom powder for 5 minutes.
- Add the tea leaves and remove from flame.
- Cover the lid and brew for 3 minutes.
- Strain and pour into cups and add almonds into each cup.
- Serve hot.

COLD BEVERAGES

Apple Punch (Fig. 7.6)

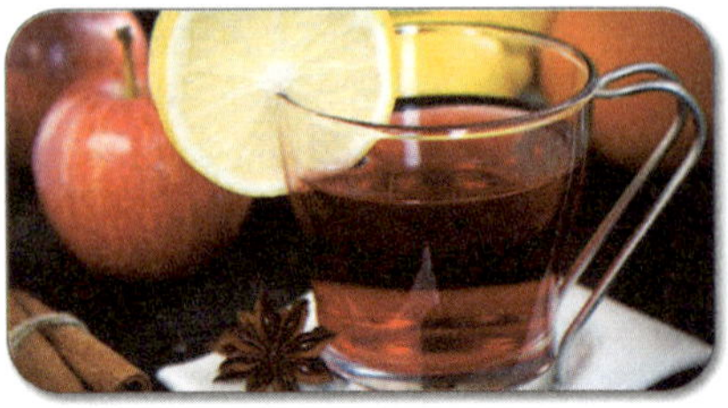

Fig. 7.6: Apple punch

Ingredients

- ½ liter apple juice
- 4 tsp lemon juice
- 2 sticks cinnamon
- ½ inch ginger cube
- 3 cloves
- Lemon string
- Mint sprigs

Method

- Add apple juice in a container.
- Then add few drops of lemon juice into it.
- Put 2 cinnamon sticks, ½ inch ginger cube and lemon strings.
- Combine the mixture well.
- Chill and garnish it with few mint leaves and serve over ice.

Thandai (Fig. 7.7)

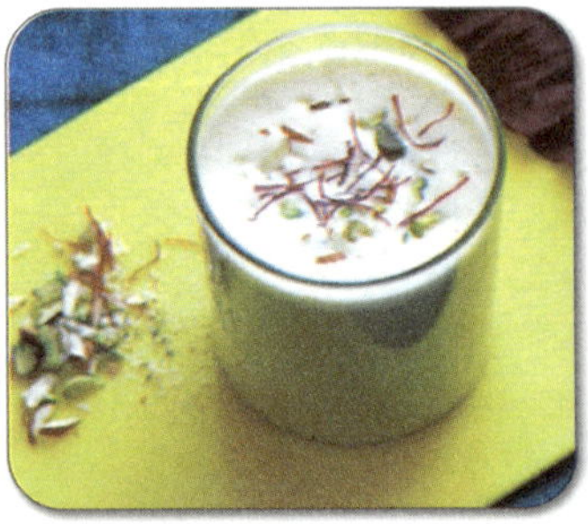

Fig. 7.7: Thandai

Ingredients

Serving 6 glasses

- ½ cup almonds
- ½ cup pistachio
- ½ cup melon seeds
- ½ cup pumpkin seeds
- 2 tsp poppy seeds
- 1 tsp black pepper
- 1 tsp fennel seeds
- 1 tsp clove
- 1 tsp edible rose petals
- 1 tsp green cardamom
- Few strands of saffron
- 1.5 L milk

Method

- In a grinder, add almonds, pistachio, melon and pumpkin seeds, fennel seeds and poppy seeds and grind into a fine powder.

- Add all the spices to the nuts and seeds powder and grind into fine powder.
- Sieve the powder to a thin powdery texture. Save the leftover pieces for garnish.
- Mix 3 tsp of this powder to the milk and mix by pouring from height from one glass to another, until it is properly mixed.
- Garnish with rose petals, crushed almonds and saffron.
- Serve chilled with ice cubes.

Cold Coffee (Fig. 7.8)

Ingredients

- Servings for 2 persons
- 1 tsp instant coffee
- ¼ cup warm water
- 1 tsp sugar or more according to taste
- 2 cups chilled milk
- 4–5 ice cubes

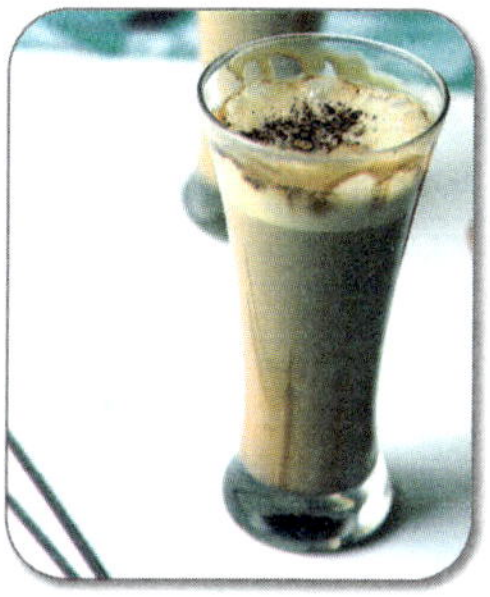

Fig. 7.8: Cold coffee

Method

- In a blender, take 1 tsp coffee, sugar, and water.
- Stir very well till the coffee solution becomes frothy.
- Pour 2 cups of chilled milk and blend once more till everything is mixed well.
- Pour in glasses, add ice cubes and serve chilled.

Aam Panna (Fig. 7.9)

Ingredients

- 1 large-sized raw mango
- 2–3 cardamoms crushed or powdered
- 4–5 black pepper crushed or powdered
- 2 tsp black salt
- Powdered jaggery or sugar almost double the amount of mango pulp

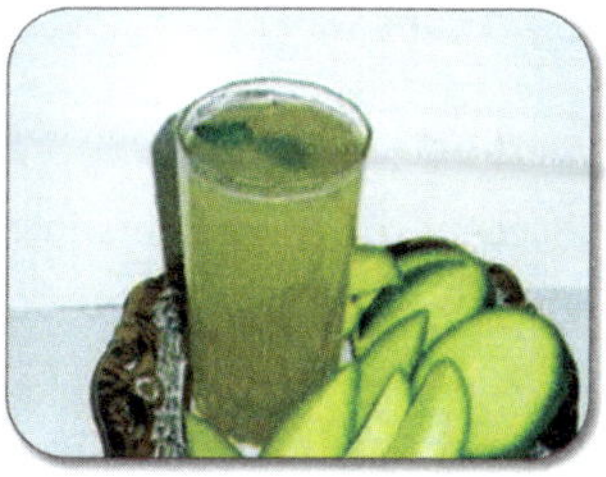

Fig. 7.9: Aam panna

Method

- Rinse the raw mango in water.
- Steam the raw mango in pressure cooker for 3–4 whistles till it becomes completely soft and pulpy.
- Remove the peel and take out mango pulp.
- Mix the cardamom powder, salt, jaggery to mango pulp.
- Mix the ingredients and blend it to smooth.
- Store it in an air tight container.
- While serving add 1 tsp of the preserved mixture to one glass of water.
- Stir and add ice cubes, serve aam panna cold.

Jal Jeera (Fig. 7.10)

Ingredients

- Cumin seeds roasted—2 tbs
- Amchur powder 1 tbs
- Lemon slices for garnish
- Fresh mint leaves
- Fresh coriander leaves
- Lemon juice 2 tbs
- Soda ½ L

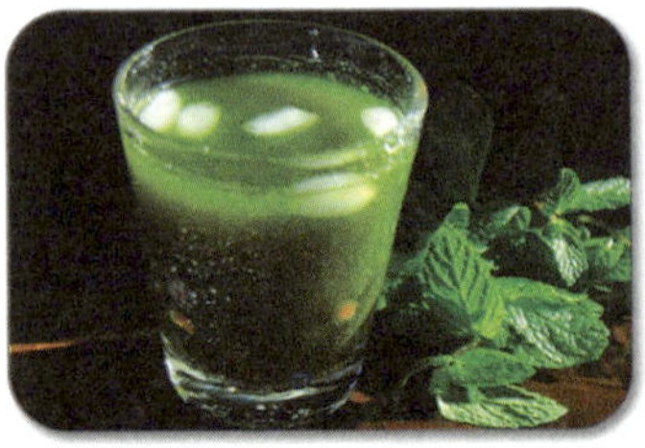

Fig. 7.10: Jal jeera

Method

- Pound the cumin seeds, black salt and amchur (dry mango powder) in mortar with pestle. Grind the mint leaves and coriander leaves with sufficient water into smooth paste.
- Add the lemon juice and pounded masala and mix well. Put the ice cubes in two tall glasses. Divide the concentrate equally and top with soda.
- Mix well, serve immediately, garnish with a slice of lemon.

Fresh Lemonade (Fig. 7.11)

Ingredients

- 1 cup freshly squeezed lemon juice
- 1–4 tbs sugar according to taste
- 1 cup crushed ice
- 4 cups water

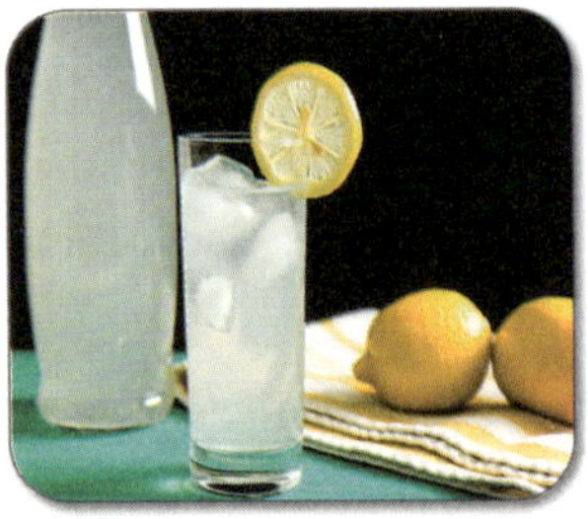

Fig. 7.11: Fresh lemonade

Method

Place all the ingredients in a blender and process until completely smooth. Serve over ice.

Mixed Fruit Juice (Fig. 7.12)

Ingredients

- 4 oranges
- 1 big apple
- 2 cups black grapes
- 1 cup kiwi pieces
- 1 tbs sugar
- A lemon wedge for garnishing

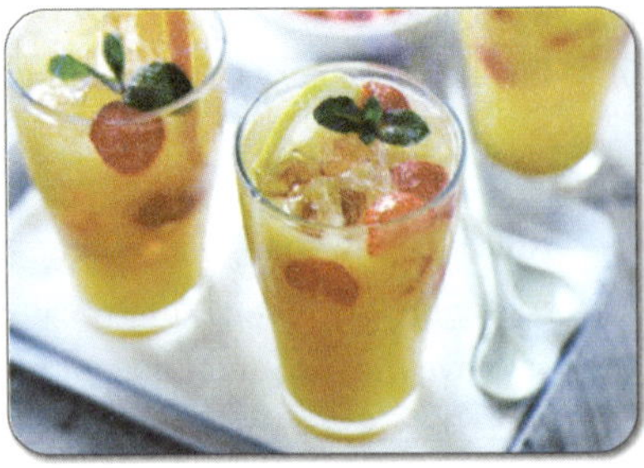

Fig. 7.12: Mixed fruit juice

Method

- Wash and rinse all the fruits and remove tough and bitter parts from them. Also remove seeds and stem.
- Chop the fruits into appropriate pieces or slices. Use seedless grapes and make sure that there is no stem lingering.
- Put the pieces of fruit in the mixer and blend for 2 minutes.
- Take out the juice from the blender and strain it.
- Refrigerate it if want you to and serve chilled or consume fresh immediately.

Banana Shake (Fig. 7.13)

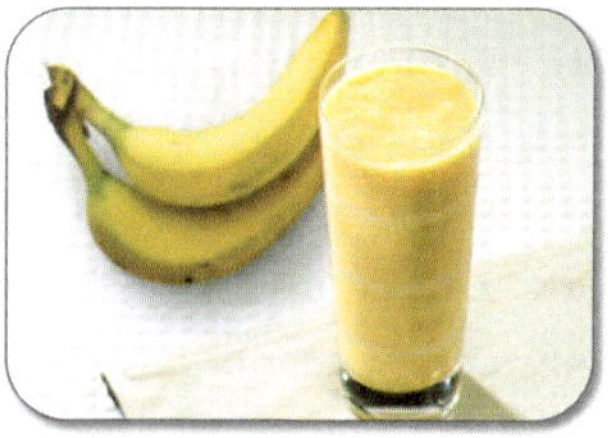

Fig. 7.13: Banana shake

Ingredients

- 1 large banana
- 3–4 cups chilled milk
- 1 tbs sugar or according to taste
- 2 scoops vanilla ice cream (optional)
- A pinch of cardamom powder (optional)

Method

- Take a ripe banana, peel and cut into slices.
- Add sliced banana in the jar of a blender.
- Add a pinch of cardamom powder (optional) and 1 tbs sugar.
- Add 2 scoops vanilla ice cream (optional).
- Pour milk over it and blend until mixture turns smooth and serve chilled.

Coconut Milkshake (Fig. 7.14)

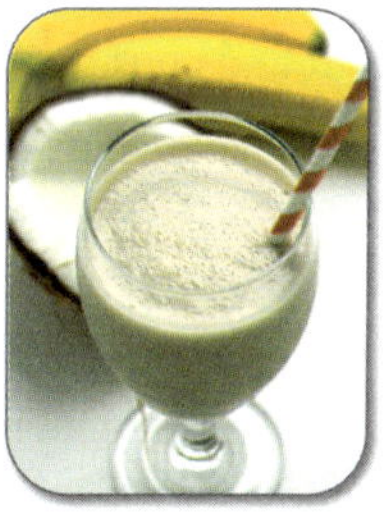

Fig. 7.14: Coconut milkshake

Ingredients

- 1 medium banana
- ½ cup coconut milk
- 1 tbs sugar or according to taste
- 2 scoops vanilla ice cream
- 2 ice cubes

Method

- Take a ripe banana, peel and cut into slices.
- Pour coconut milk into the blender. Add sliced banana, vanilla ice cream and sugar and blend it until mixture turns smooth and serve chilled.

Note: Recipe for other fruits shake is the same, use fruits like peach, mango, strawberry of your choice. Wash it, peel into pieces and add milk and sugar according to taste and blend it smoothly and serve chilled.

SOUPS

Vegetable Soup (Fig. 7.15)

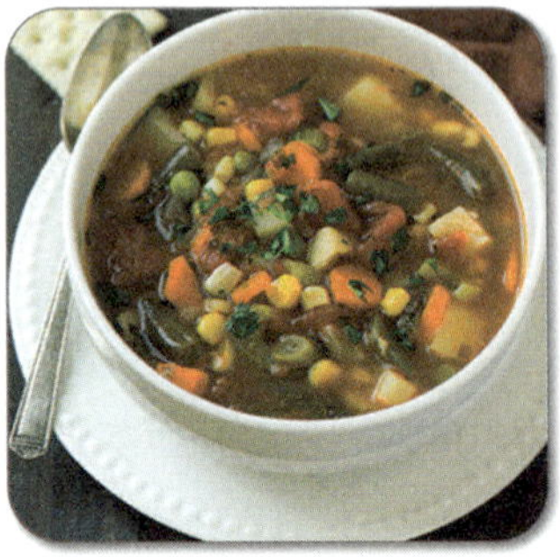

Fig. 7.15: Vegetable soup

Ingredients

- 2 tbs chopped onion
- 2 tsp minced garlic
- ⅓ cup chopped carrot
- ⅓ cup chopped green cabbage
- ⅓ cup chopped French beans
- ½ tbs vinegar
- ¼ tsp ground black pepper
- 2 tbs corn starch (white corn flour)
- ½ tbs butter or oil
- 2½ cup water or vegetable stock
- Salt according to taste

Method

- Chop all the veggies (carrot, cabbage, French beans, onion and garlic) into small pieces.
- Add 2 tbs corn starch (corn flour) in a small bowl.
- Add 3 tbs of water in the bowl and mix well.
- Heat ½ tbs oil or butter in a large heavy bottomed stock pot over medium flame. Add chopped onion and garlic.
- Saute for 1–2 minutes.
- Add carrots, cabbage, sweet corn, French beans (only for veggies).
- Stir and cook for 3–4 minutes.
- Add 2½ cups water. Stir well and bring the mixture to boil. When it starts boiling add salt.
- Add black pepper powder.
- Add corn starch and water mixture and stir continuously for 1 minute to prevent lump formation.
- Stir and cook until mixture turns thick and no raw smell of corn starch. It will take around 7–8 minutes.
- Add vinegar and mix it well and serve hot.

Tomato and Carrot Soup (Fig. 7.16)

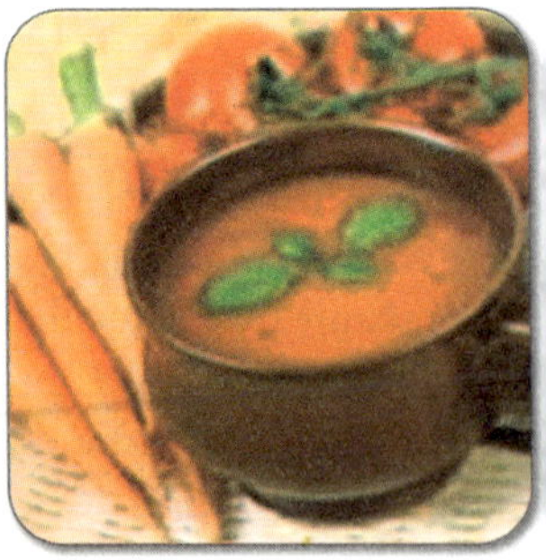

Fig. 7.16: Tomato and carrot soup

Ingredients

- 750 g red tomatoes
- 3–4 medium carrots
- Salt according to taste
- ¼ tbs black pepper
- 4 tsp butter/fresh cream to serve
- 1 tsp brown sugar
- 1 tbs chopped coriander leaves

Methods

- Wash tomatoes and cut each tomato into 4 pieces.
- Wash, peel and cut carrots into small pieces.
- Add salt in tomato and carrots. Boil tomatoes and carrots with one cup of water until they get tender.
- Allow boiled tomatoes and carrots mixture to cool.
- In a blender, transfer the mixture and blend it completely. Add more water if needed to get the required consistency.
- In a sauce pan, boil the tomato and carrot mixture for 10 minutes and add sugar and black pepper as per taste and serve hot.

Sweet Corn Soup (Fig. 7.17)

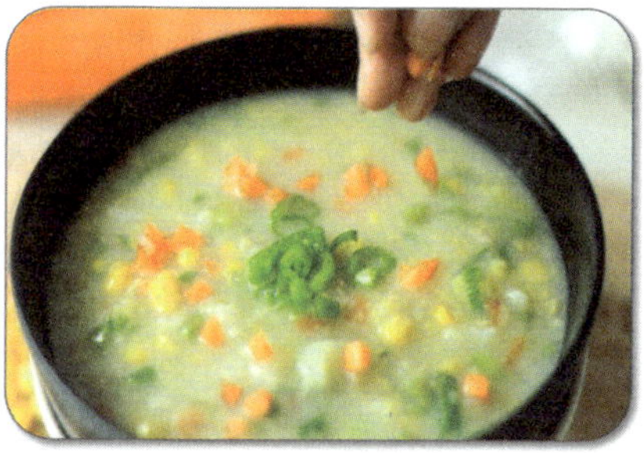

Fig. 7.17: Sweet corn soup

Ingredients

- 1 medium size corn cob (makai or bhutta)
- 1 tbs chopped spring onions
- 1 tbs oil and butter
- 2 cups water
- ½ tbs corn starch (corn flour) dissolved in 2 tbs water.
- Salt as per required

Method

Making Sweet Corn Paste

- Boil the corn cobs. Scrape the corn kernels from the cob.
- Reserve some of the corn kernels aside (about 2 tbs).
- Blend the remaining corn kernels with some water to a smooth paste.

Steps

- First boil or steam the corncobs. This can be done in a pan steamer or pressure cooker.
- Let the corn cobs cool and scrape the corn kernels from the cobs with a knife.
- Blend the corn kernels with some water in a blender till smooth. Keep aside a few corn kernels.
- Heat oil or butter in a pan. Add spring onion, saute the spring onion till they turn translucent.
- Add corn paste and stir.
- Pour water and stir again.
- Let the soup come to a boil. Add freshly ground pepper and salt and the remaining corn kernels.
- Simmer for few minutes.

Mushroom Soup (Fig. 7.18)

Ingredients

- 1 cup chopped mushroom
- 2 tbs chopped onion

- 2 tsp plain flour (maida)
- 1½ cup milk
- 2 tsp butter
- Black pepper according to taste

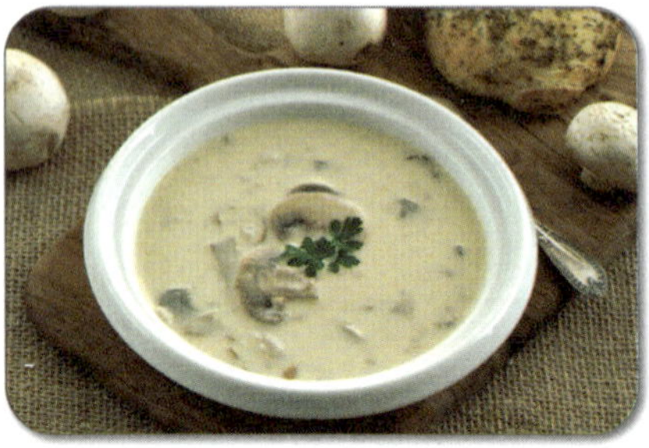

Fig. 7.18: Mushroom soup

Method

- Combine the milk and 2 cups of water in a deep pan and bring to a boil and keep aside.
- Heat the butter in a pan. Add the onions and saute on a medium flame for few minutes.
- Add the mushroom and saute on a medium flame for 2–3 minutes.
- Add the plain flour and saute on a medium flame for a few seconds.
- Add the milk water mixture gradually and cook on a medium flame for 2–3 minutes till no lump remain while stirring continuously.
- Add the salt and pepper and bring to boil.

Buttermilk (Lassi) (Fig. 7.19)

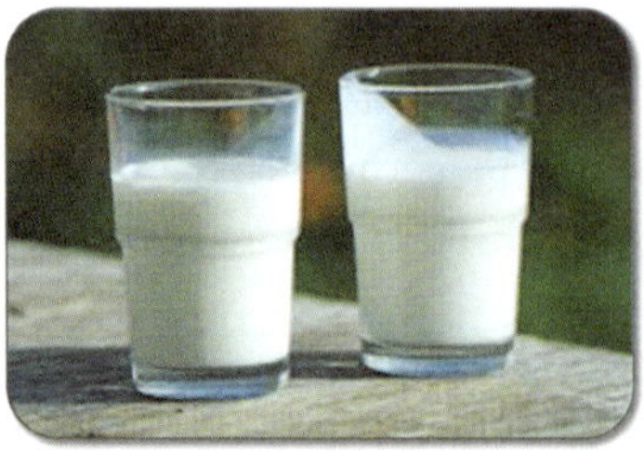

Fig. 7.19: Buttermilk (lassi)

Ingredients

- 2 cups curd
- Salt / sugar according to taste
- Water according to need

Method

- To prepare simple buttermilk, take 2 cups of curd and churn it with either wood churner or blend it in a mixer grinder.
- Add water and salt/ sugar according to taste.
- For additional flavors one can also add coriander or mint leaves.

Barley Water (Fig. 7.20)

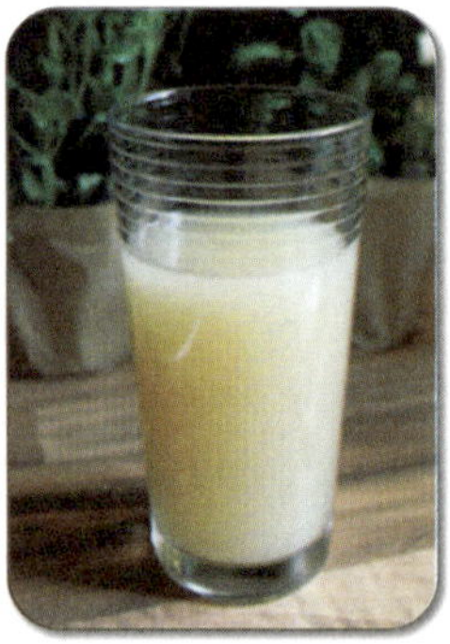

Fig. 7.20: Barley water

Boil 1kg of barley pearls until they turn soft (add 3 volumes of water to one volume of barley). Strain and collect the extract. If one does not like the taste, then add a dash of orange or lemon or brown sugar according to taste. This is a perfect solution for losing the weight.

EGG PREPARATIONS

Eggs are also known as super foods because of their multiple health benefits. Eggs not only provide high quality proteins but also are rich source of 11 vitamins, minerals, omega-3 fatty acids and antioxidants. Most of the protein in eggs can be found in egg white, while the yolk contains healthy fats, vitamins, minerals and antioxidants. Just one boiled egg contains 40% of daily vitamin D, 25% of folate, 12% of vitamin B_2

requirements, 20% of selenium requirements. Besides that egg contain vitamin A, E, B_5, B_{12} as well as iron, iodine and phosphorus.

Source: www.australianeggs.org.nutrition

Following are few egg preparations:

Egg Flip (Fig. 7.21)

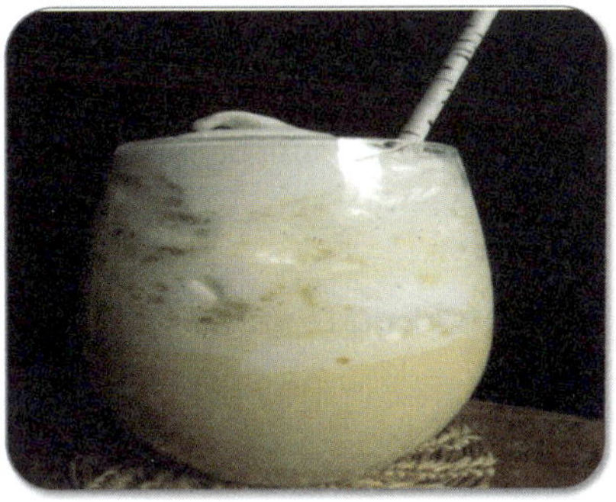

Fig. 7.21: Egg flip

Ingredients

- 1 cup milk
- 1 tsp vanilla extract
- 1 egg
- 1 tsp sugar
- Grated nutmeg

Method

- Place all ingredients in a shaker and shake vigorously or you can blend in a blender.
- Put chilled mixture into glasses and shake nutmeg on top.

Note: Raw eggs should not be served to the pregnant women, young children, babies, elderly or the person who are already sick due to dangers associated with salmonella poisoning.

Egg Scramble (Fig. 7.22)

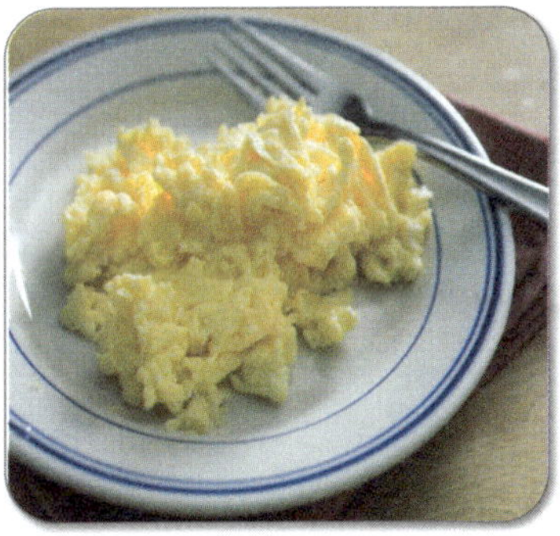

Fig. 7.22: Egg scramble

Ingredients

- 2 large eggs
- Salt and freshly grounded black pepper according to taste
- 1 tbs unsalted butter

Method

- Lightly beat the eggs, add salt and pepper in a medium bowl.
- Melt ½ tbs of butter in a medium nonstick skillet over low heat, swirl to coat the bottom and sides. Add the eggs and cook slowly, scraping them with a rubber spatula occasionally, until most of the liquid has thickened and eggs are soft. Remove them from the heat and gently fold in the remaining ½ tsp of butter. Serve hot.

Omlet (Fig. 7.23)

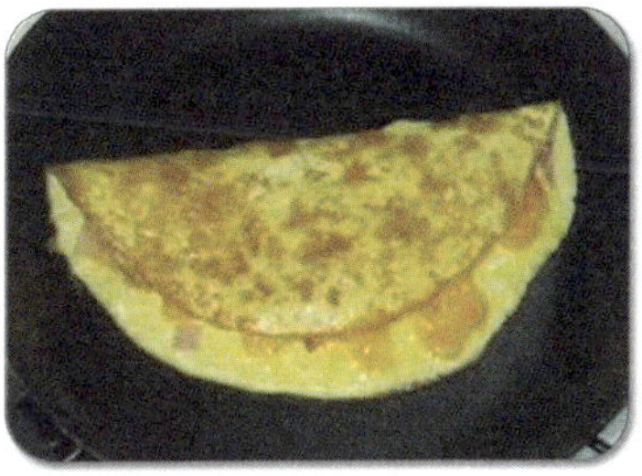

Fig. 7.23: Omlet

Ingredients

- 2 large eggs
- Pinch of salt and pepper
- 1 tsp of oil

Method

- Take the eggs and crack them into the bowl.
- Add a pinch of salt and pepper before whisking with a fork and mix the white and the yolk part properly.
- Bring pan to the high heat and add oil so that mixture does not stick.
- Pour the mixture and cook on a high heat for two minutes, making sure that mixture is spread out evenly.
- Cook the set omelet for another minute, and then loosen the edges with a spatula and fold the omelet in half and tilt the pan and slide the omelet into plate and serve immediately.

Note: Omelet can also be filled with vegetables like onion, tomato, fresh herbs, and mushrooms or with sea food like prawn.

Poached Egg (Fig. 7.24)

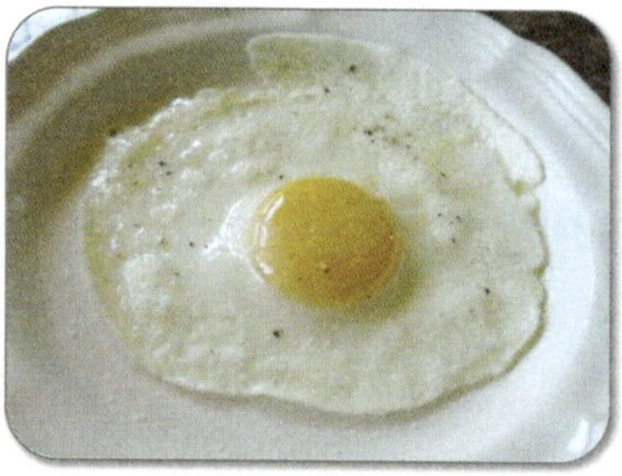

Fig. 7.24: Poached egg

Ingredients

- 1 large egg
- Pinch of salt and pepper
- Water

Method

- Fill a wide pan with boiling water.
- Bring it to simmer and add a pinch of salt.
- Crack a large egg into cup.
- Gently pour the egg into the simmering water in one movement.
- Egg begins to cook immediately. Do not worry if the edges look a little scruffy.
- To check if it is done, carefully remove it with a slotted spoon and place it on the kitchen paper to dry off.
- Serve it with the hot toast and also sprinkle sea salt and black pepper.

LIGHT DIET

Light diets include the foods that are well tolerated by patients whose digestion is impaired as a result of illness or surgery. Such foods are soft in texture, easy to chew and digest. This diet is recommended for patients who are not able to consume a full or normal diet. The following are few examples of light diet.

Porridge (Fig. 7.25)

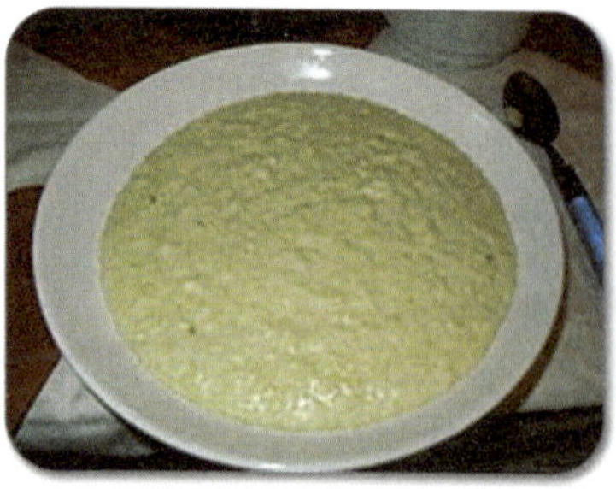

Fig. 7.25: Porridge

Ingredients

- 1 cup traditional rolled oats
- ½ cup skim or full fat milk
- Honey or brown sugar to serve

Method

- Soak oats in one cup of water overnight.

- Add some water in the soaked mixture, put over medium heat until mixture boils, then simmer, stirring for 3–5 minutes or until thick.
- Add milk and stir until heated and divide porridge among bowls. Top with honey or brown sugar and serve with extra milk on the side.

Gruel (Fig. 7.26)

It is a thin porridge made by boiling groats (the crushed grains of various cereals) in water or milk. This type of food is commonly eaten in middle ages.

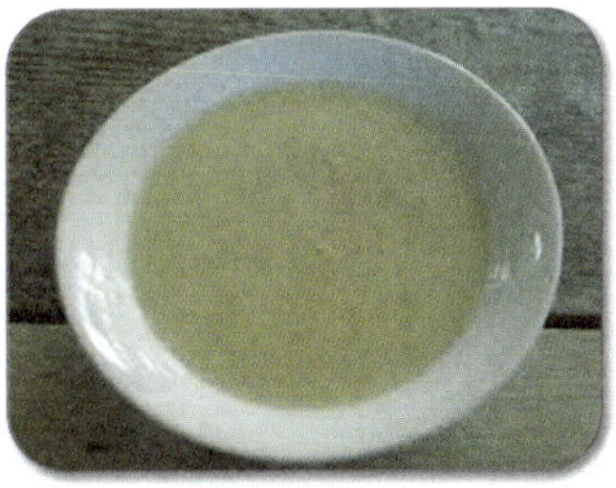

Fig. 7.26: Gruel

Ingredients

- 1 tbs of groats
- 2 tbs of cold water
- 1 pint of boiling water

Method

- First put the groats together with the cold water into a saucepan and mix together until smooth.
- Over this stirring all the time, pour one pint of boiling water.
- Now stirring frequently boil for 10 minutes.
- Add salt and black pepper according to taste and serve hot.

Khichdi (Fig. 7.27)

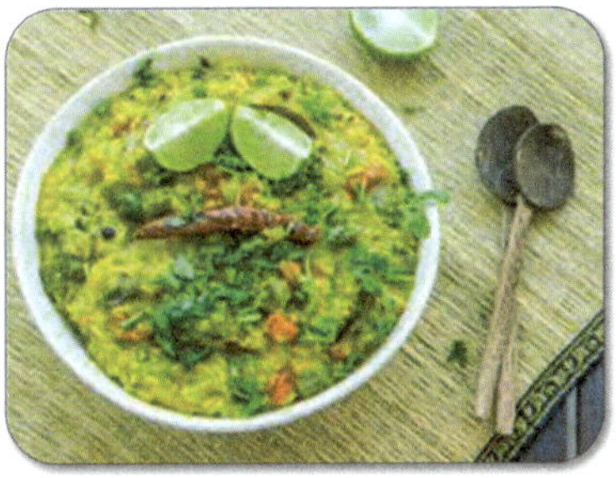

Fig. 7.27: Khichdi

Ingredients

- ½ cup moong dal (split and husked)
- ½ cup rice
- 1 small to medium sized onion—finely chopped
- 1 medium size tomato chopped
- ½ inch ginger—finely chopped
- 1 small green chili
- 1 tsp cumin seeds
- ¼ tsp turmeric powder
- 1 pinch asafetida
- 3.5 cups water
- Salt according to taste

Method

- Rinse and wash moong lentils and rice together.
- Soak both of them for 30 minutes in water.
- Heat 2 tbs ghee or oil in a pressure cooker; add cumin, when cumin splutters add onions.
- Sauté onion till translucent, then add tomato, green chilli and ginger.

- Stir and add turmeric powder and asafetida, sauté till tomato softens.
- Drain the rice and moong lentils and add them to pressure cooker.
- Stir for a minute, pour water and salt according to taste.
- Close the lid tightly and pressure cook the khichdi on low flame for 2–3 whistles.
- The consistency of the khichdi can be adjusted as per choice by adding less or more water.
- Serve moong dal khichdi hot with curd or on the top of khichdi ghee can be added (optional).

Dalia (Sweet) (Fig. 7.28)

Ingredients

- ¼ cup raw dalia (cracked wheat)
- 1 cup milk
- 1 cup water
- 1 tsp melted butter or ghee
- Dry fruits (optional)

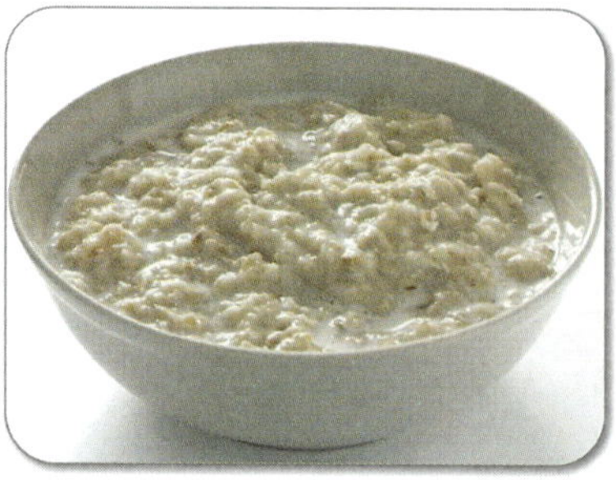

Fig. 7.28: Dalia (sweet)

Method

- In a roasted pan, add dalia and butter or ghee and roast it on a medium low heat for 4–5 minutes or till it becomes light brown and gives roasted aroma.
- Add water and mix the roasted dalia and partially cover the pan.
- Let it cook for 10–12 minutes until it becomes tender.
- Add milk, let cook it until it reaches the desired consistency.
- Add sugar according to taste and dry fruits like sliced almonds, chopped raisins (optional).
- **Note:** If you do not want to add ghee or butter, roast dalia dry on low heat.
- Dalia can also be cooked salty just like khichdi.

Kanji (Fig. 7.29)

Ingredients

- Rice–50 g
- Moong dal–25 g
- Salt–1 tsp
- Water–1 L

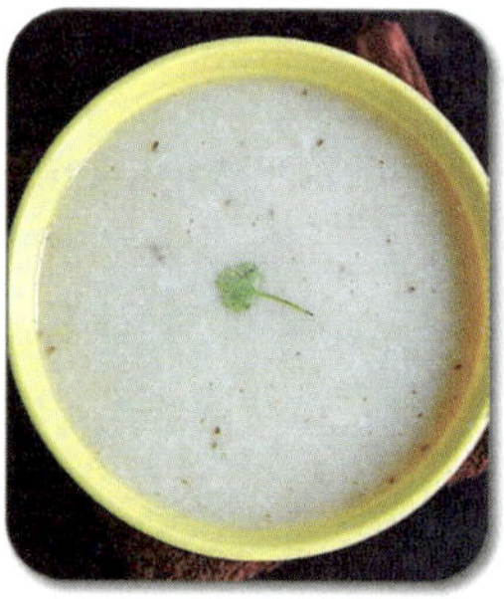

Fig. 7.29: Kanji

Method

- Grind rice and moong dal to a coarse powder.
- Boil ½ L of water in a vessel.
- Add the powder and simmer the flame.
- Cook well by mixing it with a spoon or ladle.
- Check whether the rice and dal is cooked.
- Once it is cooked put off the flame.

- Transfer to a bowl and at the time of serving add 2 cups of boiled water, salt and drink in watery consistency.

Note: It is one of the simple and easily digestible food items preferred in South India in illness especially in the fever.

Boiled Vegetables (Fig. 7.30)

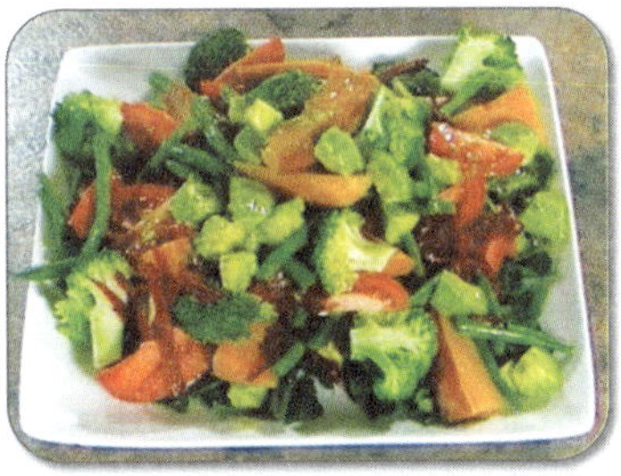

Fig. 7.30: Boiled vegetables

Ingredients

Any vegetable can be boiled or steamed depending upon the individual choice. For example, spinach, peas, broccoli, sweet corn, potatoes, turnip, cauliflower, cabbage, etc.

Method

- Cut the vegetables into equal sizes.
- Add some water (1 inch) to the pan and insert the steamer basket. The surface of the water should be under the basket.
- Bring the water to boil. Add the vegetables into steamer basket, put the vagetables which take longer time to cook first and then the vegetable which take lesser time for cooking. Then reduce the heat to medium.
- Steam the vegetables till they become tender.
- Serve the vegetables by adding some butter, salt, pepper or with a little olive oil. Lemon can also be squeezed to make it more tasty.

SALADS

Vegetable Salad (Fig. 7.31)

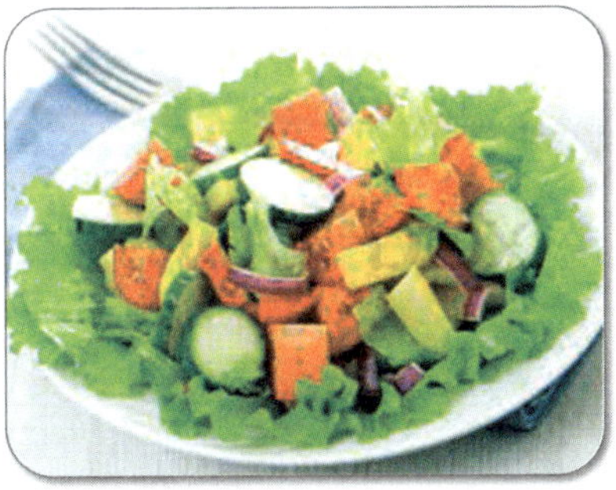

Fig. 7.31: Vegetable salad

Vegetable salad not only helps to digest the meal better but also adds nutrition to the meal.

Ingredients

- Cucumber, carrots, onions, tomato, green chilli, cabbage or any other vegetable can be used to serve in salads
- Salt, pepper powder as needed
- Lemon juice as needed
- Vinegar can also be used instead of lemon
- Mint/coriander leaves as needed

Method

Cut all the ingredients; add to a bowl or plate. Put salt, pepper, lemon juice or vinegar, mint/coriander leaves as needed. Serve immediately.

Note: To reduce the pungent smell from onions, chop them and put more lemon juice and set aside for sometime.

Fruit Salad (Fig. 7.32)

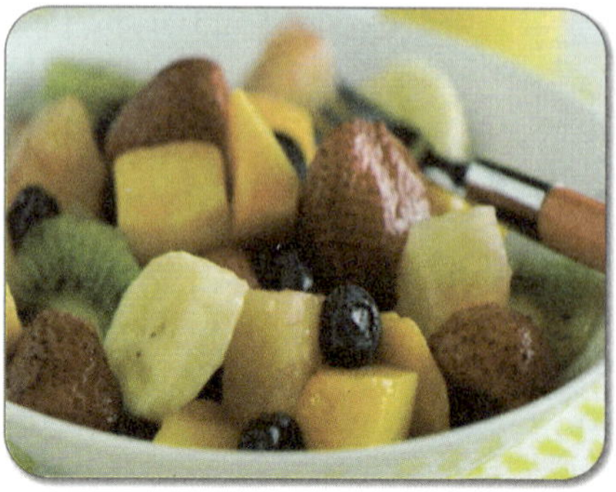

Fig. 7.32: Fruit salad

Ingredients

- 2 cup mixed berries (blueberries, strawberries)
- 1 cup seedless grapes
- 2 apples
- 2 bananas
- 3 peaches or apricots
- Lemon/orange juice
- Nutmeg (optional)

Method

- Chop berries, grapes, apples, bananas, peaches or apricots.
- Place them in a large bowl and mix gently.
- Pour some lemon juice, rock salt and stir. Serve immediately.

Mix Fruit Custard (Fig. 7.33)

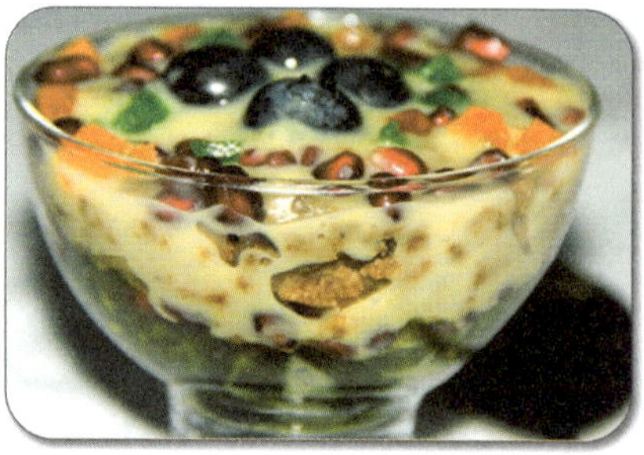

Fig. 7.33: Mix fruit custard

Ingredients

- 1 liter milk
- 3 tbs custard powder
- 3 tbs sugar
- 2 apples (chopped)
- 2 bananas (chopped)
- 1 cup grapes (halved)
- 2 small mangoes
- 2 tbs honey
- 450 g vanilla ice cream

Method

- Take 80% of milk into a pan and bring to boil.
- Stir custard powder with the remaining milk in a bowl.
- Pour into the boiling milk, stirring continuously.
- Stir in sugar and simmer until thickened.
- Remove from heat and cool to room temperature.
- Refrigerate until chill.
- Mix fruits with honey in a large bowl and mix custard.
- Garnish with vanilla ice cream and serve cold.

LOW COST HIGH NUTRITION DIET

The purpose of low cost and high nutrition diet is to provide maximum nutrients at a very reasonable cost to cater the needs of lower socioeconomic groups. These food items are not only locally and easily available but also easy to prepare.

Peanut Chikki (Fig. 7.34)

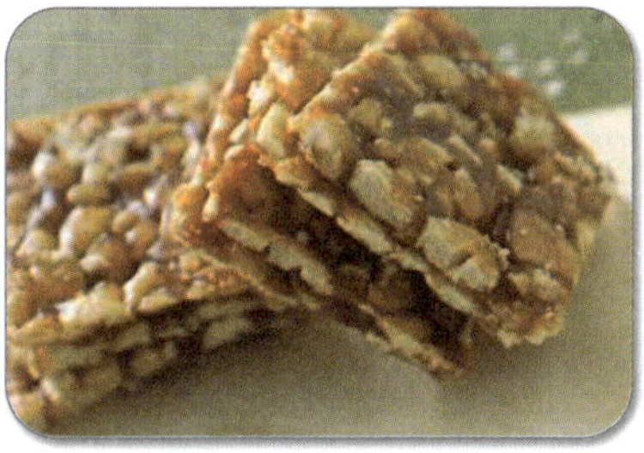

Fig. 7.34: Peanut chikki

Ingredients

- 250 g peanuts
- 200 g sugar/jaggery
- 25 g butter

Method

- Skin, roast and coarsely crush the peanuts.
- Heat jaggery with ½ cup of water until thick.
- Boil the syrup until hard crack consistency (Test its consistency by putting a drop in cold water—it should crack after taking out).
- Add the peanuts and mix thoroughly.
- Grease a tray and spread the mixture.
- Roll flat to 1 cm in thickness and cut into squares when cooled and store in an airtight container.

Note: Dry fruits can also be added in chikki

Multigrain Roti (Fig. 7.35)

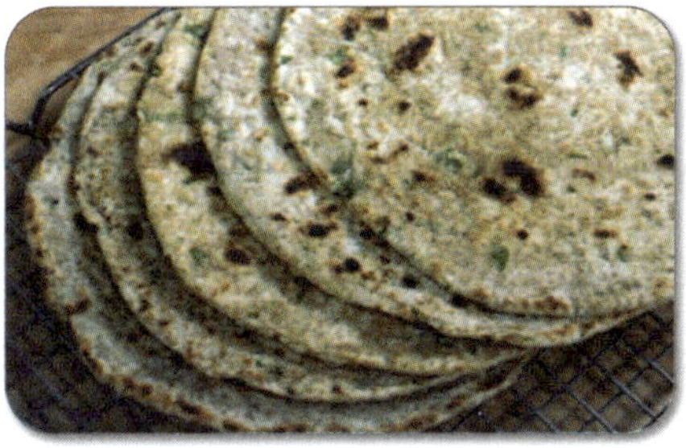

Fig. 7.35: Multigrain roti

Ingredients

- 75 g whole wheat flour
- 75 g jowar flour (white millet flour)
- 75 g bajra flour (black millet flour)
- 75 g ragi flour (finger millet flour)
- 75 g soybean flour
- 75 g makki flour (maize flour)
- 1 tbs ajwain
- 1 tbs cumin seed
- 1 tbs white sesame seed (til)
- 1 tbs salt
- 2 tbs hot oil
- 150 mL hot boiling water

Method

- Mix all the flours, seeds and salt nicely. Put hot boiling water and warm oil. Cover and keep aside for 15 minutes.

- Knead into soft dough and cover with a damp cloth for 5–10 minutes. Make small balls. Roll the balls with roller into rounds. Dust some flour while using the roller, otherwise the dough will stick to the roller. Repeat the same process with rest of the balls.
- Place tava or pan on high heat. Once it is heated nicely put flame into medium heat. Keep the roti over the tava/pan, cook roti from both the sides. Serve hot with any vegetable.

Nutritious Laddoo (Fig. 7.36)

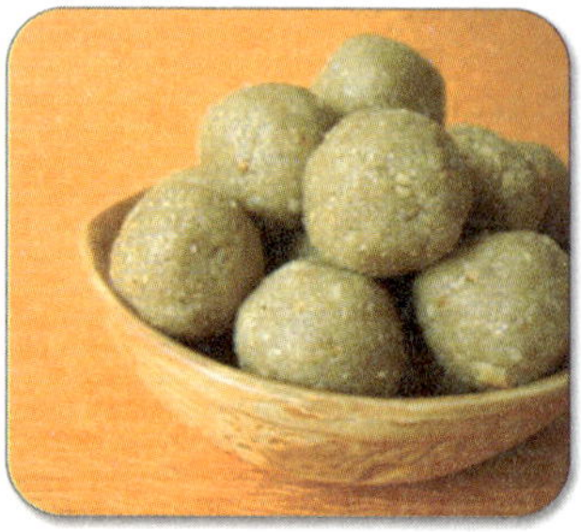

Fig. 7.36: Nutritious laddoo

Ingredients

- 100 g ghee
- 100 g wheat flour
- 150 g jaggery
- 100 g besan (gram flour)
- Roasted moong pulse flour (green grams)—100 g
- ½ bowl peanuts
- 10–15 g til (white sesame seed)

Method

- Put small amount of water in 150 g jaggery and heat it for some time until it becomes little thick (it should not be too thick). Keep it aside.
- Put ghee in a pan. Put wheat flour, gram flour, roasted moong dal flour in ghee and roast it for some time until it becomes light brown and gives roasted aroma.
- Put prepared syrup of jaggery. Add peanuts and white sesame seed. Grease a tray and spread the mixture and make laddoos from it.

Note: Dry fruits may also be added (optional).

WORLD HEALTH ORGANIZATION (WHO) NUTRITION ADVICE FOR ADULTS DURING THE COVID-19 OUTBREAK

Proper nutrition and hydration play a pivotal role to combat with any disease. People who eat well balanced diet tend to be healthier with strong immune system and low risk to catch the infectious diseases. The following points must be kept in mind while combating with pandemic.

Eat fresh and unprocessed food every day:

- Eat fruits, vegetables, legumes, nuts and whole grains like unprocessed maize, millets, oats, wheat, brown rice, milk and food from animal sources like meat, fish and egg.
- Eat at least 2 cups of fruits (4 serving) and 180 g of grains everyday, and 160 g of meat and poultry products at least 2–3 times per week.
- Choose raw vegetables and fresh fruits for snacks rather than foods that are high in sugar, fat or salt.
- Do not overcook vegetables and fruits as this can lead to loss of many important vitamins.

Drink enough water everyday:

- Water is essential for life. It transports nutrients and compounds in blood, regulates body temperature, helps to get rid of waste, lubricates and cushions the joints.

- Minimum 8–10 glasses of water must be consumed.
- Avoid too much caffeine, sweetened fruit juices, syrups and other soft drinks.

Eat moderate amount of fat and oil:

- Consume unsaturated fats that are found in fish, avocado, nuts, olive oil, soy, canola, sunflower and corn oils. Avoid saturated fats that are found in fatty meat, butter, cream, cheese and ghee.
- Choose white meat like poultry and fish which are generally low in fat rather than red meat.

Avoid processed meats as they are high in fats and salt:

- Consume low fat version of milk as well as other dairy products.
- Avoid industrial produced fats that are found in processed food, fast food, snacks, fried food, frozen pizza, burgers, pies and cookies.

Eat less salt and sugar:

- When cooking and preparing food, limit the amount of salt and high sodium condiments like soy sauce and fish sauce.
- Daily intake of salt must be <5 g (approximately 1 tsp) and always use iodized salt.
- Limit intake of soft drinks, sodas and other high sugar drinks like fruit juices, flavored milk and yogurt.

Avoid eating out:

- Eat at home to reduce the rate of contact with other people and lower the chance of being exposed to COVID-19.
- Always use face mask, wash the hands or sanitize hands frequently and maintain at least 1 meter distance while going outside.

Counseling and psychosocial support:

- Along with proper nutrition, hydration, sleep and all safety precautions people who are suspected or confirmed cases of COVID-19 also need counseling and psychosocial support to improve their mental health and reduce stress and anxiety.

Source: www.emro.who.int

Notes

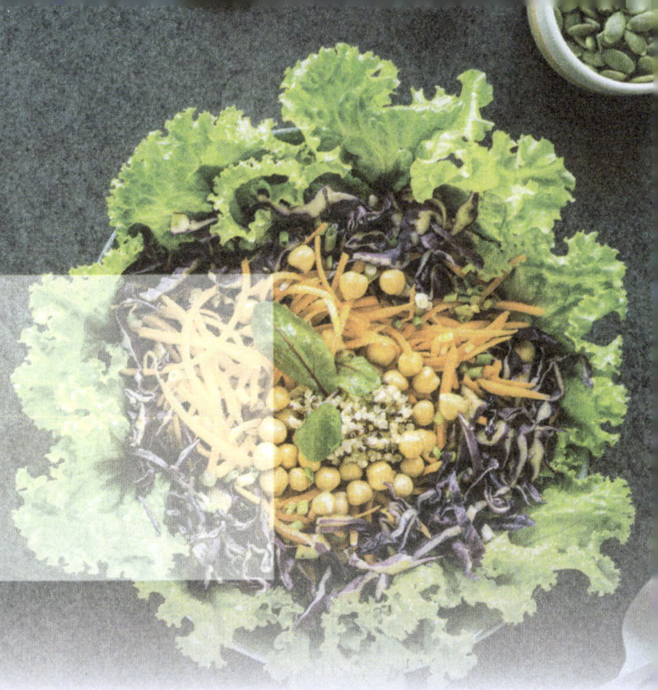

Annexure

COMMONLY ASKED QUESTIONS IN EXAMINATION

- Explain common nutritional problems in India.
- Discuss dietary sources of proteins.
- Discuss protein deficiency diseases.
- Plan one day diet for toddler.
- Enlist fat soluble vitamins.
- What are the principles of cooking?
- Describe the different factors that help a patient in acceptance of diet.
- Explain different methods of preparation, preservation and cooking of food.
- Write a short note on balanced diet.
- Explain normal dietary requirements.
- Describe factors affecting selection and planning of meal.
- Write about food hygiene and laws related to food.
- Write a short note on classification of food.
- Write down the classification of proteins.
- What are the factors to be kept in mind by the nurse while selection and planning of meal?
- Explain functions of carbohydrates.
- Enlist main vitamin deficiencies.

NUTRITIVE VALUES OF COOKED PREPARATION

Katori = 1 **Volume = 200 cc** **Diameter = 78 cm** **Depth = 4 cm**

Cooked foodstuff	App. Wt. Qty.	Raw (g)	Protein (g)	Fat (g)	Carbohydrate (g)	Energy (kcal)	Na (mg)
Chapati (thin)	One	25	3.0	0.4	17.3	85	5.0
Chapati (medium)	One	30	3.6	0.5	20.8	102	6.0
Chapati (big)	One	40	4.8	0.6	27.7	136	8.0
Rice	1 Katori	40	2.7	0.2	31.2	138	—
Wheat porridge	-do-	25	2.6	0.2	18.7	87	5.2
Dal moong (with husk)	-do-	25	6.0	0.3	14.1	83	7.0
Dal moong (washed)	-do-	40	9.8	0.4	23.9	139	10.8
Dal urad (whole)	-do-	35	8.4	0.3	19.8	116	10.8
Dal urad + chana (3 + 1)	-do-	25 + 10	8.0	0.7	20.6	123	22.5
Dal urad (whole)	-do-	30	7.2	0.4	17.8	104	12.0
Dal masoor	-do-	35	8.7	0.2	20.6	120	—
Dal malka masoor	-do-	35	8.7	0.2	25.0	137	8.7
Chana dal	-do-	35	7.2	1.9	19.6	116	25.6
Arhar dal	-do-	35	7.8	0.5	20.1	117	9.9
Rajmah	-do-	35	8.0	0.4	21.2	121	—
Dal urad (washed)	-do-	45	11.0	0.6	27.0	156	20.0
Bengal gram (whole)	-do-	50	8.5	2.6	30.4	180	18.6
Coffee-milk (30 cc) sugar 10 g	-do-	200	1.0	1.0	11.3	59	4.8
Tea-milk 20 cc sugar 10 g	-do-	200	0.7	10.8	52.4	53	3.2

NUTRITIVE VALUE OF COMMON INDIAN FOOD ARTICLES

Foodstuff	Amount	Proteins (g)	Fats (g)	CHO (g)	Energy (kcal)
Milk and milk products					
Milk toned	100 mL	3.5	3.5	5.0	66
Milk cow's	100 mL	3.2	4.1	4.4	67
Milk goat's	100 mL	3.3	4.5	4.6	72
Milk buffalo's	100 mL	4.3	6.5	5.0	117
Milk human	100 mL	1.1	3.4	7.4	65
Curd	100 mL	3.1	4.0	3.0	60
Curd toned	100 mL	3.0	3.0	4.0	55
Buttermilk	100 mL	0.8	1.1	0.5	15
Milk powder	100 g	38.0	0.1	51.0	357
Milk liquid	100 mL	2.5	0.1	4.6	29
Paneer	100 g	18.3	20.8	1.2	265
Cheese processed	100 g	24.0	25.1	6.3	348
Whole milk powder	100 g	25.8	26.7	38.0	496
Cream	100 g	1.5	40.0	2.5	385
Cereals and pulses					
Wheat atta	100 g	12.1	1.7	69.4	341
Rice	100 g	6.8	0.5	78.2	345
Maize	100 g	11.1	3.6	66.2	342
Gram	100 g	17.0	5.3	61.0	360
Porridge	100 g	12.0	1.5	71.2	346
Oat meal	100 g	13.6	7.6	62.8	37.4
Cornflakes	100 g	0.8	—	85.0	385
Popcorns (salt added)	100 g	13.0	5.0	87.0	385
Rice flakes	100 g	6.6	1.2	77.3	346
Rice puffed (salt added)	100 g	7.5	0.1	73.6	325
Suji	100 g	10.4	0.8	74.8	348
Vermicelli/semia	100 g	8.7	0.4	78.3	352
Maida	100 g	11.0	0.9	73.9	348
Cornflour or custard powder	100 g	0.5	—	86.6	345
Biscuit sweet	100 g	6.4	15.2	71.9	450
Bengal gram whole	100 g	17.1	5.3	60.9	360

Contd...

Foodstuff	Amount	Proteins (g)	Fats (g)	CHO (g)	Energy (kcal)
Grapes	100 g	0.5	0.3	16.5	71
Lemon	100 g	1.0	0.9	11.1	57
Jamun	100 g	0.7	0.3	14.0	62
Litchi	100 g	1.1	0.2	13.6	61
Lime sweet (mosambi)	100 g	0.8	0.3	9.3	43
Mango	100 g	0.6	0.4	16.9	74
Orange	100 g	0.7	0.2	10.9	48
Orange juice	100 g	0.2	0.1	1.9	9
Papaya ripe	100 g	0.6	0.1	7.2	32
Peaches	100 g	1.2	0.3	10.5	50
Pear	100 g	0.6	0.2	11.9	52
Plums	100 g	0.7	0.5	11.1	52
Pineapples	100 g	0.4	0.1	10.8	46
Pomegranate	100 g	1.6	0.1	14.5	65
Raspberry	100 g	1.0	0.6	11.6	56
Nuts and oilseeds					
Almond	100 g	20.8	58.9	10.5	655
Cashewnuts	100 g	21.2	46.9	22.3	596
Charoli seeds	100 g	19.0	59.0	12.0	666
Coconut dry	100 g	6.8	62.3	18.4	662
Coconut fresh	100 g	4.5	41.6	13.0	444
Walnut	100 g	15.6	64.5	11.0	687
Gingelly seeds	100 g	18.3	43.3	25.0	563
Groundnuts	100 g	26.2	39.8	26.7	570
Pistachio nut	100 g	19.8	53.5	16.2	626
Chilgoza	100 g	13.9	49.3	29.0	615
Butter and oils					
Butter	100 g	—	81.0	—	729
Ghee (pure)	100 g	—	100.0	—	900
Vegetable cooking oil	100 g	—	100.0	—	900
Vanaspati ghee	100 g	—	100.0	—	900
Miscellaneous foodstuff					
Arrowroot	100 g	0.2	0.1	83.1	334
Betel leaves	100 g	3.1	0.8	6.1	44
Cane sugar	100 g	0.1	0	99.4	398

Contd...

Foodstuff	Amount	Proteins (g)	Fats (g)	CHO (g)	Energy (kcal)
Honey	100 g	0.3	0	79.5	319
Jaggery	100 g	0.4	0.1	95.0	383
Papad	100 g	18.8	0.3	52.4	288
Sago	100 g	0.2	0.2	87.1	351
Yeast dried	100 g	39.5	0.6	391	320
Jam	30 g	0.1	—	18.0	73
Beer 6%	250 cc	—	—	4.0	110
Whiskey 42%	50 cc	—	—	—	140
Brandy 54%	50 cc	—	—	—	150
Horlicks	One tbs	2.4	0.1	7.0	42
Horlicks	100 g	14.0	0.8	72.0	416
Bread	100 g	7.8	0.7	52.0	245

POTASSIUM CONTENT OF VARIOUS FOODS

Foodstuff (100 g)	Potassium content (mg)
Fenugreek leaves	31
Beetroot	43
Broad beans	39
Ridge gourd	50
Lettuce	33
Radish pink	10
Cucumber	50
Snake gourd	34
Pineapple	37
Arrowroot flour	20
Rice, raw milled	70
Field beans, tender	74
Peas	79
Apple	**75**
Papaya, ripe	69
Semolina	83
Banana, ripe	88
Guava	91
Orange	93
Pear	96

Contd...

Foodstuff (100 g)	Potassium content (mg)
Milk	90
Bitter gourd	87
Maize tender	151
Rice flakes	154
Carrot	108
Radish white	138
Bitter gourd	171
Brinjal	200
Lady's-finger	103
Tomato green	114
Onion big	127
Cauliflower	138
French beans	120
Pomegranate	133
Watermelon	160
Lime, sweet malta	170
Tomato ripe	146
Curd	130
Barley	253
Wheat (whole)	284

Contd...

Foodstuff (100 g)	Potassium content (mg)
Maize dry	280
Wheat flour	315
Wheat white	284
Green gram dal	1150
Red gram dal	1104
Bengal gram dal	720
Green gram (whole)	843
Lentil	629
Spinach	206
Potato	247
Papaya, green	216
Red green tender	463
Amla	225
Lemon	270
Lime, sweet mosambi	490
Plums	247
Mango ripe	205
Sapota (cheeku)	269
Chillies dry	530
Cumin seeds	980

Contd...

CHOLESTEROL CONTENT OF FOOD ITEMS

Foodstuff (100 g)	Cholesterol content (mg)
Brain raw	200
Fish	300
Chicken, flesh only raw	60
Egg yolk	252
Ice cream	45
Lamb raw	70
Cheese cream	120
Pork	70
Butter	250
Mutton	65
Cheese spread	65

SODIUM CONTENT OF FOODSTUFFS

Foodstuff (100 g)	Sodium content (mg)
Amaranth	250
Litchi	124
Rohu fish	101
Cumin seeds	126
Melon	105
Lotus stem dry	438
Fenugreek leaves	76
Liver (goat)	73
Spinach	58
Cauliflower	53
Coriander leaves	58
Jackfruit	63
Mango	43
Lentils (whole)	40

Contd...

Contd...

Foodstuff (100 g)	Sodium content (mg)
Banana	37
Red gram dal	29
Bengal gram dal	73
Neem leaves	72
Lettuce	58
Prawn	66
Beet root	60
Black gram dal	40
Carrot	34
Raddish	33
Apple	28
Watermelon	27
Pineapple	35
Coriander seeds	32
Maize dry	16
Buffalo's milk	19
Amla	5
Potato	11
Wheat flour	20
Cow's milk	16
Tomato	13
Cucumber	10

Contd...

Foodstuff (100 g)	Sodium content (mg)
Rice	9
Yam	6
Pear	7
Jowar	9
Wheat flour refined	9
Sweet potato	6
Sapota	6
Guava	5
Oranges	4.5
Brinjal	3
Pomegranate	0.9
Colocasia	9
Lady's-finger	7
Papaya	6
Wheat vermicelli	8
Peas (green)	7.8
Plum	0.8
Pumpkin	5.6
French beans	4.3
Onions	4
Bitter gourd	2.4
Peaches	2

Source: **PGIMER manual** of diet and nutrition

NORMAL VALUES OF COMMON ELECTROLYTES

Electrolytes	Normal values (mEq/L)
Sodium	135–145
Potassium	3.5–5
Phosphorus	1.8–2.3
Chloride	98–106
Calcium	9–11
Urea	20–40
Creatinine	0.7–1.2
Magnesium	1.5–3
CO_2	22–26
Bicarbonate	24–30

Notes

Index

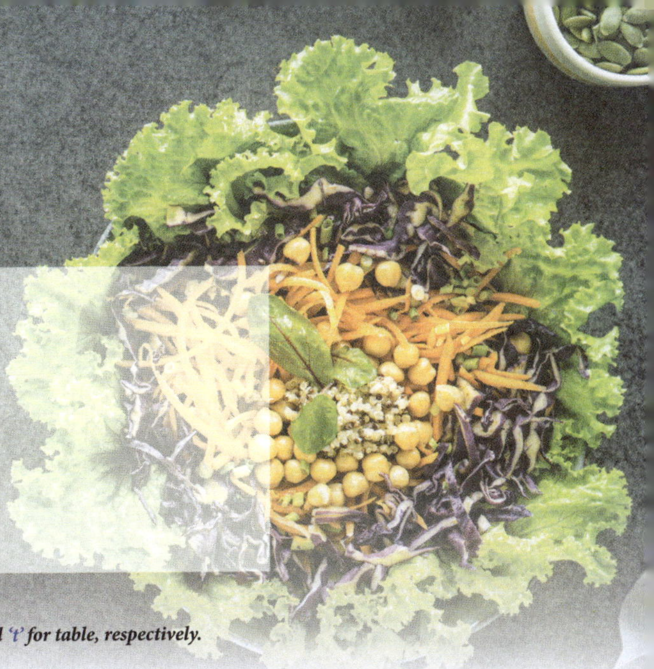

Refer 'f' for figure and 't' for table, respectively.

A

B

C